Healing
Complex Children
with
Homeopathy

ASD, PANDAS/PANS, LYME,
ADHD, AND MORE

ANGELICA LEMKE, ND

Workplay Publishing

Published by Workplay Publishing
Newton, KS 67114
workplaypublishing.com

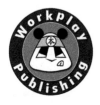

Developmental Editor: Bridget Biscotti Bradley
Interior design and layout: André Swartley
Editorial Assistant: Susan Budge
Indexer: Andrea Anesi
Cover design: Amy Gonzalez Daniel
Proofreaders: Kate Swartley, Susie Swartley

ISBN 978-1-7343946-0-3

PRINTED IN THE UNITED STATES OF AMERICA

Disclaimer: This book is for educational purposes only. The information provided herein should not be used for diagnosing or treating a health problem or a disease. It is not a substitute for professional care. Readers are advised to consult with a physician regarding personal medical care. If you have or suspect you may have a health problem, consult your healthcare provider.

"Be brave and know that you are capable. Healing abilities are not relegated to a magical few. Everyone has the ability to heal, both themselves and their loved ones."

—Heather Stewart

Contents

Introduction

by Bridget Biscotti Bradley

Soon after his fifth birthday my son changed from a brilliant, happy, healthy child to one who had such crippling anxiety that he eventually couldn't leave the house. I spent the next two years chasing diagnoses, trying to explain to friends and family that this wasn't just a discipline problem, walking on eggshells around my child, trying to put one foot in front of the other each day, and worrying about the emotional and physical toll this stressful existence took on my younger one.

I searched for anything that could help my son. I scoured Facebook groups, I pleaded with doctors for bloodwork, I bought every supplement that someone called a "game changer" for their sick child, I tried every diet, I went to specialists who didn't take insurance, we tested our home for mold and did an extensive remediation and rebuild that took seven months and more money than we could afford to spend. And he wasn't better. We couldn't get his central nervous system to calm down, he was hyperactive and would rage and hit if something set him off, he had horrible intrusive thoughts that brought him to tears every night, he had extreme separation anxiety and sensory sensitivity, he couldn't accomplish any schoolwork, and we all lived under the crippling rules and regulations that consumed him.

How did this happen? And why were there so many other parents dealing with similar, and often more challenging issues with one or more of their children? We were competing for appointments with the handful of doctors who even acknowledged that our children were suffering from brain inflammation, spending huge amounts of money on lab work and medications, and not finding much more than palliative results. Parents of children who are diagnosed with everything from sensory processing disorder to being on the autism spectrum are out there fighting for their kids every day, trying to find services, exemptions, and insurance coverage for unorthodox medical treatments, all the while dosing dozens of supplements and pharmaceutical drugs. They want to see their children thrive, but may find that working within "the system" doesn't result in the healing they are searching for.

Today's children face unprecedented health challenges. It seems as though everyday occurrences like strep infections, exposure to mold, or a tick or mosquito bite that used to be a non-event in the life of a child are now causing massive inflammation resulting in behavioral problems and learning issues. According to the CDC, 1 in 54 American children are on the autism spectrum, while about 1 in 6 children aged 3-17 have been diagnosed with one or more developmental disabilities. These numbers increase with every new report, and the list of possible culprits includes environmental toxicity, genetic susceptibility, the chemicals that we live and breathe in our day-to-day lives, the aggressive and often mandated vaccine schedule, glyphosate and other toxins in our food and water, the stripping of essential minerals from our soil, EMFs, and cell phones. It may be that the combination of these things affect some more than others but we need to be able to ask questions and demand accountability for any product that is harming our children.

I used homeopathy for many years and worked with a professional homeopath at one point in my son's journey, but I didn't really understand its breadth or power. Like many other "crunchy" moms, I knew I couldn't survive the teething years without Chamomilla and I had a few good remedies in my medicine drawer for colds and injuries but that was the extent of my homeopathic knowledge. After diets, herbs, mold remediation, and detoxing didn't help my son, I was researching other treatments to try when I stumbled upon a class that Dr. Angelica Lemke was teaching for parents of immune-compromised kids and immediately decided that I needed to take it. It's hard to describe the feeling I had listening to Angelica talk about recovering complex kids with homeopathy in that first class; I was filled with more hope and excitement than I had felt in a very long time. I instantly knew that I found what I had been looking for. I was in awe of her uncanny ability to hold space for families who needed help, at the thousands of children whose lives she had turned around, and of her encyclopedic knowledge of what remedies could heal these sensitive kids. Through her classes she inspired me to learn more, and I decided to delve deeper into the art and practice of homeopathy.

Aside from her immense knowledge and even bigger heart, what sets Angelica apart is that she empowers parents to tap into their intuition and help heal their own children. She believes that when we connect to our children with our hearts, the universe will show us what they need. As I learned more from Angelica and other amazing homeopathy teachers I began treating my son and my whole family and could hardly believe the miracles I witnessed. I was able to abandon all the supplements, all the tests, all the fear…and we began to heal. Slowly, over a year of homeopathic treatment, the layers of my son's symptoms peeled away one by one. He still has a bit more deep healing and clearing to do, but thanks to homeopathy his immune system is functioning normally rather than attacking his brain. He is once again our sweet, happy, brilliant boy and I am confident that he will make a full recovery. I realize that he is one of the lucky ones, and I humbly stand in solidarity with every parent out there whose child still struggles or for whom complete recovery is not possible.

Angelica offered a workbook called *The Book of Life* to her students and clients and when I received my copy in February of 2019 I could not put it down. It was a compilation of everything that she had learned treating complex kids and it made finding remedies for my son quick and easy. After reading it I was convinced that this information needed to be fleshed out and made available to a wider audience and I asked if I could help her do that. Thankfully, she said yes!

One of the many things that makes this book unique is that it invites parents to be active participants in the healing of their children. It is not a reference book meant only for professionals, although homeopaths and other healers will undoubtedly be inspired and further educated by Angelica's approach to treating complex children. While the book may cast a wide net, I want to address just the parents for a moment. You are probably reading this because you are also swimming upstream in the river of PANDAS/PANS, Lyme disease, and other chronic auto-immune conditions. Your arms feel like they're about to give out. I bet you've been swimming for years. Somehow, you have summoned the strength to try something new, perhaps something you know nothing at all about, because you continue to have hope that your child can heal. I want you to know that you can do this and that you are not alone. Join the conversation at www.homeopathyforcomplexchildren.com and meet other parents who are learning right along with you as we share our successes, seek advice for our challenges, and support one another.

Learning how to use homeopathy will allow you to stand in your power and find peace in your home and your heart. If you are looking for a professional homeopath to work with, find one who will respect and utilize your intuition as the parent, who encourages you to help find remedies that resonate, and who will support you as you hone your own dosing skills. Beyond treating your complex child, you will soon start to learn how to use homeopathy for your entire family for day-to-day issues like accidents, colds and viruses, tummy aches, and more. There is truly no greater gift than being able to heal yourself and your family.

The following quotes are from other parents who went down this path and saw healing that no other modality had provided. We call our children orchids and canaries in the coal mine because they are sensitive to the world in a way that many kids are not. While that can be challenging, we have to hold onto the idea that it's a blessing. These kids are the true healers. They will show us the way if we listen, and hopefully be the generation that turns the tide.

"Homeopathy has been fundamental to my family now living a liberated life: free to identify and follow our underlying soul purpose, feelings, and needs. My children are back at school after 2 years of homeschooling and part-time school due to PANS symptoms. Homeopathy has supported the physical issues from PANS and also helped them move through resistant feelings and beliefs and into more helpful states of being. We've had many 'a-ha' moments where we've given a remedy and a symptom that has been stuck for months or years just disappears (selective mutism, violent rages, stomach pains, etc.). We would definitely not be where we are now without homeopathy."

—*Katrina Horn*

"Homeopathy came into my life when everything was spinning out of control. I had a wealth of knowledge in holistic health, herbs, vitamins, and essential oils at the time. When my youngest son was diagnosed with PANDAS no one even knew what it was. I felt like every time I was giving him antibiotics I was poisoning him with a pink-filled spoon. Luckily, one of the moms in an online support group mentioned the huge results she was getting from homeopathy. That was over 7 years ago. Homeopathy not only healed my son's PANDAS but healed my entire household of numerous issues. Homeopathy has taught me patience and a deep trust in the universe. Our local basketball team, the 76's, has a saying, 'Trust the process.'

To me that is so fitting with homeopathy and healing. Sit back, try to relax, and trust the process."

—Abbe Lang

"The biggest lesson has been that nature provides what we need to heal and that we can discover it through our intuition. My child has taught me patience, that healing is a journey, and although we may see immediate improvement, comprehensive healing takes time. She taught me to have love and patience throughout the journey even in the low times."

—Anonymous

"My son was vaccine injured and had autoimmune encephalitis from the HPV vaccine. Since Western medicine could not heal him they recommended putting him in an inpatient psych program. Knowing my son was not mentally ill, we chose homeopathy instead. After 2.5 years of homeopathy, my son is in school full time again (after missing 3 years of school). He is completing high school in 2.5 years, and he received a 98% on his college board exams. Before homeopathy he was unable to attend school, leave the house, or hang out with friends and family. Homeopathy was our family's miracle."

—Christie Biesold

"Adding the intuition component to homeopathy has been a game changer. I feel more empowered, both with homeopathy and just with my life in general. I feel like less of a passenger and I have more faith in myself and the universe to provide me the answers I need. I have always struggled with decisions and trusting my own judgement, so adding intuitive meditations and muscle testing has enriched my life in so many ways. I feel like a different person."

—Anonymous

"When PANS hit my daughter, I thought she would never get better and that I had lost her forever. I tried many different doctors and approaches but no matter how hard I tried, nothing would make a difference. Thank goodness a friend suggested I try homeopathy and it literally saved my daughter's life. I just wish it had been the first thing I tried, not the last! Angelica's Book of Life *was my springboard into homeopathy and into learning about the main remedies that could help my daughter. After I got a sense of the remedies in general, I started to follow my gut instincts*

as to what remedies my daughter needed during flares as each flare would feel different to me. I allowed myself to try the remedies without any fear as I knew that the only possible 'side-effect' would be some aggravation of her symptoms that would go away in a few hours. The more positive results I got, the more I trusted my intuition and the more my daughter improved. It has been a year since our PANS nightmare started and my daughter's healing has been nothing short of a miracle."

—Flavia B.

"With homeopathy, I've finally been able to see the strength of my son's soul. He's been given labels like hypotonia, mitochondrial disease/dysfunction/insufficiency, and chronic fatigue. But in healing with him, I've been able to feel how robust he really is and that is reminding me that we are more than bodies. I'm looking at him as more than what he's able to show me."

—Heather Stewart

Chapter 1

Healing with Homeopathy

I wrote this book to empower parents, homeopaths, and healers to use their intuition, along with homeopathic remedies, to heal the growing number of today's children who suffer from a wide range of complex conditions. These children are experiencing deep levels of unresolved pain, trauma, and toxicity. Some of these "blocks" to healing are ancestrally inherited, and some are created during the gestation and lifetime of the child via exposure to environmental toxins and medically induced traumas. Homeopathy is a safe and effective system of medicine to unblock these layers of toxicity and trauma, and this book will be a roadmap that you can follow to create the highest expression of health for the next generation.

I am a naturopathic doctor and homeopath and have been treating complex children and adults for over a decade. Families come to me to assist in the healing of those who have constellations of symptoms that defy simple conventional diagnosis and a one-medication-one-disease approach such as developmental delays, autism, Lyme disease, learning disorders, attention deficit hyperactivity disorder, autoimmune and neuro-immune conditions such as PANDAS and PANS (Pediatric Autoimmune Neuropsychiatric Disorders Associated with Streptococcal Infections and Pediatric Acute-onset Neuropsychiatric Syndrome), oppositional defiant behaviors, genetic immunodeficiency disease, methylation issues, mold and chemical sensitivities, allergies, cancer, birth trauma, and more. After seeing thousands of cases, my passion is to teach parents and healers how to find the right remedies for these truly complex kids. Finding the right remedy isn't always easy; sometimes you can give many remedies and see little impact. But when you find the right remedy or group of remedies, the healing can be so miraculous that it will change your entire outlook on life!

There are so many fad therapies out there offering palliative solutions that will come and go. What I hope to direct you to are solutions that spring from your own intuition and will fundamentally accelerate your whole healing journey.

While my educational background is in Western medicine and classical homeopathy, I have found that an inclusive and open-minded approach to all systems of medicine is needed for these complex cases. For example, when I first started to practice, I would prescribe a single remedy to be dosed only once per month. While the remedy was usually a wonderful fit for the child, this classical practice of giving only one remedy once a month took these multilayered cases only so far and I soon learned that I could individualize my approach to greater effect. Some of the mothers I worked with would muscle test (see page 34) potencies and how frequently to dose the remedies to their children, and they experienced quicker progress with less aggravations. As a result, I began to incorporate intuitive practices and a more inclusive mindset recognizing that this new era of complex cases requires a creative mindset. Being inclusive means that we invite in many possibilities of treatment, however, we can focus our approach by trusting our intuition as well as incorporating new classification concepts from contemporary homeopathy, which I will be sharing in this book.

An intuitive homeopathic approach relies upon a connection to your inner knowing guiding the homeopathic remedies given and having faith in the natural healing process. Due to the sheer complexity in the cases these days, an intuitive approach, as opposed to a purely rational one, has the capacity to capture what needs to be healed in your child with breadth and depth and to gently assist your families' healing. Albert Einstein said, "We cannot solve our problems with the same level of thinking that created them." The rational scientific approach in medicine has turned into dogma that has forgotten the soul of the individual to detrimental effect. To fully embrace the power of homeopathic medicine is to let go of the requirement that all disease can be scientifically explained and diagnosed and to look instead at what is presenting on all levels, also known as an empiric approach. Instead of believing that mainstream medicine has all the answers, and perhaps giving away our power in the process, it's time to start trusting our innate wisdom and that the body can heal itself with the right energetic shifts.

Each child is unique and needs specific answers to unlock their healing. To aid this process, it will help to awaken your inner healer. As parents, this is not as daunting as it seems, because connecting to our loving heart is all we need, followed by surrendering to the great unknown with faith that there is a better way. As you connect inwards, to your heart and your inner GPS, that better way will unfold before you, step by step.

This book is designed to inspire and guide people at all levels of homeopathic knowledge, understand the various energetic expressions of children, and find remedies that fit them. Chapter 2 explains what homeopathy is and how it works, but if homeopathy is completely new to you, it will help to read some other material to create a firmer foundation (see pages 402-403). More information and cases can also be found on our website: www.homeopathyforcomplexchildren.com

Expectations for Recovery in Complex Children

What is healing? For some families it will be recovering their child from a diagnosis so they can successfully compete in school, go to a great college, and be a functional, successful adult. This happens quite often, and it's awesome to witness. For some families though, with more disabled children, it will be evolving and growing soulfully, into more love, with the child guiding the way. As you do so, solutions for every day issues will show up for you and make your life easier. For these families, the ultimate healing is finding peace with their life and their child, and ways to experience what used to be limitations as gifts. Healing may ask you to change jobs, change houses, move states, heal your marriage, quit an addiction, and ultimately look at yourself. Be open to it all. Healing is an evolutionary process and ultimately allows us to live an authentically satisfying life.

That said, once you tap into your inner healer, she/he may guide you VERY specifically to remedies, therapies, dosing instructions—the key here is to have faith and see the big picture. When you know in your heart that a remedy will serve you, you will be very excited to witness the unfolding healing that occurs. It will feel like a miracle! And it is, each healing step forward is a miracle birthed from your loving heart as a parent.

People who gravitate towards homeopathy seek greater self-sustainability, want less reliance on institutions to scaffold and support them, and tend to question authority. They understand that there are many variables—including environmental, diet, medical, and ancestral—that contribute to health. They take responsibility for their own healing, understanding that their emotional states directly impact their children. To set yourself up for success, try to see the whole story—from your family's ancestral stories to your pregnancy—and recognize key themes that show up. Also, try not to compare your family with other families. Part of the journey is releasing judgments and allowing healing to occur gently and organically. Some seemingly hard cases will unpeel many layers with one good remedy, while some seemingly easy cases will take more time than appears necessary at first. The earlier a child is treated with homeopathy the better; it is less challenging to reach complete recovery in children under the age of six who have an autism diagnosis. Surrender your expectations and create the space within to allow grace to guide you on this journey.

Working in Conjunction with Other Modes of Healing

Homeopathy is compatible with all the other modes of healing out there, and I have learned not to be dogmatically for, or against, any therapy (even pharmaceuticals, because all medicines can play their specific, needed role). But tap into your inner healer to help you to be discerning. Most children in the United States are exposed to so much in the name of education and therapy that they don't have time to just be themselves or have a fulfilling relationship with their parents. In our culture we often need to learn to do less, and in homeopathy, less is more. Once you get in touch with your own inner healer you can customize your healing approach and cut out unnecessary interventions. Excessive biomedical and pharmaceutical treatments will gradually drain the vital force and slow down the homeopathic, vitalistic, source of healing. Also remember that every supplement you are "trying" in your desire to find healing for your child has to be processed by their liver, so throwing every vitamin, probiotic, mineral treatment, herb, etc. at the problem is only serving to tax an already challenged body.

Many children treated with a mainstream medical approach have been on various types of pharmaceuticals and it's possible that your child is currently taking antibiotics, steroids, stimulants, etc. While some homeopaths say that remedies will not work while a child is taking pharmaceuticals, if a parent is dedicated to weaning a child off of them under the guidance of a healthcare professional, I will still begin homeopathic treatment. I have found that the correct remedy can still create shifts, even while on medications, allowing parents to gain the courage to trust homeopathy and wean the child off of the meds. However, heavier duty pharmaceutical treatment, particularly steroids, psych meds, and anticonvulsants, will significantly dampen the capacity of the child's vital force to respond to a remedy since the nature of the drug is inhibitory or suppressive, so the body is challenged in finding natural homeostasis. The endless "kill" mentality of taking drugs to fight infection (antibiotics, antifungals, antivirals), is also at odds with homeopathy for this same reason, and can lead to deeper imbalances in gastrointestinal flora, making the road back to health a steeper climb. Pathogens evolve rapidly and can outwit pharmaceuticals, so it's a wise game-plan to strengthen the body's innate immunity with natural medicine. If you have had a bad experience with a particular drug(s), make sure to mention this to your homeopath and read the chapter on Tautopathy.

Working with a Homeopath

If you plan to work with a professional, it is of primary importance to choose a homeopath you feel comfortable with, who listens to you and respects your opinion, empowers you with knowledge, and has a history of treating children. In my experience, all methods of homeopathy can be helpful, and I utilize

WHY MOMS AND DADS NEED TREATMENT TOO

Keep in mind that children will heal faster when the parents heal themselves along with their child. Parents and children are energetically entwined, and it is important for parents to recognize and heal their own patterns of imbalance, which are often reflected in their children as well. Children are also here to help us grow and evolve; if we adults do not evolve, the healing process can quite easily stall. Many issues that require healing are intergenerational, and healing a child may mean parents also healing the relationship and issues they see in their own parents. If you feel hate towards yourself or a parent that may need resolution for your child to feel self worth and self love. See pages 393-397 for a list of remedies that I commonly use for treating parents.

COMMON ISSUES FOR MOMS

- Anxiety/fear for their children's health and future
- Self-martyrdom/resentment. Victim orientation. Can't put themselves first.
- Unmet need for love/attention
- Emotional connection/love and issues with their mother

COMMON ISSUES FOR DADS

- Disliking work, lost passion, suppressed sense of self, low self worth
- Preferring work over being at home, over-identification with career
- Lack of emotional connection, cannot express emotions
- Lack of "belief," can't see beyond the material dimensions, no spiritual dimension
- Aggression or suppressed aggression and issues with their father

aspects of all of them (see pages 45-51 for a description of the various methods of homeopathy). In my opinion, the single most important key to healing children is for parents to listen to their own intuition about their child, find a way to access their child's internal world, and share it with the homeopath. While it's important for the homeopath to meet and speak with the child, often the most significant insight and information comes from the empathic connection shared between parent and child.

The most successful cases I have witnessed include an empowered and proactive parent who learns about homeopathy, has faith in the homeopathic process of healing, and understands the differences between suppression of illness and the homeopathic healing of illness. The work of the homeopath alone will not heal you or your child; it takes your active participation. The homeopath's job is to be a partner and coach in your healing.

Finally, understand that homeopathy is not a quick fix, but a long-term unfolding of healing that will have its ups and downs with a gradual progression towards optimal health.

Treating the deepest levels of illness in a child using homeopathy can be a long and involved process, and often it is best to pair up with an experienced homeopath. However, there is much you can do yourself with homeopathy, especially in helping to manage acute conditions that arise and specific complaints. Chapter 2 will guide you through the process of choosing potencies and dosing for acute issues, but first, let's discuss how a case is taken and start thinking about narrowing in on what needs to be healed.

Casetaking

Most homeopaths can spend several hours taking in and understanding a new patient's case. There are many questions that will be asked to try to capture the larger themes and issues that need healing. Below are questions that homeopaths will ask and reasons why they need to be considered:

1. What are the main complaints of the case? Often this is where most of the energy in the person is going, and also what is most debilitating or limiting. In children, if the greatest stress is bodily pain this is usually what first needs treatment. If there is pain, what is the sensation? Go into it—what does it look like, feel like, smell like, sound like? What makes it better/worse? How do they position their body?

2. How was the pregnancy? Experiences during pregnancy (symptoms, traumas, etc.) can be a small microcosm of the future experiences of the child. Specific symptoms or stresses during this time may continue on some level in the life of the child.
    *   What work did mom do?
    *   Any exposures or medications during pregnancy?
    *   Any strong physical symptoms, or unusual symptoms, during pregnancy?
    *   How did mom relate to friends, relatives, coworkers?
    *   Any emotional traumas before or during pregnancy?
    *   What was mom's mental/emotional state during pregnancy?
    *   Any food cravings or aversions during pregnancy?

3. How was delivery? Intense experiences during delivery can reverberate through the life of the child and any traumas from this time should be understood and addressed.
    *   Any outstanding trauma during delivery?
    *   Did mom feel supported during and after delivery?

4. How was the child as an infant?
    *   Did the child reach milestones?
    *   Did the child get sick with normal colds and flus?
    *   How many times was the child put on medications, Tylenol, antibiotics?
    *   Was the child vaccinated? Which vaccines? Any vaccine reactions?
    *   Was stool normal?
    *   Was growth curve normal?
    *   Any digestive pain?
    *   What was the personality of the baby like?

5. When was regression or developmental delay noticed? Did anything precede this regression?

6. How is the child socially? Social behaviors of children are often modeled after their parents but are also deeply impacted by their community and environment.
    *   Does the child socialize?
    *   Does the child make eye contact?
    *   Do they get along with siblings? Parents?

- How do they behave at the playground?
- How do they react when approached by another child?
- Does the child act one way in the home and another outside the home?

7. How is the child cognitively?
   - Do they respond when talked to (receptive speech)?
   - What is their speech like? Clear? Slurred?
   - How is the memory?
   - Are they learning numbers/math, alphabet/reading?
   - How do they respond to learning?

8. How is the state of the family of the child? A child is intimately impacted by the health of all family members. The state of the family needs to be understood and often the whole family needs healing.
   - Any family history of particular diseases?
   - Did the family move? Any issues with places they have lived?
   - Do they have family support? Community?
   - Does either parent have a stressful job?
   - Are parents happy? Are they fighting?

9. What are the physical symptoms of the child? These symptoms are often key in differentiating homeopathic remedies.
   - Are they in pain? Head pain? Stomach pain? Do they feel pain?
   - What does the pain feel like, if you imagine you are the child?
   - How is gross motor?
   - How is fine motor?
   - How is their overall movement?
   - Do they tend to be hot or cold?
   - Do they sweat easily or never sweat?
   - Are energy levels high or low?
   - How is sleep? Issues falling asleep or staying asleep?
   - How is the stool? Diarrhea, constipation, color, consistency?
   - How is the appetite? Food cravings and aversions?
   - Any digestive symptoms—nausea, gas, vomiting?
   - How is the skin? Prone to rashes? Eczema? Dark circles? Chicken skin?

10. What is the medical history of the child?
    • Were there major medical traumas?
    • Were there regressions after any medical treatments?
    • Are they on pharmaceuticals? Are they on MANY supplements?

11. What is the personality of the child? This is where the true individual-izing, on mental and emotional levels, of the child comes through.
    • What does the child love the most?
    • Where is the child most in their element?
    • How does the child behave when stressed? What stresses them?
    • What are their fears/phobias?
    • What are the stimming behaviors?
    • How is eye contact?
    • What is their mood—are they happy, sad, angry, moody, even?

12. Are there any unusual behaviors that stand out? A homeopath is always trying to understand what makes a case unique. Is there a "strange, rare, or peculiar" fear, hobby, behavior, or obsession that the child has? Or is there a particular physical attribute that is totally unique to the child? We can often find a remedy that fits this unique attribute. Some common ones include:
    • Lining things up: may indicate a strep infection
    • Repetitive behaviors: may indicate a viral infection
    • Spinning: may indicate candida/yeast overgrowth

Taking Your Own Child's Case

Whether you are working with a professional homeopath or not, there will be situations when you need to take the case yourself. Keeping the child's history in mind and everything else queried in the section above, write down your answers to the following questions. This will help you pinpoint what needs to be healed, and as you work through this book you can write down possible remedies that address these issues. Once you have a list of possible remedies, you can look up the materia medica online or in a homeopathic guidebook for more information. Hopefully one (or more!) will intuitively feel like a good match for your child and you can try dos-ing it. More information on dosing and case management is detailed in Chapter 2.

First, write down the strongest symptoms of the complaint, being as specific as possible. To help give you a sense of the kinds of symptoms you want to elicit, take a look at the following list:

- What does the pain or sensation feel like—don't just stop at "it hurts," find out how it hurts; does it burn, or is it like electricity? Is it achy or stabbing?
- What time of day are they better and worse? Is there periodicity to the complaints?
- Where exactly do they feel the sensation, and where, if anywhere, does it extend?
- What makes the pain/sensation/symptom feel better?
- What makes the pain/sensation/symptom feel worse?
- What other symptoms come on at the same time? For example, if the complaint is hay fever, do they become highly irritable with it where they are normally not irritable at all?
- Do they want consolation and company during the acute, or want to be left alone? This is of particular importance if what they want is contrary to their normal state.
- What times of day and night do they feel worst or best? In what environmental conditions do they feel better or worse (i.e. outside with a breeze vs. a closed warm room).
- What generalities accompany the acute? Are they hot or cold, is their stool affected, what happens to their appetite and thirst, etc.?

My Personal Intuitive Approach to Case Taking

Intuition can also be deeply integrated into the homeopathic process, from case taking to prescribing to dosing. The intuitive intake process is fundamental when treating children (and especially nonverbal kids), because case taking is primarily done via the parent. It is only through imagining what it is like to be the child that we can have great insight into their experiences and ultimately find remedies that could help them.

During my case taking, after I gather all the facts, I ask parents to close their eyes, take a few deep breaths and relax, and picture their child. I ask the parent to imagine their child at their happiest and feel what it is like to be them in this moment. I often start with asking about the happiest moment because this is an easier access point for parents to connect to. I ask the parent to empathically go into detail—what does it feel like IN THE BODY, in the heart, the feet, the muscles, the joints, the face, etc.

I then ask the parent, as their eyes are closed, what does it feel like when their child feels the opposite, the most stressed. Picture the child—what do they do, what look is on their face? What does it feel like?

When I do this style of intake with parents, they often have an epiphany about how the child is feeling in a way they had not understood before. It is therapeutic in and of itself. It also helps parents realize how much their child is reflecting feelings that they have or used to have.

This intake style is derived from well-known homeopath Rajan Sankaran's method called the Sensation Process, where the purpose is to connect to the sensations of the body and release the subconscious mind, revealing its true source or remedy state. You can listen to a guided meditation at www.homeopathyforcomplexchildren.com to help you tap into the energy of your child, or you can meditate on your own using the text below to guide you.

Some questions to ask while you are imagining your child:

- Describe what is happening in her body?
- How does this affect her?
- What does it feel like?
- What comes to mind when she feels it, what does it remind you of?
- Describe the feeling (heavy, light, pain, tense etc.) more, what does (tense) mean?
- Do you have a gesture that describes it?
- What is the opposite of this feeling?
- What makes her happiest? How does happy feel like in the body? What does it remind you of?
- What is most stressful? What does it feel like in the body? Is there pain? What does it feel like? What happens next?
- Imagine her moving—how does she look/feel when moving? What does it remind you of?
- Imagine her under social stress—how does she feel under stress out in the world/playground/work?
- Imagine you are her, you feel how she feels. Now imagine walking into nature. What shows up? What do you see?
- Imagine looking into her eyes—what is she communicating to you through her eyes?

Write these sensations down and you will see a polarity between how the child feels at their best and worst. Once completed, this is an amazing

WAYS TO IMPROVE OVERALL VITAL FORCE

- Be in nature, walk on grass, get grounded
- Get pure; detox
- Clean diet, fresh and vital green foods, living foods, fasting, eating less
- Breathing exercises/ aerobic exercises
- Yoga/Tai Chi, energy practices
- Meditation, stillness, spiritual life
- Contrast showers/ hydrotherapy/sauna/ sweating/induced fevers
- Being in touch with the heart/emotions/emotional responses
- Dancing, playing, creating

guide. It is incredible how many times I have guided parents into imagining what it is like to be their children and the result has been a revelation to them. Your child may have dozens of symptoms but imagining them at their best and worst can be an important first step in finding the right remedy. Often times what comes up in a polarity between best and worst are two related sensations. For example, a child may feel best when she feels "free" and worst when she feels "trapped," so a remedy revolving around desire for freedom and sensation of claustrophobia, such as Tuberculinum, may be helpful. Another example would be a child who feels most happy when in a quiet room alone on their iPad, and most stressed at a loud chaotic party. For them, a remedy around oversensitivity to stimuli and desire for solitude, such as Natrum mur, may be indicated.

When trying to decide what to treat, we want to understand what is MOST limiting to the child in the moment. Many parents may feel, for example, that vaccines were the cause of a child's limitations and want to immediately start by detoxing vaccines, but in the moment the most problematic issue may be sharp, debilitating stomach pains and we should instead give a remedy for alleviating that state. The meditation above may elucidate that. Any time a child is most limited by severe pain, pain should be what we understand and heal first.

We can also see the connection between the parent's state and the child's state when we put ourselves into our children's state and feel how they feel. Parents may realize that the child is expressing the same feeling that his father feels while at work, or the state that his mother was in while pregnant. Making these connections can be key.

We can take this empathic detective work even further by coming into our imaginative mind and asking the universe to guide us to, or show us, a plant, animal, mineral or some other substance that matches the sensation of the child. Sometimes I guide parents into meditation and they spontaneously see the image of a certain tree, flower, or animal. In a naturally intuitive way, the parent was using the homeopathic law of similars (see page 44) to draw to them a substance that matches and can heal the state of the child.

This is not a practice to do just one time but to continue on a regular basis, because the state of a child is constantly in flux. It is a practice that opens our hearts and connects us psychically to our children, which can be especially crucial for nonverbal children.

Once you have some clarity on what needs to be healed in your child (and ideally you have used your higher self to guide you), you can then use the charts and materia medica in this book to research and find the right remedies.

Prioritizing and Expanding Your Intuition

Most people have been, unwittingly, indoctrinated from a young age to follow the advice of authority figures, institutional wisdom, and media outlets instead of relying on our own inner sources of wisdom and intuition. I have heard so many parents bemoan the decisions that they felt "forced" into due to cultural pressures and against their better instincts. Nobody knows you or your children better than you do, and while doctors and healers may have good intentions and years of professional training, they are often too busy and burned out to see the whole picture and make decisions aligned to your best interest.

Most children also have so many sensitivities these days, with a constantly changing physiologic terrain, that daily reliance on intuition can become a necessary skill to gracefully swim through challenges with less reactivity and conflict. I was pressured to rely on my intuition because the cases I was working on were so complicated and sensitive, that I eventually had to surrender to the universe and say "I have no idea what to do here! Guide me in what to do." When we connect to our higher self, there is always a better way, a better decision, that moves us forward on the path of healing.

Everyone is intuitive, your intuition is ALWAYS available to you—you just have to peel back any layers of doubt that it isn't. The love you have for your kids will lead you. Surrender what you may think you know (release your analytical mind) and open yourself up to receiving answers from your heart, your instincts, your body, and your higher self. Solid homeopathic prescribing should always help us come more into our core sense of self and connection to intuition. And solid homeopathic prescribing IS NEVER invalidated by the inclusion of intuitive input. The following strategies for improving and expanding intuition also include remedy suggestions to help parents connect to their hearts, surrender their minds, and get in touch with their higher selves.

Heal the Heart and Express Emotions

Most parents of complex children that I work with have closed down their emotions to some degree in order to protect themselves from hurt and disappointment. Subconsciously their child feels this emotional distancing and picks up on the feeling that "there is something wrong with me." This itself becomes a layer that the child needs to heal, that somehow, "I am less than acceptable, less than perfect." Further, our culture elevates intellectual understanding and diminishes heart felt emotional expression. Children feel misunderstood when their parents are unavailable emotionally and feel judged by overcritical attitudes. Healthy expression of emotions, be it anger, fear, or sadness, help us integrate with our bodies and have healthy immune and regulatory systems. Reconnecting the parent to their emotions means healing this feeling of grief and disappointment in the heart so they can be fully present with their child and build the child's self-worth by directing unconditional love at them. Common remedies I give to parents for healing the heart are Ignatia, Natrum mur, Causticum, and Aurum.

Surrender the Mind

The majority of health diagnoses and treatments are products of the analytical mind, which tends to cut up the whole picture of the person into discrete bits of information, thereby losing the big picture. Analyzing and diagnosing a child can be a crucial piece of healing. But if we rely on only a reductionist approach in healing, we can prevent ourselves from seeing the whole picture. Usually the complexity of a child's situation is so great that despite every lab test out there it is impossible to know what the root problem is. Surrendering the mind with the statement, "I have no idea what to do," or "I have no idea what is going on," and then coming into the heart with compassion and openness is crucial for connecting to intuition. Reducing our focus on mental work and media intake and spending time relaxing, meditating, being more creative, and being more physical will bring too much "headiness" into balance. Common remedies I give to parents to help them surrender their mind are Lycopodium, Ignatia, and Nux vomica.

Get Centered in Your Power

One of the greatest challenges of healing is creating awareness of negative and blaming attitudes that keep us limited, stuck, and off balance. When we allow ourselves to be a victim of circumstance, we give our power away to something external to us. We get centered and take ownership over our lives by realizing that we always have the power to say no, the power to walk away from a situation, the power to choose joy, and the list goes on. Old traumas such as sexual abuse, accidents, violence, and even past life trauma can create stuck patterns that are hard to release. Bringing positive energies of forgiveness and love into these traumatic memories can be a crucial practice for deep healing. For people in a deeply destructive or self-sabotaging mode, having some form of inspirational practice such as regular meditation, inspirational reading, or prayer to nourish their connection to positive energy is key. To some degree, everyone has negative shadow states, and remedies that can help release them are Chlorum, Staphysagria, Pulsatilla, Sepia, Natrum mur, Oxygenium, remedies that treat parasites, and reptile remedies.

Connect to Our Higher Selves and Call on Divine Support

Our higher selves are the part of our souls that are connected to truth, divine intelligence, and universal consciousness. I also refer to our higher selves as our angels. We all have angelic guidance within, it doesn't have to be sought outside of ourselves. All we need to do to connect with our angelic selves is to quiet our minds and listen to the voice of our hearts. The act of total surrender can help with this; when we surrender the part of ourselves that is our limited ego, that thinks it knows best, we can be more receptive to our higher selves. Sometimes we have to stop trying so hard to fix a situation, get passive, and allow the answer to come to us. A powerful act of healing is saying, "Dear universe/grace/higher self, please guide me, bless me, protect me, show me more abundance, more miracles, and more love today." Remedies to strengthen our inner connection to our true selves are Carcinosin, Thuja, Silica, and remedies for suppression (see pages 366-370).

Embodied Awareness

Intuition is not accessed outside of our bodies, it requires embodied awareness from our toes on up. We direct our attention to the parts of our body that are in discomfort and pain because they have messages for us. With our intuitive hearts listening to our own bodies, with great receptivity, we interpret any sensations, emotions, or images that arise. The "issues are in the tissues," and the tissues have something to say. Developing sensitivity to our body's energy field can help discern when the body is feeling contracted and stressed, or relaxed and open. This can also help us choose the right remedies and potencies. Our physical bodies have an awareness of subtle energies and an innate intelligence to discern between them that our conscious mind does not have. Learning to muscle test, pendulum test or sway test can be wonderful ways to tap into our embodied wisdom (see Appendix). If this is daunting to you, realize they aren't required. Sometimes we know when an answer is correct because we can breathe deeper, or an answer is incorrect when our breathing tightens.

When we connect inwards and listen to our bodies, our souls speak to us through imagery, emotions, and associations. For example, when feeling head pain, you may feel a band sensation, or envision a vice, or experience a sad emotion. Everything is valid, enter into these feelings and visions as if they were a portal. Allow your creative and imaginative mind to speak to you. A deeper theme will emerge and a remedy can be found to match the resonance of what shows up. Somewhere buried in all of our DNA is an ancient shaman healer who is connected to all of nature. This ancestor has access to "the Universal medicine chest" where we can all tune into the exact substance in nature that will heal us.

Everything Has Meaning

Once you have tapped into your higher self and your energy field, you will start to realize that the universe speaks to you in numerous, creative ways all the time! Everything has meaning, and everything is connected. Life takes on more meaning—the old friend who out of the blue calls you, the animal you keep seeing run across your yard, even the weather patterns. Because you are more connected, these experiences are a part of YOU and they speak to you.

Using the tools of visualization, dreams, and imagination are powerful for navigating this realm of super-connectivity. If you have an odd dream that keeps repeating, what is the meaning and could a remedy bring meaning to this? If your child keeps showing you a certain object, or certain phrase or word, could it signify something? The key here is to stay connected, grounded, and embodied, or else we can get too "out there." If we regularly connect with our embodied intuition and invite grace to work in our lives, we can experience everyday miracles of synchronicity and abundance.

Children are Intuitive

Children are naturally more connected to their emotions, body, and source energy. This makes them naturally intuitive and we can emulate them as intuitive teachers by being in the present moment with them and honoring their inner guidance. When a child is feeling upset or hurt, ask them to close their eyes, feel into their heart, and give them the space to express themselves. You can put an array of remedies, supplements, foods, flower essences, etc. in front of the child and using intention to connect to the child's higher self, ask the child to select an item that will nurture them. The adult/parent makes the ultimate choice, but if what they select feels right to you, support them by allowing them to take it. That said, children are often operating from their own limited understanding and will sometimes make choices, such as to eat too much sugar, that we need to be discerning with. Finding the right balance and trusting our child's inner light as much as possible allows them to become incredibly self-sufficient and confident, and to stay connected to their authentic source.

SHAMANIC HEALING MEDITATION

- Relax, close your eyes, and take a few deep breaths.

- Feel into your body, what sensations arise as you connect into your body?

- Describe those sensations in detail—what additional adjectives describe the feeling you have?

- When you feel into specific areas of the body, with your eyes closed, do any images arise?

- Imagine holding the part of your body that you are feeling and that needs healing, as if it were a baby.

- Imagine walking into nature holding this part of yourself. Picture the surroundings: the sky, the earth, the sun, the breeze, the smell of the earth.

- Imagine holding this part of yourself in nature and asking nature, "Show me something in this place that will heal this aspect of me." It could be a rock, a gemstone, a tree, a flower, a source of water, a color, an object, an animal, anything! If something shows up, explore it, feel it, understand it, speak to it.

- Close the meditation by thanking nature for what it has provided to you.

- And take the opportunity to look up the homeopathic materia medica of what showed up for you as well!

The Process of Choosing a Remedy

Once a case is taken, what larger themes emerge? What is most important to treat?

There are thousands of remedy possibilities in homeopathy, so how do we target our approach and find useful remedies for each unique child? Your child may also have numerous health issues occurring, making it difficult to prioritize what to give attention to.

Decoding Behaviors in Children

The source of behaviors in complex kids can range from deep expressions of the emotional state of the child to physiological responses to bacterial, viral, and fungal infections. Decoding this behavior takes a hybrid of empathic understanding and experienced analysis. Below are some of the associations I have found to exist between behaviors and their underlying cause. These are not one-to-one correlations, but rather general trends I have observed. Knowing these associations will help you focus in on what remedy to choose.

Poor Eye Contact

The eyes are the windows to the soul. When you try to look at your child, do they look away in shame, anxiety, anger, or dreamy bliss? Knowing why is critical to understanding the symptom—we care more about why they look away than about the poor eye contact itself. From a homeopathic standpoint, improved eye contact is one of the deepest signs that a child is responding to a remedy. It indicates a level of comfort and security within the self, and often an increase in openness to the environment and desire to connect.

Delayed/Poor Speech

Delayed speech frequently indicates a degree of "system shut down," but it is not necessarily simply a matter of cognitive delay. Delayed speech can also be a sign of emotional impairment or physical pain. If a child feels emotionally suppressed, or is in constant pain, they are less likely to have the energy to be receptive to their environment and develop their speech. There is a window under the age of 5 during which rapid speech development occurs; if treatment begins after 5 then recovering this capacity in special needs children is more challenging. Speech can improve with homeopathic treatment but often tends to be one of the last things to fall into place. Many of the non-verbal children that I have treated healed all of their other issues from early childhood first, and later improved in communication skills.

One of the major challenges a special needs child must overcome is the experience of having been treated as disabled, and as a result having a lower bar of expectation as well as co-dependencies on caretakers that end up enabling them in unhealthy ways. Developing the true self-confidence needed to move beyond their diagnosis requires much love and faith.

Uncontrollable Giggling

The causes of uncontrollable giggling can vary widely. "Drunken giggling" can be a physiological response to high levels of yeast in the body. "Uncontrollable maniacal giggling" can indicate brain inflammation due to infection. Giggling at inappropriate times or awkward moments can indicate the release of suppressed emotions or even grief.

Tantrums and Rage

Tantrums are a complex and mixed display of emotional reactions and immune responses. Some children are fixated on wanting something so badly that when they don't get it, they are totally devastated, and the ensuing tantrum is rooted in a sort of extreme sadness or dismay. For others, tantrums represent a true "fight or flight" response with a deep level of fear for their very life; which is the result of a deep immune response occurring in their body, even though the situation may not seem to warrant such a response to the parent or observer. These children may also try to "escape" due to their instinctual adrenaline response to stress. Other tantrums are based on premeditated violence or pure manipulation in an effort to control their environment. Rather than just considering the tantrum behavior, it is important to understand what is at its root and what deep internal issues it is reflecting.

Sensory Issues and Pain

Many children have sensory issues that respond to deep pressure or massages in certain areas of the body, or intense movement of the body such as rough play or jumping. In general, this is in response to numbness or lack of sensation, pain, or tension in the body, or a lack of integration of the senses. Oversensitivity to sound, touch, and light can be the result of suppressed infections in the nervous system or overwhelmed detox organs.

Children may have unusual movements and behaviors in place to moderate pain or sensory issues. They may clench their teeth, push on their jaw or bang their head due to headaches, often caused by toxicity and brain inflammation. Often children with digestive issues have tummy pains that cause them to twist and turn, or push into their tummies, and there are specific remedies that can be chosen depending on the nature of and reaction to the pain.

Most parents instinctively know when their child is in pain, but a homeopath wants to know exactly what the pain feels like. Often the pain a child has mirrors the pain that a parent has, making it easier to express. But other times people don't truly understand the pain and it can be important to empathically imagine what it is like to be the child while in pain—imagining the look on their face, how they hold their body, and what makes them feel better or worse. Does it feel sharp, stabbing, cutting, aching, twisting, burning, numbing, tingling, exploding, pressing, cramping, spasming, twitching, radiating, etc.? Also, what emotion arises as you imagine this pain? And how does the pain evolve—does it move around the body? Sometimes just taking the time to be present with the pain and understand it starts the healing process.

Issues of Elimination

Enuresis (or wetting oneself), constipation, and loose stools are very common symptoms that can be challenging to treat because there are many causes. Enuresis can be caused by environmental or food allergies, excessive yeast, excessive medications/supplements, inherited kidney weakness, and even anxiety. Constipation can be an issue of slowed peristalsis, dehydration, diet, liver toxicity, not enough exercise, and more. Playing with stool or urine are behaviors that can signify the need for a nosode or parasite treatment. Homeopathy can bring up detoxification, so "peetox" and/or stinky poops can result after remedies (see pages 60-62). It is important to help identify and treat the cause, but also to recognize that elimination is how the body detoxes and these symptoms will improve with time as the body finds balance.

Fears and Anxieties

Identifying specific fears and anxieties can be very helpful for finding a homeopathic remedy. Many fears are common, such as fear of the dark, separation anxiety, or nightmares. Some of these fears stem from deeper inflammatory processes that trigger our more instinctual fears; Stramonium is a good example of a remedy that helps treat this. Some fears are more adrenaline-mediated and may come up when PTSD is triggered; the remedy Aconite often helps when a child is in this state.

Obsessive Compulsive Tendencies

OCD behaviors can vary from hand washing and lining up toys to fixating on certain objects or routines. In my experience, chronic, recalcitrant streptococcus or viral infections are a major cause of OCD behaviors. These behaviors also often provide a way for the child to control the environment and create a sense of security.

Stimming

Common stims include shaking strings, pens, or other objects in front of the eyes, vocal noises, spinning wheels, and hand flapping. Replicate the gesture that your child does and imagine how they feel. For some children, the gesture is an expression of total joy or sensory stimulation. For others, it is a release of tension in the body. An emerging possibility is that a lot of stimming behavior is the result of bacterial infection in the gut. In these cases, stimming severity may track flares in gut imbalances. Sometimes specific isopathic nosodes directed at gut imbalances can help these types of stimming.

Tics/Tourette's

Tics are usually a sign of suppressed emotions or infections that have been pushed into the neurological system. For some children, tics arise like a warning system, the first sign that there is a challenge to the immune system. Releasing the root of what is suppressed and strengthening immunity is key to treating most tics and Tourette's syndrome.

What A Child Loves or Hates

What children love not only alleviates their daily stress, it also gives us insight into the nature of the remedy that they need. What they can't stand shows us what their triggers are. I saw one boy whose favorite movie was *Cars*—he loved watching the cars race around and crash into one another, it was all he wanted to watch all day. I saw another boy whose regression into autism was literally triggered by watching the movie *Cars*. He was so traumatized by the shock of the cars crashing that he stopped speaking after watching it. Needless to say, they each needed very different remedies.

Behavior in Nature

What do your children do outside? Do they run after squirrels? Find water to play in? Gather up leaves? Listen to the sound of the breeze through the trees? Are they afraid of certain things outside, such as insects or birds? What is their "element?" Are they in total bliss when they are in water? Do they try to jump so high on the trampoline that you think one day they may just defy the laws of gravity and float away? All of these little behaviors are wonderful clues towards what remedy a child may need.

Socialization

Do your children prefer adults or younger children? Do they fixate on having one friend at a time? Do they need to be a part of the group or do they prefer absolute isolation? When stressed do they need to be consoled or do they push you away? Try to put yourself in your child's shoes, why do they enjoy or not enjoy the company of certain people? The specifics of any social or anti-social behaviors are critical clues to differentiating remedy types.

Conclusion

Helping special needs children takes a lot of love, perseverance and insight. But it can be an amazing journey as well, and we can learn so much from them. This was nicely summarized by a mother who told me, "At times at night, he is quiet and smiling and looking at me, and I say I love you and he just smiles back sweetly—and there is so much heart-to-heart conversation between us without talking. It is blissful to me. We know we love each other. In those moments he is so perfect. He is love. In these moments you see your real child. At heart he is pure, peaceful, and loving, and those are the basic qualities humans need to have. He has abundance of that and it shows. And there are a lot of people in the world who do not have that. Why does the world have to worry so much?

I have learned so much from him. This is the key— to remain positive and give unconditional love to your child and not compare your child to others. Look at your child as the only child in the world, do not compare them. This is becoming a mother in its truest sense. Otherwise life passes you by, you take mothering for granted, and they just grow up. If he did not have his diagnosis, I would not have learned this. This is how children are supposed to be brought up. By not making them conditional to what the world expects from them and accepting them perfectly as who they are. Saying to them, 'It's ok - in your time, you will be fine'. We parents try too hard to make them a part of this society and that doesn't work for all kids. These children are a lesson in love."

In the next chapter we will review the basics of homeopathy—its history, rules and guidelines, as well as case management. Getting comfortable with homeopathy takes practice and learning these fundamentals will bring you more confidence. However, don't get too caught up in worries that you are doing the wrong thing; homeopathy is both powerful and forgiving.

Chapter 2

The History and Practice of Homeopathy

Homeopathy is a holistic system of medicine founded by the German physician Samuel Hahnemann in 1796. Hahnemann's inspiration for the development of homeopathy was an experiment. To investigate the use of cinchona (i.e. quinine) in the treatment of malaria, he began to ingest regular doses and found that it produced all the symptoms of malaria, though of mild severity. In 1796 he published his Essay on a New Principle for Ascertaining the Curative Power of Drugs, laying out the framework for the "Law of Similars"—the idea that an illness could be cured by giving a medicine which, given to a healthy person, would produce similar but less severe symptoms of that same illness. Hahnemann's homeopathic methodologies were further expounded upon in The Organon of the Healing Art, which he published in 1810.

Hahnemann continued to experiment with dosing various substances at different levels of dilution and wrote down the full range of mental, emotional, and physical effects that those substances created, recognizing that the more dilute a substance the more etheric its effects. When people came down with a specific subset of symptoms that matched a substance, he would give it in very dilute form to heal them. The process of homeopathic dilution, while secondary to the law of similars, became an important aspect of the medicine and one that radically differentiated it from the orthodox medicine of the time.

Homeopathy was widely embraced by the United States in the 1800's; it offered an integrated, coherent, systematic basis for treatment and gained a wide following among educated physicians. The American Institute of Homeopathy was formed, and in response, orthodox physicians formed the American Medical Association (AMA), both of which exist to this day.

At this time, and into the early 1900's, many of the largest medical schools in the country taught homeopathic medicine, including the New York Medical College, Boston University, and Stanford University. Twenty to twenty five percent of all physicians in urban areas identified themselves as homeopaths.[1]

By the end of the 19th century there were 22 homeopathic medical schools, over 100 homeopathic hospitals and over 1,000 practitioners in the United States. Homeopathy's greatest success at the time was in treating epidemic diseases; hospital records show that death rates in homeopathic hospitals were 12-50% those of orthodox hospitals. During a cholera epidemic in Ohio, for example, only 3% of the patients in a homeopathic hospital died as opposed to 50% of patients in an orthodox hospital.[2] During the Spanish Flu of 1918, which killed 50-100 million people worldwide, homeopathy was also very successful. While the mortality rate of people treated with traditional medicine was 30 percent, those treated by homeopathic physicians had mortality rates of 1.05 percent.[3]

Competition between the two schools of thought started coming to an end after the release of The Rockefeller Foundation-sponsored Flexner report, which sought to standardize medical education with a bias towards orthodox schools and resulted in the shutdown of all but two homeopathic colleges. Homeopathy then declined for a variety of reasons, including the advent of antibiotics and large-scale pharmaceutical production, which heralded a new era of orthodox medicine. Homeopathy began a resurgence in the 1970s fueled by the lay public and dissatisfaction with mainstream medicine. In the 1970s there were as few as 100 homeopaths in the US, but by the 1980's there were over 1000.[4]

Since the 1980s, homeopathy has seen steady growth. It is included in the national health systems of many countries, including Switzerland, Brazil, India, and Mexico. In France, 36% of the public and 32% of physicians use homeopathic medicines. In Germany, 10% of physicians specialize in homeopathy. In the United Kingdom, 42% of physicians refer patients to homeopathic doctors. Homeopathy is practiced ubiquitously in India as well, where there are 125 four- and five-year homeopathic medical colleges and more than 100,000 homeopathic physicians treating 100 million people who use it as their sole medical care. In Europe, 29% of people use homeopathy for day-to-day health care. According to the National Institute of Health, over 6 million people in the United States use homeopathy for day-to-day health care.[5] Remedies are prepared by licensed homeopathic pharmacies and regulated by the FDA. The term HPUS found on homeopathic medicines refers to the regulating code book, The Homeopathic Pharmacopeia of the United States, which since 1897 has regulated the production of thousands of homeopathic medicines.[6]

The Four Fundamental Laws of Homeopathy

1. The primary basis for homeopathy is the Law of Similars, or "like cures like." Put simply, whatever symptoms a substance is found to be able to cause when given to healthy people, it should also be able to cure in those that are ill. For example, the remedy Apis is made from a honeybee, and is used to treat histamine-like allergic responses such as swelling and itching that are similar to the symptoms that occur after a bee sting.

2. The second law of homeopathy is the Law of Minimum Dose. Hahnemann discovered that when preparations are diluted (in serial steps) and vigorously shaken (succussion) between dilutions, they retain or even increase in healing potential despite a reduced (biochemical) concentration. He named this process "potentization." Unlike orthodox medicine, which generally maintains the principle that higher doses are more potent, homeopathic experience shows that:
   • Low potencies, i.e. small dilutions, have a short and superficial effect
   • Medium potencies act longer, and the range of the symptoms they effect have broader and deeper proportions
   • High potencies, i.e. the greatest dilutions, can be the deepest acting, and their influence continues long after cessation of use

3. The third law of homeopathy is the Single Remedy Law. Therapists of classical homeopathy will determine only one remedy at a time for the person—one with a symptom picture matching the whole person (all symptoms). Most homeopaths are on the lookout for the best single remedy to fit the whole person.

4. The fourth fundamental law of homeopathy is Hering's Law: "Cure proceeds from above downward, from within outward, from the most important organs to the least important organs, and in the reverse order of the appearance of symptoms."[7]

This means that a well-selected remedy will stimulate the body to heal the most important systems and organs first. Symptoms of the disease will be "pushed" outward from the deeper layers to the more peripheral ones and move downward, away from the head. Recent symptoms will also tend to heal before old symptoms. This law is important to understand when healing chronic disease to assess whether a remedy has had good effect. If after taking a remedy, a person is more mentally stable, but also has more rashes, fevers, or colds, this is considered a positive direction of healing because the mental level is considered deeper than the physical level of symptom expression.[8]

How a Homeopathic Remedy is Made

Homeopathic medicines can be sourced from plants, animals, minerals, microorganisms, and even forms of energy like x-ray and ultrasound. Through a serial (repeated) process of dilutions and vigorous shaking, the remedies are "potentized." If the remedy is made from a soluble substance, it is first dissolved in alcohol to create what is called a "mother tincture." To get a 1C potency (one part per hundred), one part of the mother tincture is added to 99 parts alcohol and then shaken (also called succussed). This process of serial dilution and succussion is repeated to create higher potencies (of increasing dilution). To get a 30C potency, you would repeat the 1:100 dilution and succussion process 30 times, for example. The dilution is then usually dropped onto sugar pellets (a stable form of remedy storage), which can be taken directly in the mouth or dissolved in water and sipped. Remedies are also available in liquid form or as creams for external application.

Insoluble substances (like many metals) can also be ground up with lactose to create a homeopathic remedy, referred to as trituration. A 1C potency is obtained by mixing one part of the substance with 99 parts lactose, and serial trituration is continued as with soluble substances to get higher potencies.

Homeopathic Methodologies

There are many schools and methodologies of homeopathic treatment. Even amongst homeopaths who practice a similar style, such as classical homeopathy, there is much individual variation. Many homeopaths eventually use their own unique combination of the methods listed below.

Classical

Classical homeopathy is the most common form of homeopathy practiced today and is based on the principles set forth by Hahnemann in his treatise, *The Organon of the Medical Art.*

In classical homeopathy, the main focus is on the whole person being treated, including elements of their disposition, personality, and "constitution" that may have existed before the disease began. Ideally, understanding the deeper constitution of a case leads to the discovery of a "constitutional remedy," which includes in its materia medica all those symptoms of the disease itself, and when this occurs these can be some of the most powerful, deep-acting prescriptions.

The key distinguishing concepts of classical homeopathy include:

- Matching a remedy to an illness based on comparing the specific symptoms of the illness to the known materia medica (symptoms) for a remedy
- Giving only ONE remedy at a time in treating the illness
- Giving the "minimal dose," meaning the lowest dose and fewest number of dose repetitions in each particular case

In my experience, most cases of complex children have many layers of illness that must be peeled away before an underlying constitution of the case can be recognized. With the degree of suppression found in today's children, there will be many blocks to the expression of a natural constitutional state, and other methods of prescribing may be necessary to progress the case. Focusing exclusively on a singular constitutional remedy that is meant to address all aspects of the case may distract us from finding remedies that address the presenting complaint.

However, if a remedy reveals itself as consistently healing a child deeply and over a lengthy period of time, this remedy could be deemed a constitutional remedy. Often this constitutional remedy covers a broad range of symptoms in a child and is associated with their physiologic structure. Examples of common constitutional remedies for children are mineral remedies like Calcarea carb, Sulphur, Phosphorus, and Silica; plant remedies such as Lycopodium and Pulsatilla; or even miasmatic remedies like Tuberculinum and Carcinosin. Defining a child's constitutional remedy can be useful because it can often be dosed during periods of stress to strengthen the child's inherent state. Regardless, situations of acute infection or trauma will arise that a constitutional will not address and other remedies will be needed.

To understand how classical homeopathy works, consider reading Amy Lansky's book *Impossible Cure,* in which she cures her child of autism. Her book and website include an index of homeopaths who practice in this style.[9]

Contemporary Group Analysis Approach

This is the idea of studying homeopathic medicines in groups based on chemical or natural similarity.[10] Examples of these groups include families of animals such as mammals, snakes and insects; or plant families such as the nightshade or rose family; and groups of chemicals such as carbon-based chemicals. Group analysis actually traces its roots to a book published in 1887 by Ernest A. Farrington called Clinical Materia Medica, which arranged medicines by their kingdom and chemical relationships. However, Hahnemann himself wasn't supportive of this approach, which is likely why it wasn't popularized until more recently by trailblazing contemporary homeopaths including Jan Scholten, Rajan Sankaran, Lou Klein, and Massimo Mangialavori.

The group analysis approach actually forms the backbone of this book. Because I personally find this approach helpful, this book is organized by chapter according to animal, plant, mineral, nosode, sarcodes, and so on. I find this approach to be essential for my capacity to capture the breadth of what is available in homeopathy, and it helps to refine my remedy selection. Each chapter has summary information on the basic themes that define each group, and this will hopefully help you hone in better on the right remedies as well.

Sensation-Style Prescribing

Sensation-style prescribing is based on the teachings of Indian homeopath Rajan Sankaran. It is essentially a different style of case taking, placing an emphasis on tapping into the sensations of the body and subconscious to find a deep-acting remedy that matches the unique "sensations" of the child. Sankaran developed an understanding of the various homeopathic remedies from this perspective of deeply felt sensations.

For children with autoimmune disorders and/or autism, this style of homeopathy can be very effective in identifying unusual remedies that are poorly described in the materia medica. However, it does require an empathic parent to comprehend these sensations in their children and communicate them to a homeopath.

Intuitive Homeopathy

My personal intuitive approach to homeopathy described in Chapter 1 is not unheard of. This approach is also recognized in Ian Watson's book, *A Guide to the Methodologies of Homeopathy* as "Prescribing from an immediate recognition or 'felt sense' of what is needed, without the intervention of the analytical mind."

In reality, most homeopaths use some level of intuition in their prescribing, whether they are aware of it or not. During the consultation, homeopaths are constantly using intuitive perception to pay close attention to the client, picking up cues from their non-verbal behavior. Often, this is done subconsciously and allows the homeopath to ask certain questions and explore certain topics, all in search of the information needed to prescribe the best-suited remedy. Intuitive homeopathy uplifts these intuitive processes to primary modes of gaining knowledge and may also integrate the use of explicitly intuitive tools such as muscle testing or pendulum testing.

It could be said that an experienced homeopath, after a few decades of seeing thousands of clients, selects remedies intuitively based on cumulative experience and a heightened ability to recognize often-seen patterns. This is certainly one form of intuition that relies on the building up of an internal warehouse of knowledge. However, there seems to be another form of accessing information whereby a homeopath senses that they are accessing information from something greater, such as the "higher self" of themselves or their clients, a spirit guide, or a connection to universal knowledge or the collective consciousness. When this happens, a homeopath may be directed to a remedy they know little or nothing about, but nonetheless have great faith in, perhaps supported by positive feedback with a tool like muscle testing. An intuitive homeopath is open to this possibility and when this inner voice speaks, it is regarded with respect and acted upon, not automatically dismissed by the analytical mind.

Isopathy/CEASE Therapy/Tautopathy

Isopathy is a method whereby remedies prepared from the same disease, drug, vaccine, or toxic material that are thought to have damaged a child are given to that child in homeopathic preparation (high dilution) in order to help detoxify those substances and promote the body's own healing immune reaction. This approach is valuable when there have been obvious shifts, bad reactions, suppressions, and also when the body's immune system has ceased responding to a particular bacteria, virus, or other intrusion.[11]

The difference between isopathy and classical homeopathy is that the practitioner does not require the materia medica of a substance to match its symptoms to the disease or the child's constitution. Rather, they give the same substance that damaged the child. For example, a child who has a bad reaction to a vaccine and develops a high fever with a pounding headache and anger may be given Belladonna by a classical homeopath, while an isopathic practitioner may give the harmful vaccine itself in homeopathic potency to try to clear the toxicity or ill effects.

CEASE Therapy (Complete Elimination of Autistic Spectrum Expression) was created specifically to treat ASD by Dutch homeopath Tinus Smits, and essentially utilizes prescriptive treatment with various isopathic remedies. You can find CEASE-certified homeopaths on the CEASE website (see Appendix).

In my own practice, I integrate classical homeopathy and isopathy. I find that the isopathic remedies do help children detoxify and better deal with drugs, infections, vaccines, and other insults that have harmed them. In combination with more holistic prescriptions that strengthen the child's general constitution and immune response, isopathic remedies can be very effective aids to healing.

Sequential

Sequential homeopathy was developed by Dr. J.F. Elmiger of Switzerland and further developed in North America in the early 1990's by Patty Smith and Rudi Verspoor of the Hahnemann College and Clinic for Heilkunst. In this method, a timeline of traumatic events is created based on a child's health history. Remedies, often in combination, are given to address and hopefully remove the effects of those traumas, starting with the most recent ones and moving backwards in time.[12]

For more information on the method and its history, visit the Hahnemann Center for Heilkunst and Homeopathy website (see Appendix).

Homeopathic Drainage

Homeopathic drainage was developed by a French physician, Léon Vannier, in the 1930s. Drainage utilizes combinations (specific formulas) of low-potency, homeopathically prepared substances to target specific organs or tissues in the body and help promote their detoxification capabilities. Popular lines of drainage formulas are the "UNDA numbers," produced by the French company Seroyal, and spagyric formulas by PEKANA. Drainage is useful for children since it allows for targeted but gentle detoxification of specific organ systems that are often weakened by toxicity, such as the liver, kidney, intestines, or nervous system.

One strategy is to start a child on drainage remedies for at least a few weeks to open detox pathways before beginning other homeopathic treatment. When there has been excessive medical intervention or toxicity, internal systems can become blocked and remedies might not work when the body is in this state. A good indication that homeopathic drainage is needed first is when all other modalities seem to aggravate the child, for example when all herbs or supplements cause a strong negative reaction. This method offers a slow and gentle detoxification on the physical plane, although you may not notice shifts on the mental and emotional levels as obviously as with standard homeopathy.

Combination Remedies

Combination remedies are formulas of multiple (sometimes many) homeopathic remedies combined into one pellet, liquid, or topical application. Most are available over-the-counter and are commonly seen everywhere from Whole Foods to Walmart. They are usually targeted at specific conditions, such as insomnia, teething, cold and flu, sinusitis, etc. By including many remedies known to be helpful for certain conditions in low potencies, combination remedies simply take a shotgun approach at homeopathy. While they may not be as effective as a well-chosen single remedy, they are frequently helpful in ameliorating the symptoms or length of an acute condition. Usually they don't help prevent the recurrence of that condition because of their generality, but on the plus side they are easy to self-prescribe and are readily available.

Homeoprophylaxis (HP)

In a general sense, homeoprophylaxis refers to the use of homeopathic remedies to prevent acute illness. In a more specific sense, some homeopaths have designed a "HP" program of dosing to replace the need for standard vaccinations. The prophylaxis protocol uses nosodes (homeopathic remedies prepared from disease material) for disease prevention by theoretically stimulating the body's natural immune reaction. Some parents may utilize homeoprophylaxis as an alternative to traditional vaccination where possible, working with a certified practitioner to follow the protocol. For more information visit the Free and Healthy Children International website.[13]

Cell Salts

Cell salts are low potency homeopathic remedies made from common minerals found in the body. They are used almost as low-dose multivitamins in helping to supply and encourage the body's healthy utilization of minerals for the support of specific body tissues. Cell salts are often available at health food stores and pharmacies with alternative medicine sections. You can readily search online for the indications of what symptoms specific cell salts help address, and they are easy to self-prescribe.

The Practice of Homeopathy

Although theories for the mechanism of homeopathic action vary widely, most would agree that it stimulates the body's natural vital force and a positive immune response. Rather than providing a material dosage of a biochemically active substance, homeopathic remedies seem to deliver a signal or piece of information to a person that is highly specific. Much like an intricate key that will only open one particular lock, a given homeopathic remedy is only useful for a very particular set of symptoms or a particular individual. Often times we give homeopathic remedies when a person becomes stuck in a repeating pattern. The more the pattern repeats or the stronger the pattern, the less the person is able to snap out of it, almost as if their own body does not recognize that it's stuck. Sometimes the effect of the remedy seems as simple as showing the body where it's stuck—just enough of a nudge to generate a response back towards balance and break the pattern before it is further ingrained.

Recognizing Suppression, Palliation, and Cure

A suppressive medicine is one that disrupts or blocks a natural immune or physiological process to ameliorate a symptom, leading to unintended negative consequences. A good example is a steroidal cream put on a skin eruption like eczema, which works by suppressing the immune system reaction. While the rash may be reduced, the suppressed immune system may also be less able to combat infection. In homeopathic philosophy, suppression can make the individual unhealthier on the whole, and may even push the symptomology deeper, encouraging chronic disease. The problem is that the body does not produce symptoms for no reason—symptoms are often the result of a necessary healing process such as detoxification, or combating infection, etc. If we block these natural healing processes, we prevent the body from doing its job to correct imbalances, and if we do this over the long term we risk compromising our health.

A palliative medicine will help get rid of a symptom without causing harm to the body but will not actually improve the whole disease or the body's ability to heal. The common use of many natural and conventional medicines fall into this category. While they may help with a symptom such as pain, they never actually cure the body of the root cause of that symptom.

A curative medicine, on the other hand, is able to reduce the symptoms of disease by treating the root cause of the disease or symptom. Homeopathy explicitly strives to achieve a curative approach, and the experience of homeopathic practitioners over hundreds of years has confirmed its ability to do just that. Other medicines can also be curative, but the practice of classical homeopathy is built around finding this solution. The main goal of homeopathic medicine is to aid in this natural ability with a gentle, but highly targeted, approach. Nonetheless, homeopathic medicines can be palliative when used in less specific or individually tailored ways, although they are rarely if ever suppressive.

Materia Medica and Repertories

The symptoms that a specific homeopathic remedy can treat are compiled into a written description called a materia medica. The materia medica for a remedy is organized into different physical areas of the body, as well as mental and emotional symptoms. For common remedies, you can often search online and find various versions of the materia medica. When prescribing a remedy, the goal is to fit as many of the symptoms a person has to the specific symptoms listed for a particular remedy in the materia medica. A second important tool that homeopaths use is called a repertory. These books list physical, mental, and emotional symptoms, under each of which are listed all the remedies known to produce or cure that symptom. Homeopaths sometimes use a computer program to enter a person's symptoms and quickly check which remedies include the most matching symptoms. Affordable repertorization software suitable for beginners can be found at www.completedynamics.com. In my own intuitive homeopathy practice, I will write down lists of remedies that come to mind as I take a case and then muscle test each one to come up with a shorter list, often finishing the process by reviewing the materia medica to come up with a final choice.

Interpreting Materia Medica for Children

Most materia medica contain some reference to how symptom pictures may show up in children, and some excellent materia medica books have sprung up for treating pediatrics in particular. Most of these books discuss common constitutional remedies, such as Paul Herscu and Amy Rothenberg's book *The Homeopathic Treatment of Children,* or for treating acute illness in children such as Miranda Castro's book *Homeopathy for Pregnancy, Birth and Your Baby's First Year.* Empowered parents who use these books as guides will do a wonderful service for their children. For special needs children, many traits remain under-represented in materia medica and can be hard to treat. This book attempts to bridge that gap.

Choosing Potencies and Dosing

There are two primary considerations once the remedy itself is chosen: the potency and the dosing frequency.

The X potencies (3X, 6X, 12X, 30X, etc.) are considered low potencies. They are commonly found in over-the-counter medicines such as teething tablets that are made of a combination of many remedies. While remedies in these low potencies can be repeated frequently, they are generally not thought to be as deep acting as higher potencies. Combination remedies in low potency can work very well, but do have some disadvantages. One remedy within the combination can reduce or antidote the effectiveness of other remedies in the combination, and there is no way to tell which of the different remedies was most helpful so that it can be used in higher potencies for greater effect.

Remedies in the C potencies (6C, 12C, 30C, 200C) are commonly used by professional homeopaths for constitutional dosing. Children can start with 30C potencies and adults can start with 200C potencies. Sometimes 6C or 12C potencies are used when a daily dose is desired, especially when treating only on the physical plane.

Remedies in 1M, 10M, and 50M potencies (still technically C potencies, but the M notation stands for 1000, so a 1M is equivalent to a 1000C) are used by professional homeopaths. When given to someone sensitive to that specific remedy, these higher potencies will often result in a deeper and stronger response than a C potency remedy. Because higher potencies are more dilute, they are often more "specific," so a person who is not sensitive to the medicine may have no response at all, whereas if given a low C or

X potency of the same remedy may have had some response. This is one of the reasons that over-the-counter combination remedies use the lower X potencies, it is more likely that a wider range of people will respond to them. Higher M potencies are extremely powerful, working on a deep, often familial/ancestral level, and can help to create a profound shift in the body and mind.

Despite these potency guidelines, keep in mind that everyone is different. Some children improve by dosing a 1M potency daily and some do well with a few drops of a 30C potency once a week. Just as a remedy is individualized to the patient, dosing is individualized as well, and the dosing process can sometimes be as difficult as finding the right remedy in the first place.

- X potencies: treats mostly on the physical plane, commonly found in combination over-the-counter formulas
- 6C and 12C: treats mostly on the physical plane with some emotional component, good for acutes
- 30C: treats all planes but is gentle, a good potency to start children with
- 200C: treats deeper on the mental/emotional plane, useful for constitutional dosing; a good potency for when there is symptom overlap between a parent and child
- 1M and higher: can be useful to move up to these potencies when a lower potency has proved itself as deeply healing; helps heal at the ancestral level; can also be useful for emergency acutes

Dosing Frequency

Depending on the situation, you may decide to dose a remedy multiple times per day, as infrequently as once per month, or anywhere in between. Deciding on potency and frequency depends on the reactivity and strength of the child, consideration of other medications being used, and also the nature and severity of the child's symptoms. In general, homeopaths start with a lower potency, perhaps a 12C or 30C, and then work up to higher potencies. As long as a specific potency works well it will generally be continued.

When the first dose of the remedy is promising, here is some guidance on what to do next:
- If the symptoms that initially improved after giving the remedy come back, dose again.

- If you see a general pattern of symptoms improving then worsening after a set number of days, you can dose on a schedule. Parents commonly report this cycle: day 1 after dosing a remedy the child is worse, day 2-4 they are better, day 5-6 are neutral, day 7 is worsening again. In such a case we would decide to re-dose once every 5-7 days, when the child gets worse.
- It is important to let a remedy continue to work as long as the child is making overall progress. In other words, one bad day with a slip in symptoms is not cause for a re-dose of the remedy if the overall pattern points to improvement.

When to Change Potency

Move up in potency only when the current potency no longer has a beneficial effect, or when the effect stops lasting as long. Move down in potency, such as from 30C to 12C, if a child is getting easily aggravated by the current potency.

Overall, remedy re-dosing and changing of potencies is perhaps one of the most difficult parts of homeopathy. Poor timing with re-dosing can result in stalled progress, while overly frequent dosing can cause unnecessary aggravations. Use your intuition, take detailed notes so that you can pinpoint any behavioral patterns related to dosing, and don't be afraid to try something new if things aren't working.

Different Styles of Dosing

Homeopaths often give differing advice on exactly how to dose. I recommend all remedy dosing to be 10 minutes away from other food or drink (with the exception of water) into a neutral mouth. I usually suggest a dose of two pellets before bed.

While it's best to keep homeopathic remedies where children cannot reach them, if a child accidentally gets hold of a remedy bottle and eats 40 pellets all at once, this is not toxic. But if the child shows signs of an aggravation, see advice on pages 62-63.

The time of day for dosing usually doesn't make a big difference—some people dose first thing in the morning, some before bed or mid-afternoon. I like to dose before bed since that allows the body to integrate the shifts while sleeping. If multiple remedies are given in a day it is ideal to space them out. It's OK if remedies are given around the same time as herbal supplements, vitamins, etc. if you are doing a frequent dosing schedule, but if the remedy dosing isn't that frequent try to give it at a separate time from other supplements or medications. A homeopath will likely instruct you on how to dose, but below are various dosing styles I have seen parents experiment with in dosing their children:

- Drop Dosing: Dissolve 1-3 pellets into 1 tablespoon of water. Using a dropper, give 1-3 drops into the mouth. Even though this seems like very little, it can often trigger a deep reaction.
- Basic Water Dose: Dissolve 1-3 pellets in 2-4 ounces of water and drink the water down all at once.
- Sip Dose: Dissolve 1-3 pellets in 2-4 ounces of water and give a sip every 5-15 minutes until the water is finished. This is often used for nosodes/clearings.
- Acute Drop Dosing: Dissolve 1-3 pellets in 2-4 ounces of water and give 1-3 drops of the solution from a dropper every 15 minutes for a certain amount of time (see below).
- Dry Dose: Place 1-3 pellets directly into the mouth and let dissolve.
- Plussing a Remedy: Dissolve 5-10 pellets into an 8-ounce glass bottle of spring water. Before you dose, shake the bottle vigorously or hit it against your open palm several times, then drink 1 tsp of the water. Keep the bottle of water in the refrigerator for up to one month. Plussing a remedy helps gently increase the strength with each dose you take.
- For extremely sensitive people, there are other more subtle ways of dosing. You can smell a remedy, hold a remedy, make an intentional paper remedy (write down the remedy and place under a glass of water or in your pocket), put a remedy on your skin, or sleep with a remedy under your pillow. There are also other potency ranges and preparations such as LM or Q which could be sought out. Some parents find that diluting a remedy in a large amount of water, such as a quart of water, and drop dosing from that solution helps with extremely sensitive children. Which method to try requires accessing your intuition; luckily people who are extremely sensitive often already know how to do this!

In most acute states, such as treating an injury, put 2 pellets of the remedy into the mouth and wait a short period to assess improvement. How long you should wait depends on the severity of the situation. If improvement occurs, wait before re-dosing. Re-dose a correct remedy again if symptoms start to return. If nothing happens, then try another remedy. You might try a new remedy within minutes in an emergency situation or wait a few hours when treating something like a sore throat. Sip dosing and drop dosing (see above) are also helpful during acutes. If the acute is severe, such as a high fever or a significant injury, you may want to start out with a higher potency immediately, such as 200C or 1M, if you have it.

If someone can't take a remedy into the mouth (if sleeping, or at the hospital) you can rub a water dose of the remedy onto the skin, especially on areas of the body that sweat like under the armpits or on the belly.

Intuitive Testing and Dosing

Classical homeopathy does not integrate or promote forms of intuitive testing such as muscle testing. However, when working with challenging populations who see alternative healers, it's common to come across these somatic-based testing methods and many families have integrated it into their daily practice. I have found that allowing families to use intuitive testing to help with homeopathic remedy selection and dosing to be empowering. This doesn't mean that we dismiss materia medica, but that we integrate the intuitive into the rational decision-making processes. The result of this is more engagement in the healing journey, as well as less aggravations and trial and error with remedies. It is especially helpful for very sensitive and reactive children.

For beginners, an easy place to start is with sway testing. To do this, stand up and imagine that there is a plumb line at your center. Imagine your heart is in the center of that plumb line. Hold an object (supplement, food, remedy, etc.) in both hands at your heart center. Say to yourself, "I have no idea if this will help me, my heart will guide me with a yes or no." If your body/heart/plumb line sways backward, away from the object, your body's answer is no. If your heart is attracted or pulled to the substance, your body's answer is a yes. It's incredibly simple, just as most decision making is meant to be!

Other families make regular use of muscle testing or pendulum testing to help with remedy selection and dosing. The body does not lie. This is how lie detectors work—they sense the tension that arises when the body lies, and the relaxation in the body when truth is told. There are online sources for teaching this, but overall muscle testing and pendulum testing should not be complicated. Ultimately, we have to find that aspect of ourselves that feels the truth. One person I worked with always expressed a little giggle when I spoke aloud the name of a remedy that had resonance for him. For myself, I always feel my lung/throat catch when something feels wrong, and I feel my breath/lungs relax and more joy in the heart when something feels right.

And let's not forget that children are highly intuitive beings. Children can be given a remedy kit and asked to let their heart choose a remedy for a given ailment; you may be surprised to find that a child chooses a remedy with materia medica to fit the complaint!

Purchasing Remedies

Homeopathic remedies can be found in supermarkets such as Whole Foods, natural pharmacies, and from online retailers and pharmacies. Stores generally carry the popular remedies for acute illnesses in low potencies as well as various combination remedy formulas. There are several online pharmacies that carry more unusual remedies and higher potencies that anyone can buy from. There are also professional dispensaries that you can gain access to by working with a homeopath, and sometimes that is the only way to get specific remedies that you might need, such as nosodes.

Because single remedies are generally inexpensive, it is wise to order several potencies of each remedy up front. Often you will start with a 30C, for example, but quickly move up to a 200C and then a 1M or even 10M if the remedy works well for your child.

For anyone embarking on treating their child themselves, I strongly suggest ordering a homeopathy kit that contains 50 or 100 remedies in either 30C or 200C potencies. Kits are an upfront cost, but having the right remedy in the house makes it much more likely that you will be

MAKE YOUR OWN REMEDY

Sometimes there is an infected bodily fluid, environmental allergen, or other aggravating substance that can be made into a remedy to help the body react in a more balanced way or detox that material from the body. Example substances are saliva, mucous, urine, dust, mold, cat hair, pollen, or a medication.

- Put 1/4 tsp of the material in a small jar with 4 ounces of water
- Put a lid on the jar and shake 100 times
- Dump the water out, which will leave a few drops on the inside of the glass of the jar
- Add another 4 ounces of water
- Cover and shake 100 times
- Do this 6 times for a 6C, 12 times for 12C, 30 times for a 30C, and so on
- You can use a previously made dilution, for example a 12C, to make a higher dilution such as a 15C for the next dose (for example, you could continually increase the potency, such as doing 5 additional dilutions per day and re-dosing)

able to avoid trips to the ER or doctor's office for everything from injuries and flu to allergies and autoimmune flare-ups. Building your library of remedies will pay off in the end; this is truly a situation where more is better. Remedies essentially never expire if stored properly and each small vial will last months or years when you are dosing one or two pellets at a time.

Storing Remedies

Remedies should be kept dry and stored out of direct sunlight. Exposure to extreme heat or cold should be avoided. Keep remedies away from essential oils and anything else with strong scents; storing them too close together can negate the effects of the medicine.

Once you establish a large collection of remedies, you may want to look into storage options to keep things organized and easy to find. The simplest solution is to place the envelopes or vials in a box alphabetically. Plastic drawers sold for organizing make-up or crafts also come in handy for finding the right remedy quickly.

Case Management

The nuts and bolts of case management may be the most challenging aspect of homeopathy. Knowing when to redose, when to back off, when to dose a higher potency, when a remedy has acted and is no longer needed, and when an aggravation is occurring are all things that a professional homeopath can help you with. That said, I have worked with many parents who are able to help manage cases in their own children by understanding homeopathic guidelines and tapping into their intuition.

How Do We Know a Remedy is Working?

A good remedy will stimulate the immune system, cause detox reactions, create more comfort with being in the body, and improve sleep and energy. According to Hering's Law, deeper neurological symptoms and suppressed emotions may heal before physical ones do.

When a remedy is working well, we will see a combination of:

- Slow and gentle reduction of symptoms
- A detox reaction such as rash or stinky poop
- An immune reaction such as a fever

- Sleepy or increased need for sleep
- Dreams that are vivid, feel significant, or are memories of the past
- Comments from the child on memories of the past
- More energized after dosing
- Emotional release, such as crying, expression of anger or more joy
- Memories and issues from the past coming up, an attempt at healing old traumas
- Better eye contact, more sociable and confident
- With time, a gradual shift out of that state, as if peeling off a layer, and into another state

Managing Healing Reactions

Healing reactions such as fevers or discharges may arise after taking a good remedy. Sometimes dosing a correct remedy will result in a short aggravation followed by a healing response. A general naturopathic approach can be helpful managing these reactions and additional homeopathic remedies can also be supportive as well, especially if your child has moved into an "acute" state. Remember that healing reactions both detoxify and strengthen the body and should be supported, not suppressed. Naturopathic support that can help include increased fluids, activated charcoal, antioxidants, greens powders or chlorella, Epsom salt baths, sauna, bentonite clay, and a light diet with no sugar.

Fevers

Fevers are a positive sign that signify the remedy has triggered a healing response. Steady fevers between 99-103 degrees are normal and healthy reactions of the body's immune system. The purpose of a fever is multifold, with most infectious pathogens unable to survive the higher temperature of the body. Fevers should ideally be supported and not suppressed, in fact there is a proven correlation between autism diagnosis and the use of acetaminophen for inflammation and fevers.[14] Anti-febrile medications are often suggested out of fear that if a fever spikes too high and too quick, it will cause a seizure and subsequent brain damage. This is a rare outcome, and there are homeopathic remedies to help prevent it.

Ideally, we want to let a fever run its course while giving electrolytes, keeping the body comfortable with cool drinks, taking sponge baths, optimizing rest, and ingesting broths and soups. If a fever is causing discomfort and spikes too high, dose a remedy in 30C potency once every 1-3 hours until the fever subsides. Some remedies well known for fevers include:

- Aconite: After sudden onset of a fever, especially if after exposure to cold or wind; with fever there is anxiety, restlessness, palpitations, and thirst; pupils may be contracted.
- Arsenicum album: Prolonged chilly phase with shaking, even during fever; thirsty for small sips of water; anxious and restless.
- Belladonna: Sudden, intense fever; dry, burning fever without chills; face and body hot while hands and feet are cold; craves lemonade; throbbing headache with fever; glassy eyes; pupils dilated; delirium.
- Chamomilla: Fever in young children, especially if teething; long-lasting heat; one cheek red, the other pale; inconsolable; desires to be held and carried.
- Ferrum phos: Fever with few other symptoms; dry heat without chill; early stages of a fever.
- Gelsemium: Fever with weakness, trembling, chills running up and down spine; sleepy and weak, with drooped eyelids; occipital headache; pupils constricted; heaviness of body.
- Nux vomica: Chills and shakes with fever, worse uncovering and drafts; desires a lot of heat and warm drinks.
- Rhus tox: Terrible aching with fever; stiffness in body; feeling restless and anxious.

Rashes

Rashes arising from detoxification or immune reaction are usually not problematic and will pass without needing to do much. Occasionally, with the dosing of a nosode such as Streptococcinum, Candida albicans, or a viral nosode, there will be a subtle non-irritating rash that is a manifestation of the body responding to that pathogen. This is different from rashes that arise from allergy reactions that are itchy and swollen and may need remedies like Uritca urens or Apis. Rashes from the healing of a viral infection ideally will move down the body and outwards as it heals.

Increased Urination

Also called "peetox," increased urination is a common detoxification reaction. This may come with or without increased drinking. Often there is an accompanying different odor, such as a stronger ammonia smell. In general, not much needs to be done for this, but if it becomes problematic, you can support the kidneys with a sarcode, drainage remedy, or herbal support.

Smells

Changes in smells of the body's sweat, ears, breath, nose, bowel movement, or urine can signify detoxification or infection. If there is a quality to the smell that is sour, acrid, salty, sweet, fetid, rotting, or so on, make note of this as these smells are sometimes represented in homeopathic materia medica for certain remedies.

Sleep

An increased need to sleep may occur after taking a good remedy, and this likely will happen in cases where there has been a chronic deficiency of sleep. Sleep is when the body resets and heals, so if children are needing sleep to heal, they should be given this time and not be forced to wake up.

Die-off Reactions

When certain pathogens are killed, such as candida and parasites, the death of these pathogens will create sets of symptoms in the body such as headaches, fatigue, and body aches. These are ultimately healing reactions as the body is clearing that dead pathogen out. Homeopathic treatment generally doesn't result in strong die-off reactions, but they do sometimes occur. If this does happen, other remedies may be needed such as Natrum mur for a headache, or Carbo veg for gassiness. Some parents find that sip-dosing (see page 56) the remedy that brought about the die-off reaction, especially if it's a nosode, helps to clear it out faster while also supporting the body with activated charcoal, plenty of fluids, and other naturopathic supports.

Aggravations

An aggravation means that the symptoms a remedy is intending to heal get temporarily flared right after taking that remedy. For example, if I chose to dose Apis 1M for a bee sting and the child then gets very heated and restless, this may be in response to too high a potency and the child is aggravated by the remedy. Usually the symptoms will decrease soon afterwards. Aggravations are generally due to dosing a remedy in too high of a potency than what was needed, temporarily amplifying the state. You can either wait it out, or you can choose to slightly change the potency of the remedy by dosing an "aggravation zapper," which reduces the intensification of symptoms and brings on a quicker healing response. Follow these instructions to make your own "aggravation zapper":

- Dissolve one pellet of the remedy in 4-6 ounces of water (you can put it into a bottle and shake it)
- Pour 99% of the water down the drain, leaving a few drops of water in the bottle
- Add another 4-6 ounces of water; shake the bottle a few times
- Pour 99% of this water down the drain, leaving just a few drops in the bottle
- Add another 4-6 ounces of water, shake the bottle a few times...
- Do this process of pouring out water, adding water, shaking, then pouring it out again 8 more times for a total of 10 times
- Give 1 tsp of this water one time only OR sip dose 2-4 ounces of this water
- If any life threatening situation should ever arise, such has asthma that is not being managed effectively at home by either medication or natural medicines, seek professional help or go to your nearest urgent care provider.

What to Do After Dosing the Right Remedy

There can often be a honeymoon period right after you find a good remedy where many things improve. In most cases, however, this doesn't last. The state that was there previously will want to creep back in. The healing journey often becomes a process of two steps forward one step back, like a tango. Be patient and aware, with correct re-dosing you can keep moving forward. Also be mindful that if a remedy stops working, it may be because the child has switched states and no longer needs it. Some guidelines to follow after dosing a remedy are:

- If you see improvement: watch and wait, don't change remedies
- If you see improvement that then plateaus: redose the remedy
- If a remedy is working for a while and stops working: move to another potency
- If you see mixed symptoms, some things better, some things worse: ask more questions and consult Hering's Law. Are deeper symptoms improving first?
- If you see aggravation of current symptoms with a deeper layer improving: give a lower potency
- If you see an aggravation of current symptoms with no improvement: do the "aggravation zapper"

- Is another layer emerging? Do you need a different remedy? Is the overall picture different?
- And you can always watch and wait, give more time, or consult a homeopath.

How Do We Know When a Remedy is Not Working?

Most likely when a remedy is not working, nothing happens. And that is one of the great things about homeopathy—if you chose the wrong remedy and it doesn't resonate, you are none the worse.

However, very often people will say "nothing happened" when many shifts happened and they just didn't realize it due to focusing on the negative, not recognizing the change, or needing an outside observer to see the difference. Sometimes, when an issue heals, the person forgets about it all together and thinks "nothing happened." This can also occur when someone takes a remedy but doesn't believe in homeopathy, which I often see when people treat their spouses. This is why seeing a professional homeopath can be quite helpful because they may notice changes more than you can. However, most parents I work with are very sensitive and astute to shifts so this tends not to be a problem for them.

Remedies also are not working if after taking a remedy there is the development of symptoms that are new without deeper improvements that signify a true healing process. This may be termed a "proving."

What is a Proving?

If a person develops new symptoms that weren't there before and have no deeper improvements, then they could be "proving" a remedy. An example is taking the remedy Sulphur and developing the symptom of hot feet, whereas before you didn't have hot feet. Proving symptoms are generally mild, although some people who are sensitive have the tendency to prove remedies more than others. Proving symptoms can arise when remedies are taken too frequently or in too high a potency.

When proving symptoms happen, it doesn't always mean that the remedy is incorrect. Sometimes a remedy may be helpful and improve a deeper neurological symptom while manifesting a proving symptom that is new. For example, if I give Tarentula to a child with seizures, and the remedy eliminates the seizures but at the same time the child develops a proving symptom of mild sound sensitivity that they hadn't had previously, this is still a helpful remedy because we rank the importance of symptoms according to Hering's Law. In this case, the seizures were a deeper and more important symptom to heal, and the manifestation of sound sensitivity was secondary. As a homeopath I trust that the sound sensitivity will improve with time, or with the next prescription.

A challenge in case management is to differentiate between possible proving symptoms and a deeper layer arising. It's important to ask whether this symptom is something the child has ever had in the past. It is very common for old symptoms to re-emerge after taking a remedy, suggesting that a layer has been peeled away. Also, a new symptom can emerge that is simply a physical manifestation of detoxification, such as a rash, wart, stye, discharge, etc. These are not necessarily proving symptoms. What I usually see are people who develop proving symptoms on a subtle, behavioral level—such as a certain fear of heights or cats—that they didn't speak of before. When the remedy associated with that fear is stopped, and possibly a new remedy is given, that behavior should recede.

Sometimes people who experience proving symptoms that feel unpleasant do not want to wait for the symptom to recede and choose to antidote the remedy, which means rendering it inactive in the body.

Antidoting

When a remedy is having a strong effect on someone, possibly causing proving effects, it can be antidoted to stop or subdue the reaction. To antidote the remedy, you might smell strong menthol or drink a strong cup of coffee. Another option would be to follow the instructions above for an aggravation zapper.

There are other things that weaken our energy field and have a subduing effect on our whole system and the remedy state, such as EMF, Wifi, petrochemicals, and pharmaceutical medications. Some homeopaths say that people should not drink coffee at all while taking homeopathic remedies, but I feel that remedies can work if someone has a daily habit. What coffee does do, which can be a detriment to the healing process as a whole, is redirect internal energy reserves outward and upward, making us more stuck in our thoughts. So quitting coffee can be beneficial for the purposes of healing. However, if you drink coffee, do not use it as an excuse not to try homeopathy—the right remedy can still work!

Is Homeopathy Not the Right Modality in My Case?

Homeopathy is amazing but it isn't always the answer. Stay open to all possibilities. In general, I find that something other than—or in addition to—homeopathy is needed in the following types of cases.

- When enough remedies have been taken to create change and we just need more time to allow shifts to take place.
- In strong deficiency states that require supplements, diet repair, herbs, glandulars, etc.; cell salts can also help here.
- When there are dental issues such as cavities, for which holistic dental work is needed.
- When a good diet is not in place, such as too much reliance on carbohydrates when yeast overgrowth is a problem.
- In emergency situations such as a broken limb or life-threatening asthma attack (remedies can help in both cases but other medical intervention is also needed).
- When there is a heavy load of parasitic infection that requires pharmaceuticals.
- When family issues or parental issues are continually impacting the child.
- When a person does not want to wean off pharmaceuticals or an addictive substance that is suppressing their healing.
- In cases with high exposure to environmental stressors such as cell phone towers or mold in the home or at a school and the child needs to be moved from this environment.
- When there are spiritual issues such as no desire to heal, lack of faith in healing, self-blame, a need to feel "punished" by the universe, a strong attachment to the disease state, Munchausen syndrome, rebellion against parents, need for boundaries from parents trying to "fix" them, a need to release judgment, or fear of judgement. This list can go on and on!

Moving Forward

The following chapters provide detail on groups of remedies. The purpose of grouping them as such is because each group has overall themes to help you understand and choose remedies with more accuracy.

This book is an attempt to provide you with a wide array of possible remedies to help the broad range of complaints that complex children have. All of the remedies listed in this book have significantly more materia medica available than what I am able to include, so you can also research a chosen remedy online and through other detailed materia medica books such as Frans Vermeulen's *Concordant Materia Medica,* Roger Morrison's *Desktop Guide,* or Robin Murphy's *Nature's Materia Medica.*

Chapter 3

Miasms

A miasm is a homeopathic term that refers to an underlying infectious disease agent which may prevent a chosen remedy from acting, or a cure from sticking, because an inherited disease was not addressed in the previous generation. It coincides with the idea of a state being "chronic," so that all acute symptom exacerbations are really expressions of a deeper chronic disease tendency.

Hahnemann announced miasm theory in 1828 in his book *Chronic Diseases* and it was immediately controversial.[1] It was conceptually difficult for the medical world to grasp—he was ahead of his time—mostly because germ theory (the connection with germs and disease) hadn't taken hold yet. The three main miasms proposed by Hahnemann were psora, sycosis, and syphilis. Tuberculinic miasm was proposed at the end of Hahnemann's life. The cancer miasm came into being in the late 19th century after homeopath James Compton Burnett made a nosode of breast cancer (Carcinosin), despite the fact that the tissue wasn't of a specific infectious material. The miasms of cancer, tuberculosis, syphilis, sycosis (related to the disease of gonorrhea) and psora (related to scabies infection) are well established in homeopathy and are covered in depth in this chapter.

To this day, the concept of miasms is controversial and different homeopaths have varying perspectives on the concept. My perspective is largely colored by homeopath Rajan Sankaran's expanded work on miasm theory.[2] He developed nine miasms that signify how people feel and react to most major stresses and problems in life. Sankaran argues that their overall attitude and perspective is reflected by the diseases that they develop. For example, he created the acute miasm, whereby every stress is reacted to through fight or flight reactions such as seizures, as well as the malarial miasm which corresponds to the periodic complaints of worms and malaria. It is my sense that a new group of predominant infectious diseases could theoretically be called miasmatic—these include strep, candida, Lyme (borrelia, babesia, bartonella), herpes strains, and more.

A child's miasm is often the miasm of the parent and is inherited and reinforced by the patterns of family behavior. It cannot be overemphasized how much children reflect their parents AND their ancestors, and it can be of great help to intuitively feel into what side of the family a child is taking after in his or her expression of disease. Investigating the constitutions of the child's parents and grandparents and unlocking passed-down patterns in a child is the true value of deep homeopathic healing. Beyond even just suppressed infectious disease agents, shocking and stressful events within a family such as genocide, sexual abuse, murder, traumatic death, and suicide make their impacts multiple generations forward. Homeopathy offers us a pathway of releasing these deeply patterned traumas.

In some cases, a miasmatic pattern will seem persistent and fixed. For example, when cancer is strong in a family the remedy Carcinosin, as well as remedies known for treating cancer, may be of assistance over a long period of time. In other cases, miasms can shift rapidly, especially as we dose remedies to "clear" miasms. Using Rajan Sankaran's expanded use of nine miasms, below is an example of constitutionally treating an ASD child with rages through shifting miasms. Note that not all remedies known for treating miasms come from infectious diseases; many are plant medicines.

- First layer: Belladonna (for acute miasm) to treat the acute fight or flight rages from deep seated inflammation
- Second layer: Carcinosin (for cancer miasm) to treat suppressed immunity
- Third remedy: Thuja (for sycotic miasm) to treat suppressed viral infection
- Fourth remedy: Cina (for malarial miasm) to treat parasites
- Fifth remedy: Psorinum (for psoric miasm) to treat suppressed skin infections

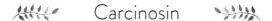 Carcinosin

Carcinosin is a remedy that treats the cancer miasm and is frequently prescribed for immune deficiency and dysfunction. Children needing Carcinosin are extremely sensitive, easily overwhelmed by chaotic situations, often clingy with their parents, highly dependent on the mother, and plagued by many fears. They attempt to compensate for the fears and anxieties by exerting control over their environment but are easily thrown into panic or even tantrums when that sense of control is lost. Other common characteristics include perfectionism, empathy, great love of animals and nature, and often a level of intellectual and emotional sophistication or precocity that surpasses other children their age. Perhaps for this last reason, they often get along well with adults. They can either be extroverted or shy, and are often quite imaginative or artistic, which is another aspect of their sophistication. As one mother explained, "He has bad separation anxiety, has to know where mom is and be with me. That umbilical cord is still there. Adores mom beyond the normal, needs to be with mom, where he feels safe and secure. Also has fears—going up escalators, he breaks out in a sweat. Fear of falling. LOVES the ocean. Gets wet head to toe. Totally connected with animals, dogs don't bite or fear him. He is determined, and can be quite fastidious but can also wreck a room in five minutes."

On the physical side, they tend to have highly suppressed immune systems. Many are sick constantly and can't kick an illness. Others do not exhibit typical cold and flu symptoms at all. In these cases, I often find a history of illness earlier in life, which became suppressed by the overuse of allopathic medicines such as antibiotics and anti-inflammatories. Instead of manifesting a normal immune reaction of mucous membrane inflammation during acute illness, these children instead show up with worsening emotional liability or tics, a deeper layer of inflammation and illness. When Carcinosin children do develop tics, they are often able to control the twitching during school because they want to please their teachers, then "let them all out" after school in the safety of their home. It's another example of the anxiety, control, and suppression that is found throughout the remedy.

After treatment with Carcinosin, it is common for a child to develop a fever; sometimes prolonged for several days. This is referred to in homeopathy as a "healing crisis." In these children, it is a sign of the immune system reawakening. Occasionally, after treatment with Carcinosin, these children may even express old grievances that they had kept bottled up; perhaps sadness from a loss or trauma, anger at someone, etc. They may also begin to express more acute illness (runny nose, fever, etc.) than they had before. In the most general sense, a child treated with Carcinosin should begin to show a stronger sense of self; standing up for what they want, pushing back more with siblings or friends who pick on them, becoming stronger emotionally, sometimes even exhibiting something like a "terrible twos" stage that perhaps they never really went through before. They are developing better boundaries (immune system, emotions) and ego. Whereas before they were terrified of getting in trouble at school, they may begin to show more resilience and brush off such things.

Carcinosin can also be called for when there has been significant family history of cancer at young ages or autoimmune disease. Children needing Carcinosin often have "type A" mothers who are in high stress jobs (or a high stress home!) during or after pregnancy. This kind of stress often creates a state of self-suppression in women; they suppress their emotions and the physical needs of their body for the sake of fulfilling the demands and expectations put on them by the outside world. They may feel as if they are juggling many balls and if they drop one, everything will fall apart. Another common etiology for Carcinosin children is a mother with a history of emotional trauma that she bottled up, such as suppressed grief and anger due to an abusive situation.

These inherited family patterns of behavior, along with the family history of cancer and autoimmune disease, are collectively known as the cancer miasm. Sankaran writes in his Schema that the keywords for this miasm include: control, perfection, fastidious, beyond one's capacity, superhuman, cancer, great expectation, chaos, order, stretching beyond capacity, loss of control, and self control.[3] Likewise, the pathology of cancer and autoimmune disease itself is a loss of control wherein the body loses the ability to effectively identify its own cells versus the cancerous or pathological cells. It then mistakenly attacks its own cells, or allows pathological cells to proliferate. Connecting this to the emotional level, it is the lack of appropriate boundaries and an inability to draw the line between self and others; you take on more than you can handle from outside, and at the same time suppress your own self. When we treat a mother and child, or even a whole family, with Carcinosin, we are trying to address this general miasm in the family. We are trying to redraw appropriate boundaries and strengthen the sense of self. In so doing, Carcinosin can help prevent autoimmune disease, cancer, and emotional and physical suppression.

Common Symptoms Indicating Carcinosin
- Children who've had only 1-2 fevers as infants/toddlers, and then no longer experienced fevers during illnesses when older; as if the body loses the ability to mount a fever.

- A consistent history of poor sleep; particularly during infancy.
- A family history of autoimmune disease or cancer (especially at a young age), or prolonged illness in the mother or child where they can't seem to kick the infection (such as mononucleosis or Lyme disease).
- A strong sensation that there is chaos in the outside world, which reflects an inner state of chaos as well, and a resulting need to exert control over their environment and themselves.

When a parent of a Carcinosin child also needs Carcinosin, it can be very challenging. These parents are some of the most likely to be anxious about the homeopathic healing process, and often have a hard time committing themselves to the path of homeopathy. They can be prone to submitting to the pressures of mainstream medicine, and it can be hard for them to find the faith in themselves to follow an alternative path of healing. Or Carcinosin parents will seek out and try all alternative options, never really deeply believing or following one path, which can lead to overtreatment with too many supplements and therapies that they feel strongly reliant on. The most successful cases I see are parents who learn about homeopathy, develop faith in it, and become empowered to step away from mainstream demands and participate as a healer in their child's illness.

The cancer miasm includes other, overlapping remedies with Carcinosin-like traits. Children who appear to need Carcinosin may start off needing one of these related remedies or may move into these states after treatment with Carcinosin. The most common of these for neuro-immune children include: Anacardium, Anhalonium, Argentum nitricum or Argentum metallicum, Arsenicum album or Arsenicum metallicum, Aurum, Carcinosnum cum cuprum, Conium, Cuprum metallicum, Ferrum metallicum, Germanium, Ignatia, Natrum muriaticum, Opium, Phosphorus, Physostigma, Ruta, Sabina, Silica, Staphysagria, and Zincum metallicum.

More unusual remedies similar to Carcinosin for treatment of children include: Lac caninum, Lac equinum, Lac delphinum, Lac maternum/Lac humanum, and Placenta.

If a Carcinosin child becomes even more deeply suppressed and the pathology reaches a level of inflammation within the central nervous system and brain, they may be moving into needing remedies such as Stramonium, Belladonna, and Hyoscyamus; all of which exhibit more extreme fight or flight states, violent reactions, and seizure activity. After successful treatment with Carcinosin, children may move to a large variety of healthier remedy states, such as Sulphur, Arsenicum album, Lycopodium, etc.

Children needing Carcinosin may require simultaneous treatment with a variety of other nosodes and/or vaccine remedies to help them clear any damages or imbalances. The nosodes I use most frequently in combination with Carcinosin include Strep (various subtypes), Medorrhinum, Pneumococcinum, Mycoplasma, MMR vaccine, DTP vaccine, Influenzinum, and Candida albicans. Carcinosin itself can also be a great remedy for parasites, and I have often had children expel roundworms after taking this remedy alone (without herbal or pharmaceutical antiparasitics).

Tuberculinum

Tuberculosis (TB), associated with myobacterium tuberculosis, is one of the most deadly infectious diseases on the planet. The CDC states that one fourth of the world's population has TB and in 2017 there were 1.3 million TB deaths worldwide. The incidence of TB is much higher in developing countries like China, India, and Indonesia than in Western countries like the United States, Europe, and Canada. Still, TB has had a strong impact on Western culture, and tuberculosis is a major reason why many immigrants in the United States pushed westward from over-populated east coast cities seeking better health and vitality. This helped to create the underpinnings of the health-seeking culture of the west coast. Despite TB's grim statistics, the vaccine for TB (BCG) is not considered sufficiently effective according to the CDC, and is not used on a wide scale in the United States, where the incidence of active TB cases per year is less than 10,000 annually.[4] The United States employs a different prophylactic approach for TB, which is routinely testing people for the disease with the PPD skin sensitivity test; if people test positive for the disease they are kept in home isolation to prevent its spread.

Because of the deep integration of this disease in the evolution of humanity—there is a fundamental archetype that fits the TB miasm—you can presuppose that in most families, there is likely an ancestor at some point who has suffered from TB. TB is generally slow progressing; once diagnosed, people can still live life while knowing time is short. In fact, in 90-95% of cases TB remains latent in the body, and in the other 5-10% it becomes active, especially when there is immunosuppression. This leads to a description of the TB miasm by Sankaran as, "There can be feelings of suffocation, being caught or trapped in the situation with no way out, being compressed, of the gap narrowing, and in reaction one wants to break free, to get out, to escape. There may also be the feeling that time is short and one needs to escape before things get too oppressive, and for this one works at a hectic pace, and puts in all efforts to make a change or to get out. There may be violence and destruction in these actions, especially as the situation becomes too oppressive."

Likewise, the tubercular miasm is fundamentally at the heart of a large percentage of immunodeficient children; many ASD and PANDAS cases, at root, have a predisposed weak, tubercular immunity which made them more susceptible to vaccine damage and other opportunistic infections.

Physical Symptoms Indicating Tuberculinum
- All types of lung symptoms, asthma; longs for open air
- Allergies, food and environmental; dairy and cat allergy
- Fungal infections, tinea, eczema, itching
- Low energy and stamina, weak, chilly
- Poor immunity, frequent colds
- Poor weight gain despite good appetite
- Teeth grinding

The physical structure of tubercular kids is generally not broadly built, robust and strong, but more refined and slim. It feels as if they are balanced towards the "vata/air" aspect of being, with a nervous constitution, and are more cerebral and lacking in a grounded, rooted, earth element. Kids can even have large heads and smaller, less developed bodies. There are often structural defects in tubercular children such as scoliosis, dental abnormalities or a pectus excavatum (caved-in rib cage). Other remedies that may assist with this are Calcarea phos, Calcarea fluor, and Staphysagria. It can also be key to give these children extra calcium/magnesium minerals to support bones and help ground their bodies.

One tubercular case I treated was the child of a corporate media businesswoman who flew on a plane her whole pregnancy, all over the world—it seems to have impressed upon her child a restless flightiness, desire for travel/movement and a certain lack of grounding in his body. This lack of grounding also seems to correlate with a poor ability to detoxify, to move toxins down and out of the body. While these children may love travel, their stamina is low and they will easily pick up infections while traveling. Their nervous constitution may make them desire change and stimulation, which they fearlessly seek out. But they will also go overboard towards excess overstimulation leaving them wired, frazzled, and underslept. As a parent whom I worked with described it, "He wants to express his frustration, his words are not fast enough, so he screams, and this is fun too/naughty. Feels like he can't stop moving/talking, going 100 mph, heart is beating fast, his little body wants to move a lot. A struggle where he is inside of it, and doesn't want to be in this quick moving body, he wants more control but feels like he can't control it. He also gets a thrill from moving so fast, like he might be not in his body but it is thrilling, the experience. It also feels like I cannot ground him literally…I will try to grab him right when he wakes up for a hug and he wants to fly away, moving, running…but happy about it. Still loves flying and airplanes, that is what he is the most thrilled about."

Tubercular kids have a tendency to develop lung-related pathology including deep, persistent coughs, bronchitis, and asthma, which further weakens immunity and manifests in poor boundaries with their environment. The top allergies that can really debilitate a tubercular person/child are: cats/animal hair/dander, mold, milk, and pollen and dust. Their allergies can manifest in asthma or wheezing or central nervous inflammation including rages, destructive tendencies, dilated pupils, tics, and twitches. Tuberculinum will be a key remedy to treat the underlying weakened immunity in these kids, while there are other remedies that can bring certain allergic traits down such as:

- Blatta for dust allergies resulting in asthma
- Agaricus for allergies related to molds/foods, intense itching
- Apis for heat, swelling, redness, inflammation with some anger
- Phosphorus for persistent dry cough, repairs poor boundaries
- Spongia for dry barking coughs
- Histaminum to help manage excessive histamine levels
- Arsenicum album for acrid, watery, runny nose with burning sensations
- Euphrasia for eye symptoms from allergies
- Mixed mold (Helios) to help desensitize mold
- Nux vomica for sneezing and runny nose on rising from bed

While tubercular kids may tend towards food allergies, they are rebellious at following dietary restrictions and will often cheat on restrictions placed on them. They may either be extremely picky about food or will eat voraciously without putting on weight easily. Like hummingbirds or racecars, a tubercular child may need lots of calories to fuel their turbo brains and activity levels. The great tendency is for them to rely on sugars, which leads them to develop a lot of yeast and ringworm.

Mental Symptoms Indicating Tuberculinum

- Defiant and rebellious
- Mean streak—will say mean things to try to undermine someone else's confidence
- Will do things that easily hurt themselves psychically and physically
- Hardness, destructive alternating with a sensitive/kind openness
- Adventurous/dare devil
- Intelligent, curious, gets bored easily
- Tends to feel trapped and restricted, creating restlessness
- Dissatisfied; something always feels off—never satisfied or at peace, driven by a need for move/change

Mentally, tubercular children tend to be confident and precocious with a desire for some level of worldliness—they may like to dress stylishly at a young age with their own creative ideas for dressing (like wearing one sock different from the other sock or asymetrical hair). I have found many tubercular kids like scissors and cutting, they really want to cut paper or the hair of their dolls. At heart, a tubercular child is open and optimistic, they take in a lot of the world around them which helps develop their precocity. This can conversely show up as shyness because they are so open they feel everything. If these kids are well cared for and sheltered, this openness will be preserved. However, if these children are raised in an over-stimulating environment, such as a city, they will close up/harden up, and can act out in destructive, cynical ways with a surprising ability to make cutting remarks that may be true but are cruel nonetheless. Tuberculinum kids/people also naturally want to break down societal rules, which they view as restrictive. Rules are made to be broken for TB people. Their natural rebellious nature creates early teenager-like behaviors and fuels cultural movements like anarchy and punk rock.

One parent of a child I treated summed up her destructive yet allergic child in this way: "Between the ages of 2 and 3 years old, he had a tendency to destroy things. For example instead of playing with the puzzle, he would tear the box apart. He could be very destructive. He would tear pages out of books on purpose. He had a very low frustration tolerance early on and a tendency towards aggression. He totally gave up naptime at 2, but I would try to have him at least rest in his room but he would get very angry and throw things, totally destroy the room. He also got terrible reactive airway with colds from age 9 months to 3 years and we gave him many nebulizer treatments and also inhaled steroids at the time. We took him for allergy testing and found an allergy to corn (made him aggressive) and decided to also eliminate wheat. We also found out he had dust mite/coachroach allergies (we encased bedding, added hepa filters to room and whole house), all of these measures seemed to give his immune system a rest."

Because the tubercular child is mentally open and quick, they can develop advanced skills in math, music, language, etc. But the downside is that they can also direct their mental hunger towards obsessive video gaming, which becomes a toxic addiction. It's important for parents of tubercular kids to recognize the capacity for a child to go deep with a hobby and direct them towards healthy ones.

There are also tubercular cases of greatly mentally deficient children. This is partly because tuberculosis also has destructive action on the central nervous system and brain. Wheeler and Kenyon state in their *Study of Tuberculinum,* "Tuberculinum should always be considered in the treatment of mentally deficient children. Where there is arrested development, mental or physical, for example delayed dentition, it is a particularly valuable remedy. Many cases are recorded wherein a backward child has been stimulated to normal development following the administration of Tuberculinum." The picture of this type of child on the autism spectrum will show limited language or cognitive skills, but can have a loud, high energy, restless body which tends to dominate the room, and can even be abusive to their caretakers/loved ones.

Many animal remedies are at core tubercular in nature, because animals also have the overlapping sensation that, 'life is short, so live it up" with fears of being trapped/restricted. Tuberculinum may open many cases but eventually constitutional prescribing will move towards animal remedies, particularly the birds (flighty/ungrounded), spiders (neurologically oversensitive), insects (busy, inflamed, ungrounded), fish (poor boundaries), and cats (stylish, picky, refined). Mineral remedies that have a strong tubercular picture are those that impact the lungs, such as Phosphorus, Antimonium tart, Antimonium met, and Stannum; those that are more open and neurologic, such as Argentum met/nit and Zincum; and those that impact the thyroid and glands, such as iodum, chlorum, and bromium. Also, metallic constitutions in general in the silver, lanthanide, and aurum series can be very tubercular underneath.

A key in prescribing Tuberculinum for a child is to look at the lifestyle of the parents. Most of these families either love travel for the joy of it, travel for work, or travel out of an inability to find the right "home." I've treated some very tubercular children whose parents were in the Peace

Corps, were diplomats, or were corporate jetsetters. Another tendency I have seen lead to a tubercular prescription is a strong history of smoking in the family, which weakens the lungs and creates a hardening of emotions and spirit. Kids from these families may be emotionally insensitive and very environmentally sensitive at the same time. For very ill families with tubercular children, they find themselves choosing to live in R.V.s or mobile homes because every house they move to has some issue—typically mold—and the family prefers change to stability. And lastly, many families who emigrate to a new country can develop a strong tubercular connection, especially when the immigration is paired with escaping an oppressive environment, including everything from physical peril to overcrowded cities or oppressive family structures. The stress of immigration and the subsequent "unrooting" from culture and country can lead to unrecognized effects on our energy systems and it can help if a family can learn to identify with and love the land/nature/plants of their new surroundings.

When we begin dosing Tuberculinum in these families, they feel ready to settle down, or even build their own house. It is important to realize that settling down can bring up ancestral family patterns that comes from "rooting." Often families are constantly moving to keep distracting themselves and to escape the patterns that inevitably arise that we inherit from parents. After treating with Tuberculinum, many kids and families may move to the miasms of either Medorrhinum (a bit more robust than Tuberculinum) or Carcinosin (suppressed and hypersensitive). The strep remedies, and their oppositional/defiant nature make it somewhat indistinguishable from Tuberculinum as well; the self-hatred and OCD of strep however isn't really a keynote of Tuberculinum.

There are several varieties of Tuberculinum nosodes available. Some are sourced from animals (Tuberculinum avis and Tuberculinum bovinum) and some are sourced from human tissue (Tuberculinum koch and Bacillinum). The standard materia medica of Tuberculinum is built around Tuberculinum bovium, which is most commonly prescribed, but I often use Bacillinum when there is ringworm present.

Medorrhinum and the Sycotic Miasm

Medorrhinum, the nosode from gonorrhea, is similar to Tuberculinum. Both are adventurous, confident, impulsive, rule-breaking, and fearless. There is also a sensitive openness that allows them to be artistic and empathic, but this alternates with a streak of hardened coldness that can come out, especially around their loved ones. However, Medorrhinum is generally the more robust of the two with much better stamina and a physical structure that is broader. While both would jump at the chance for a backpacking adventure to a far-flung location, it is more likely tuberculinum who will suffer the consequences by catching an infectious disease. Medorrhinum is the earthier of the two, thriving off sensorial impressions and enjoying life in an almost hedonistic way. Being derived from a sexually transmitted disease, medorrhinum seeks deep connection with people (sexually and otherwise), and that is ultimately how the disease rules its host to manifest its own spread among people.

The majority of medorrhinum cases I have seen were when I worked in the tri-state area and in New York City. There is high impact sensory engagement in big urban centers like New York or Los Angeles that attracts both medorrhinum and tuberculinum types. Medorrhinum parents abound in cities and their kids will be fashionable, tough, urban dwellers. However, medorrhinum people can go extreme and offbeat and you can also find them in the jungles of Brazil or running ultramarathons in the desert.

Does it sound like fun being a medorrhinum? Here's the downside: medorrhinum represents what is known in homeopathy as the sycotic miasm—this is a pattern where people tend to hide what is going wrong with them. Life is too good to be spoiled by a symptom or diagnosis, so the medorrhinum person will tend to ignore it or pretend it doesn't exist—they are tough cookies who don't complain or fret over a small symptom. And there are emergency rooms and pharmaceuticals for when things truly do go south. These people are literally rockstars, celebrities, and athletes who run themselves into the ground and die at an early age. Or they develop such a collection of symptoms that when the ship is sinking, it goes down fast.

The essence of the sycotic person is, "I have a disease that I can't get rid of, it just stays with me, in response, I cover/hide my disease/weakness to give the impression of wholeness which leaves me open to be constantly in interaction with my environment. I show off to the world that I am perfect, strong, capable by hiding my weakness, keeping the weak (infected) aspect of me a secret. I rely on others liking me to get by in the world."

Another chief remedy representing the sycotic miasm is Thuja, a remedy also well known for treating vaccinosis (see page 325). The essence of Thuja is that some disease has been impressed into you, giving you a feeling there is something wrong, and you hide it. But you are not quite yourself. You become who you think you need to be—hiding/denying the sick part of yourself. It's a kind of split. In Thuja you can see this with split urine, split nails, etc. I probably dose Thuja twice as much as Medorrhinum for the sycotic miasm in complex kids.

Physical Symptoms Indicating Medorrhinum
- Various sexual and urinary disorders
- Affections of the joints and the mucous membranes
- Worse from damp weather and by contact with the sea
- Warts
- Bronchitis and asthma
- Enuresis, cystitis, all types of genital issues
- Diseases that are spread through "me connecting with you" – like sexually transmitted diseases
- Hot in their bodies
- Intensity of symptoms, burning, pain, itching, discharges
- Fishy, green, strange discharges
- Can be burned out, exhausted

Mental Symptoms Indicating Medorrhinum
- Excessive desire for life/doing/going
- Many ideas, passionate
- Shuns responsibilities, loves the forbidden
- Fear that someone is behind you and going to get you
- Excessive love of pets but sometimes cruel to them
- Can be shy or extroverted

Medorrhinum children are similar to tuberculinum children—they want to be engaged in life, are precocious, artistic, athletic, and both can have rages. I once treated a medorrhinum child of a single mother and she was completely exhausted by her child who was oppositional, over-emotional and wanted to be a hip hop artist. Another mother explained her child as having no fear in life. "He is not afraid of heights, will climb and jump right off a diving board. Athletically he is ahead of the rest... freakishly strong... lifted up the couch leg at age 2 to find his toys. If he can't win he will quit. Likes to be the best with everything. Fights with his sibling, has to be smarter than her. His job in life is to make people laugh. His timing on jokes can be hysterical. He's like a 4-foot adult." These kids are extroverted and love play dates, affection, and attention and will ignore a phlegmy cough so they can keep playing sports with their friends.

Other remedies that tend to overlap with Medorrhinum cases are:

1. Viral nosodes—the Herpes nosodes, Coxsackie, Influenzinum, etc.
2. Carcinosin is a remedy that Medorrhinum can move into. Likewise, patients treated with either Carcinosin or Tuberculinum can move towards needing Medorrhinum
3. Strep nosodes, especially when strong oppositional and perfectionistic behaviors are present
4. Other sexually-transmitted nosodes should be considered as well, such as Chlamydia, Syphilinum, AIDS nosode, etc.
5. Remedies for the full passionate energy that overlaps with Medorrhinum are Sulphur, Belladonna, and Lachesis

Syphilinum

Syphilinum is known as the most destructive miasm, derived from the STD syphilis which can cause sores, rashes, aches/pains and eventually blindness and mental illness. As a remedy, it covers diseases of the nervous system, and the blood and skeleton, as well as a range of psychological disorders including alcoholism, depression, suicidal impulses, insanity, loss of smell and taste, blindness, deafness, and ulcerations. It is also associated with heart conditions, vesicular skin eruptions and diseases that have a nocturnal periodicity.

This deep destructive tendency may not be obvious on the outset—syphilitic people don't necessarily stand out in society and can make all the appearances of fitting in. But with deeper investigation, the core feeling of a syphilitic person is hopelessness, and this can make the path of healing all the more challenging. As one of my clients described her symptoms: "I have extreme OCD and extreme paranoia that have developed over the years. A few years ago things suddenly got VERY BAD and I developed ulcers in the right side of my body. I am extremely paranoid. I can feel so severely brain fogged. I feel like I have pressure around my skull so when I look at you I am not looking at you and it makes me feel disconnected from the world. I am terrified I will eat something that will make me sick, make something catastrophic. I wear plastic gloves…smells, transdermal stuff causes reactions. I have a lot of ritualistic behaviors, random fear of rabies, millions of checks coming in and out. Cramping, burning in stomach—physical contortions to look under the bed that makes me sicker. One thing triggers the next, I need to avoid everything."

For true syphilitic cases, the healer is required to boldly hold a torch of hope and optimism for them. Homeopathy can be the key to turning their hopeless case around, but it requires serious commitment to rise out of victim mentality and possibly even spiritual work, helping them to build momentum towards healing through forgiveness, gratitude, self love, and surrender to a higher power.

Physical Symptoms Indicating Syphilinum
- Deep bone and joint pains, curvatures of spine
- Ulceration
- Great weakness

Mental Symptoms Indicating Syphilinum
- Negative, victim mentality
- Hopeless, despair of recovery, deeply depressed
- Fears infection, hypochondriacal, always washing hands, compulsive checking
- Family history of alcoholism
- Confined to home, antisocial due to fear
- Ritualistic and obsessive
- Worse at night

The core sensation of the syphilitic child is, "I am alone in this disease, no one understands, no one cares, so my life is hopeless." Many syphilitic children stay contained to the home in their bedroom, often addicted to electronics. While many children are attached to their screens, true addiction to electronics and video games where social connection is rejected reflects a syphilitic tendency.

I have heard anecdotal evidence from other homeopaths who will often prescribe Syphilinum for ASD, but it is not a remedy I have used with great frequency for children. It can be helpful for deep Lyme disease-associated psychosis in children, but I tend to find other Lyme nosodes of greater help. I once treated an adopted child whose biological mother had syphilis, and while we tried Syphilinum for him, it didn't have as much of an impact as other constitutional remedies (he needed Rattus, strep nosodes, and Sulphur-associated remedies). When I do use Syphilinum it tends to be more with adults, especially those with a history of alcoholism or Lyme disease. It can heal a long-term alcoholic tendency in adults.

For complex children, however, there are remedies that fall under the syphilitic miasm that I have found on the whole more commonly useful, including:

- Reptile remedies for anger, rage, and destruction (Lachesis, Elaps, Crotalus, etc.)
- Lyme nosodes, especially Bartonella, for psychosis
- Chlorum for deep victim-minded negativity, as well as other stage 17 mineral remedies (Fluorine, Bromine, Iodine) for thyroid disorder
- Heavy metal remedies such as Aurum, Mercurius, Plumbum, Alumina, Bismuthum, etc., for emotional heaviness and loss of power
- Acids such as Nitric acid, Fluoric acid, Sulfuric acid, and Carbolic acid for sensation of cracking, burning destruction
- AIDS nosode and Aurum arsenicosum for extreme paranoia and germaphobia

Psorinum

The Psorinum nosode is produced from the scabies mite and reflects our body's primary breach of boundaries: infection through the skin. Hahnemann called 85% of all disease attributable to psora, the remaining 15% due to suppressed syphilis or gonorrhea. Skin diseases, allergies, hemorrhoids, dysfunctions of the organs, asthma, ulcers, jaundice, etc. are all fundamentally psoric manifestations according to Hahnemann (essentially all nonvenereal diseases are psoric). The use of suppressive skin ointments like steroidal preparations end up pushing the disease inwards and creates the psoric manifestation. The homeopath Kent equated psora to when man left the Garden of Eden and the ensuing misery when needing to fend for oneself. So effectively, all humans are, at their core, psoric.

The feeling of the psoric person is, "I am in a constant state of deficiency in life (energy, money, food, support) and I am constantly anxious because I need to make up for this constant loss." All people have this sensation to some extent, it's our basic state, but how much do you base your life on it? One mother described her situation using highly psoric language: "I got pregnant—but I didn't have a job, my child's dad worked in a restaurant as a busboy. I didn't know how I would support her. I was really, really stressed. And my boss made me stressed. It was bad. I worked as a cashier and if $2 was missing he took it from me—or if I was too slow he yelled at me like I was a little kid. I was not happy at all. I was always scared to work for him, didn't want to go to work on Mondays. But I needed money to buy stuff for her. Not easy finding that job, so I clung to that job for some time. We had roaches and bed bugs in the house at that time, so night was crazy and very itchy. Stuck in a bad place. We sold everything, lost family, to start from scratch. She would not get services back home though. Big rashes since Jan—worse with hydrocortizone or Benadryl. The doctor said she has scabies. Have to give her Benadryl at night. WHOLE BODY—really itchy. Right now I give melatonin—it doesn't help. She wakes up from the itching."

Physical Symptoms Indicating Psorinum
- Deficiency state, empty, loss, lack of, cold, weak, weak heart, weak structure, weak memory
- Deep back pain
- Always hungry, ravenous appetite
- All sorts of skin symptoms, itching worse at night, eczema in folds of skin/ears
- The skin boundary has been breached
- Worse cold
- Frequent acute illnesses
- Feeling inexplicably well the day before they get sick
- Cough and fatigue better from lying down on back with arms spread out

Mental Symptoms Indicating Psorinum
- Anxiety that something isn't right
- Feeling forsaken, can be suicidal
- Pessimistic
- Wearing extra clothes, layers for protection
- Collecting things to make up for lack
- Poverty mentality

The personality of the psoric child is, "I am insecure and not 'enough,' why am I falling behind, or can't get ahead." This is something that most children on a fundamental level feel, and in many cases when layers are peeled away, the base layer is a psoric one. This does not mean that Psorinum is the remedy of choice. Like Syphilinum, it is not one that I have found too commonly needed. But under the larger category of the psoric miasm, there are many psoric remedies that can be used as constitutional remedies that help address this underlying deficiency state.

⸙⸙⸙⸙ Conclusion ⸙⸙⸙⸙

The classic miasmatic remedies in this chapter can treat deeply inherited patterns in children and are some of the most commonly prescribed remedies in homeopathy. A miasmatic remedy may end up being a child's most important constitutional remedy that they take over many years in a full range of potencies (30C through 10M), or it may be useful when dosed only once or twice. Cases may also progress from one miasm to the next as the symptom picture evolves, ideally towards less destructive patterns.

In addition to addressing inherited patterns, miasm theory is used by homeopaths as a categorization tool. Various remedies fit under the meta-pattern of certain miasms in part because of their ability to heal that disease pattern. Below are keywords that may show up in a case for the miasms discussed in this chapter, as well as key remedies within that miasm. (Note that if you dive into research on this topic, homeopaths do not always agree on which remedies should be classified under which miasm.)

Cancer Miasm/Carcinosin
- Keywords: perfection, fastidious, superhuman, chaos, order, loss of control, self-control
- Key remedies: Agaricus, Anacardium, Argentum nit, Arsenicum alb, Bellis perennis, Cadmium, Carcinosin, Cuprum, Euphorbium, Ignatia, Opium, and Staphysagria

Tubercular Miasm/Tuberculinum
- Keywords: hectic, suffocation, trapped, closing in, freedom, defiant, oppression, desire for change
- Key remedies: Abrotanum, Antimonium tart, Bacillinum, Bromium, Calcarea phos, Coffea, Drosera, Ferrum phos, Natrum phos, Phosphorus, Spongia tosta, Stannum, Tuberculinum, Zincum met, as well as most spider, insect, and bird remedies

Sycotic Miasm/Medorrhinum
- Keywords: covered up, hidden, secretive, warts, avoidance, confident, assured
- Key remedies: Cannibis indica, Digitalis, Gelsemium, Medorrhinum, Natrum sulph, Palladium, Pulsatilla, Sepia, Thuja, and most Lac/mammal remedies

Syphillitic Miasm/Syphillinum
- Keywords: destruction, suicide, impossible, hopeless, despair, lie, outcast
- Key remedies: Alumina, Aurum, Bartya carb, Chlorum, Echinacea, Fluoric acid, Lyme nosodes, Mercurius, Platina, Plumbum, Plutonium, Syphillinum, and most reptile remedies

Psoric Miasm/Psorinum
- Keywords: deficient, weak, itching, poverty mentality, great sensitivity to cold
- Key remedies: Arsenicum album, Calcarea carb, Carbo veg, Causticum, Graphites, Kali carb, Hepar sulph, Lycopodium, Mezereum, Natrum mur, Nux vomica, Petroleum, Phosphorus, Psorinum, Silica, Sulphur, and Zincum

Keep in mind that miasms are just a start! Complex children often have immune systems that are dysfunctional due to layers of inherited disease patterns, which are further suppressed by mainstream treatments. The Nosodes chapter details many other remedies to treat disease patterns that we commonly see in modern children.

Chapter 4

Animal Remedies

The remedies discussed in this chapter are made from the tissues, milk, blood, venom, hair, feathers, ink, or bones of animals. They represent the archetypal energy of the animal as a whole, in addition to the more specific energetic effects of the particular substances. For example, milks have a nurturing theme and hormonal effect, while venoms may treat sepsis or tissue decomposition. Homeopaths often prescribe animal remedies when the heart of a patient's issues center on survival-oriented behaviors, such as striking out when threatened or panic attacks when feeling trapped.

Animal remedies can help treat quirky behavioral patterns in children, like an unusual stim that seems animal-like (such as writhing like a snake on the floor) or an unexplained fear. I once treated a young girl with an irrational fear of Styrofoam packing peanuts. When her mother pulled a peanut out of her bag in order to demonstrate this reaction of hers, she screamed "bug! bug!" and ran to the outer edge of the room with her back to the wall, looking terrified. I realized that she needed an insect remedy— and based on her other symptoms, prescribed the remedy Butterfly. The child moved through her survival-based fears while taking this remedy for several months, which were also limiting her integration in the classroom, and she began to socialize with more ease. In another case requiring some interpretation, I treated a boy who would demand that his best buddy walk behind him as they circled around a neighborhood block while pulling a wagon. This was an odd behavior and to help interpret it I called on associative memory and imagination. The mother and I both felt he was acting much like a horse, and I ended up prescribing Lac equinum, the remedy from horse milk, which he took for over a year. The remedy helped him mainstream into a standard classroom.

Children, especially under the age of seven, are learning to inhabit their bodies and acting out animal behaviors actually helps them integrate on the earth plane. If a child is deeply impressed by a particular animal and acts out its behaviors in an obsessive way, it may be a good indication to try that particular animal remedy. Early in my practice I treated a boy who insisted that he was a rat in a human suit. He would walk on all fours and had a rat name that he insisted everyone call him. I thought that giving him the rat remedy was too obvious, but as I investigated further, I found he had keynote behaviors which showed up in the provings for the remedy Rattus norvegicus (Norwegian rat). I ended up giving the remedy and it was a key step in helping him normalize from an Asperger's way of socializing to becoming a star on his high school football team. In fact, I have used animal remedies to treat many complex cases in which kids had very quirky behaviors that kept them from advancing socially. I once treated an obstinate, strong-willed girl who loved dinosaurs so much she thought she had a dinosaur tail, and if she sensed that you accidentally stepped on it, she would roar at you. She would call all her friends at school terrible names and was gaining a reputation as a bully. I prescribed a remedy that was made from the bone of a T-Rex and it calmed her tyrannical ways.

Another boy with an Asperger's diagnosis that I treated was a gifted artist who mostly kept to himself perfecting his art projects. He had many fixations and fears and would lash out regularly at his siblings. With some intuitive questioning he was prescribed Lac felinum (cat milk), which helped soften his aggressive behaviors, improved his eye contact, and allowed him to socialize more easily. At some point in his treatment he started rummaging through the kitchen cabinets at night for any form of sugar. It was a major problem as he would wake everyone in the house by clanging around in the kitchen. This continued for a while and I didn't find the right remedy until I had the mother imagine what it was like to be him, and we realized he needed the remedy from the mouse, Mus musculus. After giving this remedy his nighttime sugar-hunting behavior stopped!

It can be hard to believe, but when these cases present and you give the remedy and see the effects, it is truly astounding. If your child is acting in a certain animalistic way, write those behaviors down and look them up in a repertory to see if you can find remedies with matching symptoms. (You may need the help of a homeopath who has access to a wide range of in-depth materia medica.)

Animal remedies help to heal the state of survival in the brain. Sometimes the etiology of being in a deeper state of "survival mind" can come from a traumatic birth, high inflammation such as encephalitis, or medical injury. Interestingly, many of the animal prescriptions I've given were to kids whose parents were immigrants from other countries, possibly because of greater survival pressures in those countries. Also, immigration—unrooting and leaving your social fabric behind and adjusting to a whole new environment—triggers a state of survival mind. This largely goes unrecognized in American culture which expects immigrants to overcome all odds with hard work and conforming. This has the potential to negatively impact children and I have found that many immigrants have special needs kids.

It is important to note that there is a difference in the materia medica of wild vs. domesticated animals. The provings for the domesticated horse and dog, for example, show a deep suppression of the true instinctual self. For dogs there is deep shame, low self-worth, and an almost complete loss of sense of self. A horse (similar to the remedy Carcinosin) has the feeling of holding back from passionate desires. This makes Lac caninum (dog milk) and Lac equinum (horse milk) great remedies for those with suppressed immunity or a family history of abuse. In contrast, the remedies Lac lupinum (wolf milk) or Lac leoninum (lion milk) will express intense energy, anger, and dominance, and can be great remedies for rage.

On the physical plane there are slightly different qualities for different groups of animals. In general, they are:

- Mammal: hormones, suppressed immunity, milk allergy, headaches, digestive issues
- Insects: swelling, histamine, itching, UTIs, burning reactions, rashes, allergies, asthma
- Spiders: sensory sensitivity, tics and twitches, cardiovascular, palpitations, nerve pain, abdominal pain
- Birds: chest pains, teeth/jaw sensitivity, autoimmunity, sharp stabbing pains, shoulder and neck issues, food and eating issues
- Molluscs: water regulation, hormonal stagnation, dryness, fungal issues, coughs, milk allergy
- Fish: brain, memory, sensory dysregulation, environmental sensitivity, malnutrition
- Reptile: blood sepsis, tissue decomposition, liver disorders, hemorrhage, bacterial infection, cardiovascular, hormones

A single animal remedy may support a child for a long period of time. However, many cases do well with shifting to other animal remedies, as different layers arise. Additionally, there are remedies from outside of the animal kingdom that can complement animal remedies. For example, remedies that have to do with acute panic, survival, or even jealousy, such as Aconite, Stramonium, Belladonna and Hyoscyamus, may be useful alongside animal remedies in some cases. Or remedies that release suppression, such as Carcinosin and Thuja, can be helpful complements in some cases already using animal suppression-related remedies like Lac caninum and Lac equinum. Many categories of animal remedies, including birds, insects, spiders, and cats, have an underlying tubercular taint, with a fear of being trapped and sense that life is short. A deep-seated fear of being trapped with a desire to be free is often indicative of an animal remedy. In such cases the remedy Tuberculinum may be a useful complement.

Questions to Ask to Help Find an Animal Remedy

When is your child in their element?

A child who needs a remedy from a fish may need to be swimming in a pool daily. A child who needs a bird remedy may find riding on her scooter daily gives her the sensation of flying through the air. A child who needs to hide regularly in a little fort on the playground may do well with a mollusc remedy.

Imagine your child on the playground—describe the general movement of the child, their overall "gestalt?"

Some children dart around quickly and mischievously, which could indicate a spider remedy. I once visited an ASD girl who slowly moved towards me, crawled on my lap, wrapped her legs around my waist, and squeezed. I gave her the snake remedy Boa constrictor. Children may also want to wear colors or designs that give them the appearance of a certain animal.

Has an animal in the wild or at a zoo ever made a strong impression on the child or appeared in their dreams?

I have seen multiple children who needed Lac delphinum (dolphin milk) who have had dolphins swim up to them in the wild or at an aquarium. Remedies that children need can also show up in dreams or as intense fears. Often people with strong fears of snakes or insects can use a remedy from a snake or insect. Animal remedies that people need are often from animals present in their local environment.

❦ Mammal Remedies ❦

Humans are mammals! It's not hard to remember our monkey origins when a child is literally climbing up your back and clutching onto your hair. What is most distinctive about mammals is how they care for their young. They are nurtured for long periods of time closely by a mother who provides them with milk, and in response the baby imitates their mother and plays with siblings to learn how to survive. This desire for nurturing can be found in children who deeply care for dolls, stuffed animals, or pets, and will imitate their own mothers closely. Many mammal remedies are made from the milk of various species and these can treat hormonal imbalances well. Overlapping with these mammal remedies are the matridonal remedies made from human milk, placenta, vernix, and umbilical cord (see pages 312-316).

Mammals are territorial with boundaries to defend, and many live within a herd where they find safety and protection. As humans we follow "herd-mentality" (going with the group), and we should realize that this stems from our animal needs. One mother that I treated with the remedy Lac equinum (horse milk) would get really upset if people encroached on her in the checkout line at the grocery store and had numerous incidents where she would ask people to "back away."

Another child I treated with Lac vaccinum (cow milk) was very stressed when her group of friends made comments about her behind her back and made her feel like she wasn't "part of the group." Mammals are social but also create hierarchies. Many of our human behaviors reflect our mammal-ness: from cliques in schools, to competitive sports, to a need to care for pets. Children who need mammal remedies may show awareness of these groups and hierarchies, and will feel protective of their friends or clique.

While insect, spider, and bird remedies tend to be tubercular in nature, most mammals fall under the sycotic miasm, which means they will be outwardly confident and at ease but have a need to hide a part of themselves. An example of this is a secret desire to smell our body odors; it's not something we do openly but it is a natural instinct we get from being mammals. Many needing mammal remedies are also within the cancer miasm with a deeply suppressed side of themselves (usually the most instinctual animalistic side!). However, those who confidently tap into their natural animal energy can be very unique, creative, and powerful people. Temple Grandin, a woman with Asperger's who revolutionized the treatment of cattle by imagining what it is like to be them, is a great example of this.

For people who tend to suppress their animal sides, remedies like Lac caninum (dog milk) and Lac equinum (horse milk) can help them find their true selves. Lac caninum, in particular, is an important remedy for cases with a history of any form of abuse, where the sense of self gets deeply suppressed creating a sense of shame and feeling of "dirtiness" about one-self. Lac equinum is more proud but feels constrained by life and has a great desire to break out and be true to their passionate desires. Lac vaccinum (cow milk) is also for a suppressed sense of self, with many fears and anxieties. I have given it to immunosuppressed children with frequent colds, upper respiratory tract infections, and enuresis. Lac vaccinum can also improve tolerance for dairy products.

There are also mammals who live in the water; two of the most well-known sea animal remedies are Lac delphinum (dolphin milk) and Ambra grisea (whale bile). Lac delphinum is a wonderful children's remedy and strongly fits the themes of the mammals; there is an intense playfulness, sociability, and warmth to dolphin people who are very empathic and aware. Ambra grisea has the qualities of being silly and playful like dolphins, but has a streak of shyness leading them to be easily embarrassed by their silly behaviors.

Natural Mammal Behaviors

- Most evolved and intelligent of the animals
- Strong maternal instinct
- Connection with one's immediate family, especially father, mother, siblings
- Learn by imitation
- Most give birth to live young ones
- Nourish their young ones on milk
- Have hair on the body
- Highly adaptable and often modify their behavior to suit changing circumstances
- Importance of communication, especially with sounds, amongst members of their own species
- Safety within the group; theme of the self versus the group; being leader of the group; fight for the dominant position
- Guarding their own territory, territory is encroached

- Flight, fright, escape, freeze
- Submission versus dominance
- Belonging to a group, herd, or pack
- Fight to the finish is not a common association with mammals

Notable Mammal Features in Complex Children

- Imitating the behaviors of their friends very closely, "copy cats;" can actually take on the whole look of another person
- A love of babies, want to take care of babies, seek them out
- May have quirky behaviors so they don't fit in, but they really want to be a part of a loyal group of friends
- May have strong obsessions, stuck behaviors, and love collections
- Feel terrible and embarrassed if criticized by one of their friends; can't stand the idea of being disliked or an outcast
- May have milk allergy/lactose intolerance
- May have had issues with breastfeeding or bonding with their mother, issues of abandonment, separation anxiety
- A dislike of people being in their space, can get claustrophobic and trapped feeling with people encroaching on them
- Easily nauseated, a regurgitation feeling of food coming up
- Very aware of their appearance, wanting to look attractive to the opposite sex; like to wear animal prints; feel rejected by their partner if they aren't sexually appealing
- Like to smell certain areas of their mother's body, love to feel their mother's breasts
- A very strong liking or fear of a particular animal
- Very cuddly and affectionate, love to play, tackle, wrestle
- History of abuse, particularly sexual abuse, on mother's side of the family; passive behavior
- Can be very wild and fearless or more suppressed and fearful, depending on the animal
- Can secretly feel really bad about a part of themselves and not reveal that to others, a feeling of shame/dirtiness
- Can be extremely creative and imaginative, love dress up
- Like to take care of pets, a great desire for pets
- Very animated and all over the place when talking, not linear in conversation; can use sound effects when talking

Ambra Grisea (Whale Bile)

Cases of Ambra grisea are naturally introverted but force themselves to connect and become too extroverted, acting silly or hysterical with poor boundaries, and then become embarrassed of their behavior and turn inwards again, often second-guessing what they will say. For example, a nonverbal ASD child who is attempting to speak but is very embarrassed and awkward when they try. They may feel awkward about their body or size, or throw their body around recklessly in a flopping manner with no body awareness. They have an odd sense of proportion and may write or draw very large. Ambra grisea can help when there is a history of abuse or deep emotional suffering; perhaps all their problems started after experiencing a deep grief from the loss of a parent or divorced embittered parents. They hold their suppressed emotions and suffering inside and have a deep inner world with strong interest in music and animals. They may come across as moody and misunderstood or odd and eccentric. Physical symptoms include asthma, jerks, twitches, heaviness, sleeplessness, one-sided complaints, big appetite, and fast weight gain. Ambra grisea may help with speech, concentration and conceptual thinking. This remedy is like a combination of Natrum mur, with its inward timidity, and Argentum/Platina with its outwardness and concern about what people think of them.

Lac Caninum (Dog Milk)

Outgoing and connecting, these children can go outside of themselves and be totally adaptable, even doing uncanny imitations of other people. Some have an intense love of dogs and go straight to their level, petting and kissing them, while others have an intense fear of dogs due to a history of a dog bite. They may also have a phobia of snakes or vomiting. Often there will be a history of verbal or physical abuse in the child, or simply benign neglect, resulting in feeling "bad" or "dirty" about themselves, so they put themselves down and secretly suffer from self-loathing and low self-worth. They will feel very guilty and down on themselves if reprimanded. Despite this inner worthlessness they still long for the acceptance of others, dislike being alone, and present to the world a sweet enjoyable personality. Kids who need this remedy may have various odd fixations and quirks such as an obsession with windchimes, or American flags. Lac caninum can treat sore throats, tonsillitis, profuse salivation, and symptoms that change from side to side such as ear infections that alternate from ear to ear or migraines that occur on alternate sides. It also treats spacey, floating feelings in the head, vertigo, bedwetting and nausea with fear of eating, bulimia or an insatiable appetite. This is a common remedy for PANDAS with a history of strep infection and immune-suppression, feelings of failure, and use of statements like, "I hate myself," or "I look ugly." Compare to Carcinosin, Cannabis indica, Pulsatilla, Staphysagria, or Phosphorus.

Lac Delphinum (Dolphin Milk)

These are playful and amorous children but can have poor boundaries leading them to easily get sick. Oversensitive, empathetic, and generous, they like the idea of being a part of a "pack" (like a wolf pack), enjoy teamwork, and are creative with many hobbies. There may be a history of abuse that is deeply suppressed; they can withstand terrible pains and physical issues with a happy face. Lac delphinium can treat environmental and chemical sensitivities, insomnia, very sensitive digestive systems, colic, and backbone pathology. The sympathetic and social nature of this remedy makes it comparable to Carcinosin, Palladium, Phosphorus, and Staphysagria.

Lac Equinum (Horse Milk)

This remedy is for children who are aloof and sensitive, who want to be free but feel constrained and trapped by life's circumstances. This desire for freedom is expressed in a frequent need to go for walks, to run, move fast, let loose emotionally, be passionate, dance or be creative. They also like the closeness of a loyal group of friends or one best friend, essentially someone they can trust. But they also have a need for personal space and do not like it if people overstep their boundaries or disrespect them. Often competitive and wanting to do a good job, they can be dignified and dutiful and not want to disappoint or fail. Physical symptoms include hypoglycemia/diabetes, lung issues, muscle tone/musculoskeletal issues, and poor coordination. Compare with Calcarea carb, Carcinosin, Ignatia, Natrum mur and other remedies.

Lac Felinum (Cat Milk)

Lac felinum is the most tubercular of the mammal remedies, so lungs are their weakness. This remedy may heal those suffering from chronic asthma and allergies, including cat hair allergies. Many cases of children who need this remedy will have large eyes with long lashes, make great eye contact, but have eye issues (keratitis, eye pain, styes, photophobia), with fear of sharp objects and eye injury. They may even have visual synesthesia, for example seeing colors as numbers. While they can be affectionate and clinging with their mother to the point of having separation anxiety, they come across as aloof or contained to other people, sometimes acting quirky or lashing out. They can also get very absorbed in their interests which are often artistic and refined, such as a love of fashion and performance, as well as an empathic interest in the healing arts. Compare with Silica, Tuberculinum, Medorrhinum and Phosphorus.

Lac Leoninum (Lion Milk)

Lac leoninum is similar to Lac felinum, with being empathic and intuitive. However, it is a much more dictatorial, argumentative and competitive remedy. They want to be the best, and want to be able to show off strength and dominance. They are hot in the body, physically restless and have a tendency to anger, jealousy, and suspicion, but also demonstrate leadership qualities. They are also sensitive to injustice and will show great anger when contradicted. It is possible that during pregnancy, the child's mother was unjustly treated causing great suppressed anger. Like many animal remedies, they can also feel caged or trapped by the expectations of others, with a desire to escape, mock, or talk back rudely. They may suffer from backaches, insomnia, allergies, tics and twitches or itching skin. Compare with Carcinosin, Medorrhinum, Lachesis, Sulphur, and Aurum.

Lac Lupinum (Wolf Milk)

This is a remedy for incredibly energetic, wild, and unconstrained children who can tap into their inner primal force. They may suffer from ADHD or be aggressive; they sense a hierarchy between others and are competitive with siblings. There is a strong "alpha" attitude, although they desire teamwork and have a strong fear of exclusion or being left alone. They may excel in sports. They often play the role of the "bad" child—it's them versus society. They may also be tapped into very strong, protective paternal/maternal instincts. Compare with Anacardium, Veratrum alb, Sulphur, and Medorrhinum.

Lac Ovinum (Sheep Milk)

Children who need the remedy from sheep are natural followers who need someone to take care of them. They lack a sense of identity, are always looking for a boss or someone to imitate, are often chaotic and in a panic, and are innocent and naïve. Confrontation or aggression makes them feel rejected and they will sacrifice themselves to keep the group or family together. There may be immune issues leading to rheumatoid arthritis, constipation (that improves with fat intake), or variable symptoms that constantly change making this remedy somewhat similar to Pulsatilla.

Lac Suis (Pig Milk)

Helpful for stubborn, messy children who tend to hoard toys and other possessions and are affable and opinionated. They may resist authority or like to be the authority figure but don't really take on a leadership position. The family unit provides a safe space and they will often express their indignancy freely. Physical symptoms include pelvic pain, sinusitis, cellulitis, vertigo, and floating sensations. Compare with Sulphur or Magnesia sulph.

Lac Vaccinum (Cow Milk)

This is a key remedy for treating strong cow milk allergies, low immunity, and immune dysfunction (such as CVID). Due to the heavy use of antibiotics in the dairy industry, dosing the nosode Streptococcinum intercurrently with Lac vaccinum may be useful particularly when there are skin breakouts, digestive issues, low self-esteem, or depression that shows up after drinking milk or eating beef. These children present as environmentally sensitive, anxious, fearful of closed spaces but also fearful of the outdoors, listless, depressed, and indecisive. They have a long list of fears and are often afraid of insects, they cry easily, and they may suffer from headaches, poor digestion, joint pains, great thirst, frequent urination/enuresis, vertigo, white ulcers on the tongue, sinusitis, and otitis media. Lac vaccinum defloratum is skim milk and similar to the above; it's notable for neutropenia, anemia, malnutrition, headaches, milk allergies, and stomach pain. Lac vaccinum butyricum is buttermilk and good for mucousy ears, "damp spleen," and loose stools with lots of gas. Compare with Carcinosin, Natrum mur, and Silica.

Moschus (Deer Musk)

Primarily a female remedy, these girls have imaginary sufferings and may make up their illness to get attention. They are possibly over controlled and pampered by their parents. They are easily frightened to the point of fainting and are afraid that something bad is about to happen. They have a tendency to hysterical or spasmodic reactions such as spasmodic constriction of the larynx, sudden spasmodic cough, whooping cough, hiccoughs, trembling of the whole body, one cheek red and cold and the other pale and hot, immoderate uncontrollable laughter and even convulsions with alternating tonic and clonic spasms. Moschus is useful for asthma with anxiety, especially when paired with alternating moods. Digestively there may be nausea with oversensitivity to smells, aversion to food, gas and bloating. Compare to Agaricus, Pulsatilla, Ignatia and Zincum.

Mus Musculus (House Mouse)

Skittish and fearful, children who need this remedy have low eye contact, startle easily and back away from anything that intimidates them. They may also crave sugar and have an insatiable appetite. Compare to Natrum mur, Aconite, and Calcarea carb.

Rattus Norvegicus (Rat Blood)

Children who need Rattus have a delusion that something is watching them and that they are being pursued. They hoard and collect piles of junk and have itchy rashes but they also desire to hunt and love knives and swords. There is deep self-loathing with an aversion to society; these kids feel estranged, are often secretive, and like to be by themselves. Compare to Sulphur and Syphilinum.

Spider Remedies

Just watch a spider make its web and attack its prey and you'll get the sense of what qualities spider remedies help treat, which according to Sankaran include "intense hyperactivity, always busy and moving, mischievous, rhythmic." The most important feature to understand is that spider remedies help treat an overly sensitized, overwhelmed, and/or damaged nervous system, which is very common in special needs and especially PANDAS and chronic Lyme. This can show up as tics, twitches, oversensitivity to sounds and touch, chorea, and even seizures. These kids are in constant motion and too much sun, mold exposure, or a loud bang can set their nervous system off, triggering tics/twitches or rage.

While it may seem like all complex kids could use a spider remedy, there are more nuanced characteristics that are important. A unique spider remedy trait is the desire for, or interest in a regular rhythm, such as with music and dance, to help regulate their overstimulated nervous systems. This "dancing" may show up more like regular stimming movements, tapping, or banging. I once treated a mother who needed a spider remedy, and she told me that during her pregnancy she strapped a device that played heartbeat music to her belly daily. As far as I could deduce, this "educational device" simply reinforced a strong spider state in her ASD child who was constantly banging out rhythms.

Speed, impatience, and the short life span of spiders puts them into the tubercular miasm and you will often see in spider cases a family history of weak lungs, weak immunity, allergies (to dust, mold, etc.), asthma, and smoking. Bird and insect remedies, which are also tubercular in nature, can overlap. Like Tuberculinum, people who need spider remedies can be social, adventurous, and the life of the party with a capacity to see larger patterns in life (how everything is connected), and may even be clairvoyant.

The spider remedy most commonly prescribed is Tarentula hispanica, which is generally a cunning, mischievous, ADHD child sometimes prone to violence. However, I have had cases of very sweet children who want to please and have some sort of neurological issues and/or spider bite etiology that still benefit from spider remedies. In some spider cases a child who has had extensive brain inflammation will be slow, dulled, and may have a lot of head or joint pains. One such child I treated spent most of his time in the family garage doing nothing but listening to music. A few of the kids I treated with spider remedies had large, hydrocephalic heads from chronic brain inflammation, which reduced in size after taking their remedy.

Many people with Lyme disease who have neurologic sensitivities and are confined in their homes, depressed and exhausted, will also do well with spider remedies. The etiology "worse since a bug bite or spider bite" can often suggest a spider remedy (also consider Ledum or Lyme nosodes). Lastly, I have had many cases where either the mother received a spinal tap during delivery, or the child received lumbar punctures as an infant, and this seemed to predispose them to the neurological damage requiring a spider remedy to heal.

Natural Spider Behaviors

- Intense pace, speed, hyperactivity
- Busy, always moving
- Quick and constant movement; patterned, rhythmic movements
- Short life span
- Territory is defined and can be invaded/encroached/intruded upon
- Periodicity and rhythmicity
- Caught and trapped
- Deceit, cunning
- Impulsive violence, impulsive aggression

- Suddenness, sudden urges, short bursts
- Sudden death, sudden fear of death
- Prefers to hide in the dark, light aggravates
- Kill and hide
- Devours their food
- Miasm: predominantly tubercular

Notable Spider Features in Complex Children

- Always active, constant movement, ADHD, restless, jumping from one thing to the next, fingers and hands always busy, full of boundless energy; hurried and impatient
- Impulsive, can't keep hands to themselves; like to jump on people's backs
- Attention seeking, mischievous, teasing; lash out suddenly, attack, and then hide
- Will lie or make up an illness for attention; manipulative; lying and deceitful; kleptomania
- Out of a sense of victimization, can blame and complain
- Feels forsaken, parents may be too busy to give them attention, but they require a lot of attention
- Head-banging, dancing, tapping, drumming, spinning, jumping, which helps to regulate/calm the nervous system
- Tics, twitches, chorea; jerks during sleep
- An attraction to strong colors, patterns, certain shapes
- Abscesses and boils that erupt on their own, or around bug bites
- A need to listen to music, especially rhythmic music, and will move to the beat (Latin, hip hop, and rap music); loves to dance
- Head swelling, hydrocephalus, large head size
- History of lumbar punctures
- Can lash out and be violent, attack, stab; interest in knives
- Destructive and rebellious, somewhat suspicious
- Like to balance on the edge of things (e.g. walking on the curb)
- History of bad insect bites including sensations of stinging and swelling
- History of bad spider bites in the mother
- Strawberry birthmarks and angiomas
- Desires to be attractive, likes bright colors
- Urinary incontinence, frequent urination or a history of UTIs
- Hyperlexia, interest in letters and linguistics; can be nonverbal or loquacious

- Can be very cerebral and academically advanced, or have poor concentration and memory
- Can be very social or can isolate oneself; may have low attachment to parents
- Likes acrobatic performance, circus, slackline, trampoline, ninja, monkey bars
- Can have a history of visual or auditory hallucinations
- VERY sensory sensitive, sensitive hearing and sensitive to touch; auditory processing issues; delusionary hearing, sensory system overwhelmed and needs time outs
- Prefers juices and sugar over solid food; appetite disorders like anorexia and bulimia
- Prone to seek out smoking, drugs, sex
- Takes a long time to fall asleep
- Mothers who are busy, workaholics, empaths, travel a lot, and/or smoke
- Similar remedies: Tuberculinum, bird and insect remedies, Zincum met

Aranea Diadema (Papal Cross Spider)

Aranea diadema is a more emotionally sensitive spider remedy, with fear of disapproval of others creating perfectionism and workaholic tendencies, but there is still an inner sense of rebellion with desire to be recognized as an individual. They may be sensitive to dampness and feel cold to the bone. There may also be family history of lung cancer, lung issues, hemorrhaging from wounds or slow healing of wounds, neuralgia or tingling in the extremities, and joint troubles. The abdomen may feel distended with a desire to press into the abdomen with a closed fist. These complaints may come in regular intervals.

Ixodes (Deer Tick)

This spider remedy is the most "parasitic" in nature with outward hostility, lack of motivation, oppositional behavior, and mood swings if they don't get their way. This child will be self-absorbed while uninterested in and critical of others. When at their worst they are emotionally robotic, acting more like an alien than human. They will manipulate to get out of responsibility and speak offensively to anyone. Deep inside there is low self-worth, feelings of wanting to die, and exhaustion. There may be a history of Lyme disease with weak lungs. Compare with Lyme nosodes.

Latrodectus Mactans (Black Widow Spider)

A child who needs this remedy may come from a family where there has been life or death situations causing shock resulting in fainting or pains around the heart, such as angina, feeble or rapid heartbeat, or cramping pains in the chest. This child will be very sensory sensitive with love of constant movement. There may be a history of suicide in the family.

Loxosceles Reclusa (Brown Recluse Spider)

Helpful for kids with a history of wounds, skin ulcers, itchy rashes, or bites that are destructive and take a long time to heal. This remedy also treats a history of anorexia and bulimia in the mother that shows up as easy gagging and food refusal in the child. There may also be an accompanying dark aspect to the case with history of betrayal, forsaken feelings, despair, or apathy leading to a suicidal tendency. Like all spiders, a child needing this remedy will be oversensitive, with body jerking and need for constant movement and jumping.

Mygale Lasiodora (Black Cuban Spider)

Mygale is used to treat chorea in upper parts of the body or when there is constant motion of facial muscles or the entire body; chorea is worse in the morning and from motion, better during sleep. There is tendency to lymphangitis, or red streaks along lymphatic channels. These children are intense, competitive, combative, restless, and may also show strong sexual impulses. Compare with Agaricus and Stramonium.

Tarentula Hispanica (Spanish Tarantula)

This remedy is commonly prescribed for kids whose overactivity leads to overstimulation and oversensitivity. These kids can be fun with boundless energy, laugh constantly, and have mischievous attention-seeking behaviors that entertain along with impressive physical skills. They spend their days running, jumping, and kicking, and they will love karate, parkour, gymnastics, and dance. These kids love and are improved by music and movement, using the steady beat or singing to regulate and release the nervous system. For release they will toss their head, mouth things, slam into furniture, and take off their clothes. However, they overdo it. It's possible these kids have an inner feeling of being abandoned or they aren't getting the attention they desire, so they lie or fake an illness to get attention. They can also be rude and talk back. Their nervous system gets overwrought and they may have rages, violence, chorea and tics, seizures, sound sensitivity, restless limbs at night, sensitivity to touch, and involuntary urination.

In time, immunity will deteriorate with intense and continuous coughs, a dulling of intellect and memory, and worsened behavior during infection. Compare with Tuberculinum, Zincum, Belladonna, Stramonium, and Hyoscyamus.

Tarentula Cubensis (Cuban Tarantula)

Tarentula is a good remedy for anxious, obsessive, fretful kids who fear death, but who are also sensitive to others, empathetic, and have feelings of responsibility for the family possibly causing hypervigilance. They like to keep busy, such as doing nonstop housecleaning, and are always in motion. Physical symptoms include ulcers, recurring abscesses, and boils that can progress to cellulitis. They can get hysterical and oversensitive to pain with poor emotional control, drama, and lashing out.

Theridion Curassavicum (Orange Spider)

This is often prescribed for very talkative, restless kids with extreme sensitivity to noise where every little sound makes them jump. Sounds seem to penetrate the whole body, especially the teeth. They are also sensitive to light, worse from touch and pressure, and have great sensitivity between the vertebra. This remedy can treat motion sickness with vomiting or a tendency to eating disorders such as bulimia. Compare with Agaricus.

Insect Remedies

Think of an insect bite and you understand the symptoms they help to treat, such as swelling, stinging, burning, and heat. Children who need insect remedies have chronic high levels of inflammation making them highly sensitive to their environment. This inflammation may show up as seizures, asthma, allergies, sore throats, swellings, red skin rashes, and high histamine levels. Insects have a short life span, often completing their whole life cycle in one season. With this in mind you can understand why someone needing an insect remedy is busy, hurried, organized, and mostly focused on basic needs. These kids tend to have a big appetite and constant hunger, while also battling many food allergies that cause redness, swelling or pains. This combination of being busy and inflamed can create a fiery personality that is intense, active, easily angered, and has sudden impulsive behaviors. The classic remedy that fits this profile is Apis (honeybee), which

I give often to special needs kids. Some cases have terribly red, inflamed eczema, and some have a strong fear of buzzing noises. One Apis case I treated was very environmentally sensitive and had asthmatic reactions to chemicals, car exhaust, and plastics.

While the mammal remedies can be affectionate, often kids who need insect remedies dislike touch, are tense, rigid, and wound up, and can even be antisocial. Many cases I have seen of insect remedies are kids who have annoying behaviors like making loud noises or pinching/poking people and touching strangers, which worsen when they get dysregulated or over-whelmed by chaos. In general, they are highly sensitive, especially with their hearing, and may also have fears or sensory issues around loud noises, bugs, certain textures, and lights. There are many similarities to the spider remedies, however there are also key differences. Insect remedies tend to cooperate and work with the group while spider remedies want to over-power others and exert their will over others. Likewise, the insect remedies tend towards conformity and following orders while the spider remedies want to stand out and are rebellious and creative. Insect remedies have inflammation that creates an inner heat in the body while spider remedies tend to be cold and chilly to the bone. Insects also have a low sense of self, feeling demeaned and even despised, while spider remedies have big egos and will want to show that they are better than you. While both spiders and insects can be competitive, jealous, high strung, and violent, some insect remedies can have softer, gentler personalities with a desire to care for others, like Butterfly and Ladybug. The idea of change, transformation, and metamorphosis is also a key theme in insect remedies like Butterfly.

Hyperlexia, or the ability to learn how to read and write at an early age, is something I have noted in many kids needing insect remedies as they often have a capacity to understand and recognize shapes easily (spider remedies can also be very hyperlexic). This makes sense, given that is what insects are constantly doing—recognizing flowers, patterns, and colors. Likewise, these children can be very detail oriented and good at artwork and writing. Some may be quite perfectionistic. Butterfly kids often love making collages and have a wonderful sense of color. Urinary issues seem common in insect remedies and may be linked to the allergies and hista-mine issues they have. Often either the child or the mother has a history of urinary tract infections or enuresis.

Words that parents may use when describing a child who needs a rem-edy from an insect are: agitated, burning, itching, irritating, buzzing, flit-ting, going from place to place, busy, fast, swollen, and hot.

Natural Insect Behaviors

- Small, short life span focused on the basic needs of food, reproduction, and sexuality
- Organized, busy, industrious
- Suddenness, restlessness, hyperactive
- Constant, intense activity; a lot has to be achieved in a short time
- Territory is defined and can be invaded/encroached/intruded upon
- Going through stages of metamorphosis

Notable Insect Features in Complex Children

- Environmentally sensitive
- Prone to allergic reactions—red, itching eczemas; flares; swelling; inflammation
- Chronically high histamine levels causing heat and reactivity to everything
- Emotionally and physically reactive, short fuse, easily triggered or annoyed, feels agitated, and prone to sudden rage
- Can have a lot of internal heat
- Strong reactions to insect bites
- Tendency to urinary issues or UTI's (also in mom); bed wetting
- Hyperlexic; interest in shapes, patterns, letters
- Hyperactive, busy, ADHD, always doing something
- Can be open, social, and happy or quiet and introverted
- Creative in expression; interested in bright colors, patterns, and movement
- Obsessive compulsive about certain organizational things
- Fear or love of bugs. Fearful of injections and haircuts.
- Bothered by buzzing noises and loud voices; can feel the sensation of buzzing inside
- Stimming by shaking strings, or playing with strings
- Fear or obsession with specific lights and sounds
- Fear of suffocation or violent death or attack
- Violence and sudden attacks, impulse to kill, sudden fears
- Similar remedies: Sulphur, Phosphorus, Argentum nit, Histaminum, Tuberculinum

Apis (Honeybee)
Apis is a commonly used remedy for all types of swelling and

inflammation including histamine reactions, hives, rashes, red-hot eczema, edema, and even seizures.

People who need it are busy, restless, and almost "buzzing" around; they like organization and to do a job well. They may also be competitive, easily reactive and quick to anger with knee-jerk reactions. Sometimes they can have an unexpected all-out rage with a red screaming face. It is a useful remedy for environmentally sensitive kids who have allergies and are prone to eczema and asthma. It can also be given in acute situations for bee stings, anaphylaxis, sore throats with marked redness, shingles with swelling, angioedema, congestive headaches, cystitis causing edema, inflammation and swelling of the eyes and fever with thirstlessness. All complaints are worse from heat, sensitive to touch and better from cold. Compare with Belladonna, Sulphur, and Lachesis.

Blatta Orientalis (Cockroach)

For kids who are particularly sensitive to moldy damp places, mildew, or rotting leaves, causing asthma and allergies with wheezing or short, dry, hacking coughs.

Butterfly

Butterfly is a common remedy useful in treating restless, hyperactive, agitated children with some spaciness, low concentration, and poor memory. They "flit" from one thing to the next. According to homeopath Patricia Le Roux, "They tend to be patients who are delicate and fragile. Slim with an insubstantial backbone—they love to dance and move about restlessly but prettily, wearing bright colors...they tend to wrap their arms around themselves. It's as if they are trying to defend their fragile bodies from danger." These kids have a knack for "metamorphosis," loving costumes, fairy wings, dressing up, and face paint. Butterfly carries the theme of caring for the disabled or genetically impaired, and children who need this remedy will also be nurturing towards dolls, animals, and other children. They will feel stressed when their loved ones are ill and spend more time at the bedside of a sick elder than an average kid. They are likely easy going, talkative kids who everyone loves, but also highly emotional and cry easily. Physically, this remedy can treat recurrent burning urination, eczema and itchy rashes, floating sensation in the head, and pulsating back pain.

People who need this remedy may have a feeling of abandonment or lack of structure during childhood, causing an aimless wandering of interest, a lost feeling, and a deeper desire for structure as with Calcarea phos and Tuberculinum. Compare with bird remedies, Phosphorus, Pulsatilla, and Ignatia.

Bombyx Processionea (Processional Caterpillar)
Similar to Butterfly, but with an added feeling of abandonment, possibly due to an absent father. It is a useful remedy for urticaria with much stinging/scratching and can also be an emergency remedy for a twisted testicle risking castration.

Cantharis (Spanish Fly)
Burning pain is the keynote of this remedy, and it is commonly used for sunburns, kitchen burns, urinary tract infections, bladder infections, cystitis, burning gastritis, and even burning in the brain. As a deeper acting constitutional remedy, it may assist with rage, irritability, and even sexual mania. Compare with Belladonna, Hyoscyamus, and Stramonium.

Coccinella Septempunctata (Ladybug)
Coccinella acts mostly on irritation of nerves of the head, teeth, gums, and mouth as well as facial tics (tic doulourex). It can also be used for throbbing toothaches with an accompanying cold sensation in the teeth and mouth. They tend to be shy, reserved people who fear that the world is full of dangers. They have many phobias and desire protection. Likewise, they may also want to protect and care for other children and animals.

Coccus Cacti (Cactus Bug)
This remedy treats stringy, ropey discharges and spasmodic coughs ending in the vomiting of mucus. During pregnancy there may be night waking with gagging and vomiting of copious mucus. It also treats asthma with a constricted feeling around the lungs and chest with much mucous congestion, worse dairy. Constitutionally, this is likely to be a happy, go-with-the-flow child who gets along with everyone, with an underlying layer of sadness and perfectionistic tendencies that make them apprehensive. Compare to Phosphorus, Silica, Carcinosin, and Pulsatilla.

Culex Musca (Mosquito)
This remedy can treat strong histamine reactions including allergic asthma, dermatitis, and allergies in general. Personality-wise, these are angry, cursing children who argue but deep down they have massive insecurity, very low sense of self identity, and hatred toward themselves. Their

frustration with their body may show up in a desire to cut themselves. They may hit, pinch, poke, or curse at you or their teachers, and then try to get away. They are always moving, have poor impulse control, and may randomly touch strangers. They may desire to be the best and can be perfectionistic but are too tired or lazy to do their schoolwork. Culex is like a combination of the low self-esteem of Anacardium and the inflammation of Sulphur.

Doryphora (Colorado Potato Beetle)

Doryphora treats very weak kidneys with inflamed ureters, frequent urination, inability to control urination, and the involuntary touching of genitalia. Kids who need this remedy will have sensitive nerves (even a simple touch can cause pain), migraines, as well as fear of high pitched noises and a need to block them out. Irritated nerves may also be expressed as angry, irritated, attacking behavior. While they may be talkative and hyper within the home, in school they will be in a "shell" and less hyperactive, giving one-word answers to teachers. Like many insect remedies, the child will have red hot ears and cheeks after eating certain foods. Compare with Apis, Tarentula, and Cantharis.

Lumbricus Terrestris (Earthworm)

Lumbricus works well on blocked or congested tubes, such as eustachian tubes, difficulty swallowing with reverse peristalsis, anorexia, bulimia, constipation, and stiffness in the spine. It relieves acute pain from injuries on the spine, and can clear congestion and restore organ function by stimulating the lymphatic system. Compare with Calcarea carb.

Mantis Religiosa (Praying Mantis)

Cases of Mantis revolve around a history of abuse or domination of the mother by her spouse, creating deep anger. This may manifest in the child with violence towards themselves or others with a desire to cut or stab; they feel dirty and low within. There may have been shame of the pregnancy with a desire for abortion resulting in the child feeling rejected; deep down this child wants validation and connection with their mother. The child will feel hurried and impatient with internal stiffness and tension causing awkward movement. They may have a grayish hue to their face. Compare with Anacardium and Staphysagria.

Bird Remedies

Bird remedies embody the desire for freedom. For a bird case, if I ask when the child feels most happy, the parent often says, "when they feel free." Asked when the child is most in her element, the answer may be, "when they feel weightless, when they feel like they are flying." These kids love jumping off of things, feeling "up in the air" with swings or trampolines, and may literally run and flap their arms while making high pitched sounds. They often love speed and riding on scooters or bikes; they dislike the feeling of being impeded or blocked. Other words that parents use when describing a child who could use a bird remedy include light, open, sky, connecting, lifted, ungrounded, travel, trapped, and caged.

Restriction of freedom is what stresses someone who needs a bird remedy the most. These kids may panic when held down, strapped into a carseat or locked in a room. An adult who needs a bird remedy may feel trapped by the responsibilities of life and caring for their family and frequently seek out travelling opportunities. Mothers who resonate with bird remedies tend to be idealistic, soulful, and spiritually seeking. They often choose professions in healing, music, dance, or media. Birds have the tradition of being spirit guides, symbolizing our connection to the heavenly realms and spiritual guidance. Giving these remedies can unite someone with their higher self or help incarnate someone who focuses too much energy on their spiritual development and disregards their physicality.

The child who needs a bird remedy also desires to please and has a natural gift of making others happy. As empaths, they feel sad to be around others who are down so they work to raise the vibration of a group; they may be constantly singing, making up music, and also love to dance. This sensitivity may be why they often complain of inexplicable sadness, and they tend to have a wide emotional range, although they are rarely aggressive. Music often helps to channel their emotionality. Because they are airy and flighty, they may also have a hard time completing tasks that require them to sit down and focus. In school these kids will understand concepts and are curious and creative, but they can have memory complaints, problems with focusing, get overstimulated, and have a hard time sitting in their seats or completing linear tasks. Birds feel the needs of the group and many bird remedies include keynotes about anxiety when alone; likewise kids who need bird remedies can get neurotic, wound up, and have intense separation anxiety. Water bird remedies such as Ardea herodias (heron) and

Cygnus (swan) help when there is a picture of deep grief, and Haliaeetus (eagle) helps with great despair.

Like spiders and insects, bird remedies are also considered tubercular, especially with their desire for change and travel and an inner restlessness. This tubercular quality shows up as a sensation of constriction, trapped, heaviness, or suffocation in their chest. There may be heavy or stuck sensations around the sternum or xiphoid area. They tend to pick up infections easily, especially viral ones, from all their travel and poor boundaries, which can lead to obsessive neurologic behaviors. Herpes viruses, mononucleosis, and influenzinum are common nosodes that can help people who need bird remedies. The most well-known bird remedy of all is Anas barbariae, better known as the Boiron flu remedy Oscillococcinum, which has been shown in clinical trials to help reduce the severity and shorten the duration of flu-like symptoms. It can also assist with obsessive compulsive tendencies, fear of germs, anxiety, and desire for control, similar to Carcinosin.

Physically, kids who need bird remedies can have oversensitivity to lights, sounds, and noises leading to tics and twitches. They also have particular sensitivity around their teeth and may hate having their teeth brushed. Kids who need these remedies often have a high metabolism with a strong, immediate need to eat before their blood sugar drops, and their energy comes in spurts. They may have a hard time sitting at the table and will pick at their food. Some remedies like Haliaeetus (eagle) and Tyto alba (owl) can help with visual problems such as lazy eye, inflamed eyes, or issues with depth perception.

Natural Bird Behaviors

- Fly, free, take off, to rise, openness, wind, escape, floating, light, soaring, buoyant, weightless, desire to go to high places and heights
- Air and sky, bound and free; desire for freedom and travel
- Closed, shut, caged, shackled, bonded, chained, trapped, lured, confined
- Connection to mountains and sea; travel, migration, horizon
- Perfected skills, like a falcon hunting

Notable Bird Features in Complex Children

- Loves music and singing, may compose their own music
- Very emotional/emotive, very happy or very sad, large emotional range
- Desire to please, give gifts; shows gratitude

- Feels energy of the group, empathic, may want to be a healer
- Loves travel, especially air travel/airplanes, globetrotting. Travel helps break repetitive behaviors and OCD patterns, improving concentration/awareness and relieving sensory issues.
- Unique fears, like afraid of patterns such as polka dots or thunder
- Easily anxious, separation anxiety, afraid of being apart from group/mother, afraid of being alone; high strung; hypochondria
- Loves to swing, jump, trampoline, be up in the air; dislikes feeling of gravity; ungrounded
- Deep obsessions with certain activities, interests, celebrities, songs; an ability to hone in and specialize on an interest/talent. Obsessed with flying machines, space ships, rockets, etc.
- Sensitive immune systems and liver; seem to react to everything
- Gut kid with easily upset stomach; strong appetite with high metabolism; picky eaters; can't sit at the table—takes food then runs away
- Suffers from many viral infections such as herpes, influenza, coronavirus, EBV, etc.
- Extreme sensitivity to strong smells (easy gag reflex), light, weather, and air quality
- High energy fluctuating with exhaustion
- Skin picking due to anxiety; preening; dislikes being dirty; easy bruising
- Clenching the hands tightly, likes to "perch" on things or clench onto mother's neck
- Flapping, finger stims like flapping, clawing at things; running while flapping
- Fear of being trapped or blocked; claustrophobic; likes close contact or being held but not constrained
- Sensation in the sternum/xiphoid/chest area, like weight or constriction; grief in the chest; desire to scream coming from the chest; trapped, suffocated, heavy in chest; sensation of heart beating fast in the chest, like it could burst
- Desire to be in the flow, not feel impeded; finding the shortest distance between two places; riding bikes/skates, etc. for grace and speed; may be fast and agile and love jumping off things, or awkward and out of body
- Dry irritation of eyes and ears, fear of blindness, all kinds of vision issues
- Desire for sun, sunlight, staring into lights
- Sensation of something stuck in the throat, difficulty swallowing, constriction, sore throat
- Desire for music, singing, and dance

- Sharp, stabbing, or stitching pains in the chest, desire to breathe deeply; sharp back and shoulder pains/stiffness causing headaches
- Delicate vibrations, light yet intense, nervous restlessness, trembling; sudden rush of adrenaline feeling
- Similar remedies: Phosphorus, Calcarea phos, Staphysagria, Aconite, Carcinosin
- Compare with Tuberculinum for history of weak lungs, poor boundaries, craves bacon

Anas Barbariae Hepatis et Cordis Extractum (Barbary Duck Liver and Heart Extract)

Anas barbariae is the active ingredient in Oscillococcinum, a proprietary product produced by the French homeopathic pharmacy Boiron, which is used as a preventative for acute influenza or flu-like conditions. Migratory waterfowl, such as the barbary duck, are a natural reservoir of influenza viruses, including H1N1, however most of these birds are immune to them. Waterfowl have also been found to host parainfluenza viruses (related to mumps and measles), enteroviruses, adenoviruses, reoviruses, herpes viruses, parvovirus, and hepatitis B virus. Therefore, a preparation of the liver and heart of the wild duck, dosed homeopathically, can possibly prevent a whole host of infectious disease. Originally this medicine was developed as a treatment for cancer, and there are many overlaps between the symptoms of Carcinosin and Anas barbariae, including fastidiousness and need for control. This is a key remedy for the prevention of epidemics, and its mental symptoms include impatience that improves when one is busy, cannot bear disorder, fixed ideas and obsessions, fear of contagion with the urge to wash hands often, fear of shaking hands for fear of contagion, fear of thunderstorms, and anxiety without clear cause. Physically, someone who needs this remedy is likely to be sensitive to cold; needs fresh air, warmth, and rest; and has mucus or obstruction in the ears, nose, and sinuses.

Anas Platyrhynchos (Mallard Eggshell)

Like a mallard bursting out of its shell, people who benefit from this remedy want to bolt and break free; they're defiant and rebellious, impatient, and desire movement. They clench their jaws out of a restricted feeling of being caged and confined. This is a remedy for metamorphosis, the desire to transform and emerge into something new and it can bring a feeling of patience, calm, lightness and liberation. Physical symptoms include noise sensitivity, chewing movements, a need for oral gratification, and desire for movement and running.

Anser Anser (Wild Goose Feather)

Being in a flock brings about feelings of loyalty, a desire to work hard for the group, and striving to be responsible and caring towards others. Goose is oriented to the group so there is a fear of being excluded as well as fears of exams, competition, and anything that can create a sense of exclusion. The "silly goose" types who benefit from Anser anser want to be fun, artistic, and creative but they are also obsessive about cleanliness and hygiene and feel responsible about the environment. They are acute and alert, have sensitive feet, and may suffer from headaches.

Ara Macao (Macaw Feather)

Ara macao can help joyful, colorful, family-oriented people who want to be individuals and speak their truth rather than fit in with the group. There may be a tension between individuality versus the group and a feeling that they are giving in a relationship but not getting back. It can help bring about acceptance of a situation, calm nervous sensations and loquacity, and help with general awkwardness. Compare with Sulphur and Phosphorus.

Ardea Herodias (Heron Feather)

This remedy suits complex children, particularly autistic kids, as it helps with hypersensitivity of the senses, being overly absorbed in one's own thoughts, and a sensation of being alone. The provings of water birds often have a deeper theme of grief; for Ardea the chest feels heavy with grief like there is no space to breathe, and they feel better from crying and assurance that they are not alone. There may be some issues with water—either trauma from being in the water causing panic and trembling or a deep love of bath time and showers. Compare with Ignatia, Carcinosin, and the lanthanide elements.

Buteo (Hawk Feather)

Most people feel a duty to be responsible to their families, but those who benefit from Buteo naturally want to care for them and can feel exploited by them at the same time. They have an aversion to company and freedom while exhibiting great amounts of energy, power, will, anger, irritability, periodicity, sadness, and depression. I have seen several parents of autistic children who needed this remedy; it is similar to Aurum and Ignatia.

Calypte Anna (Hummingbird Feather)

Children who respond well to Calypte anna tend to be "high vibration," meaning they are light in their bodies and get overly excited, easily manic, tense, and wound up. It's possible they are the children of women who have experience with spiritually "high" experiences such as through the use of ayahuasca or meditation. These high-strung children have strong cravings for sugar and may have an unquenchable appetite for sweet liquids and fruit, which gives them energy, but later they crash out of sheer exhaustion. Alternating between being hyperactive and depleted, these kids can get "outside of themselves" easily and may have difficulty incarnating or staying in their bodies. There can be a lack of masculinity in boys, and they are always on "high alert" with their hypersensitive senses. It can be a useful remedy in autism or "twice gifted" cases where a child is brilliant in one or more areas but unable to utilize their skills in a way that society recognizes; there may also be a lack of desire to socialize with others. When in a blissful state of daydreaming they may hum without realizing it, but then a noise or thought will quickly snap them back to reality. Compare with Phosphorus and Platina.

Cathartes Aura (Vulture Feather)

This remedy treats strong fears of germs and hypochondriacal states in hypersensitive people who have many environmental and food allergies. There is a theme of "decay" and death in the remedy, where a person feels they are in the final stages of life and all structure has broken down. There may be many scabs and pimples on the scalp or face, with self-mutilation by picking hairs out of the head. There will be weakness in the throat with frequent infections, swollen glands, and the head subluxated forward. It can help with the inability to purge toxins and detox the body creating the feeling of being filled with garbage; purging or vomiting feels "cathartic" (hence the name of the bird, Cathartes). Compare with Arsenicum album, Sulphur and Syphilinum.

Columba Palumbus (Dove)

The soft, sweet children who respond well to this remedy tend to rely heavily on their mothers to protect them. It can treat deep heartbreak and a history of sexual abuse. While there may be awareness of sexual abuse, the trauma of it causes this person to seek out of body experiences and find solace in a spiritual or religious life. Compare with Staphysagria and Carcinosin.

Corvus Corax (Raven)

The core themes of Corvus corax center around the voice and loss of identity. These children have a fierce need to protect their core self at all times and feel that their individuality is not recognized. They struggle with self-doubt and a constriction of the voice, and may even feel abused as if those close to them don't respect their boundaries. There can be talk or issues of death, dying, suicide, murder, killing, and trickery. Corvus corax treats borderline personalities, drug addictions, and cases that include extreme anger, screaming, outrage, and yelling. Compare with Stramonium, Medorrhinum, Belladonna, and Opium.

Cygnus Cygnus (Swan)

This is a remedy for the kind of grief that envelops and cripples a person's day-to-day life; their grief is at the forefront of their mind and does not fade over the years. Unable to connect or communicate with others, they often fall into a deep depression and can become quite aggressive.

For a special needs child this may show up as fear of new things, withdrawal, fear of open spaces, and a need to feel protected. This eventually builds into a feeling of being ostracized for being different or not wanted by others, similar to the Hans Christian Anderson tale "The Ugly Duckling." It's possible that a child who needs this remedy was unwanted by their mother.

Sometimes these cases will have a history of sexual violence such as rape or abuse. As in many cases of grief, there may be chest and throat issues such as a feeling of constriction and difficulty breathing. Compare with Ignatia, Staphysagria, and Natrum mur.

Falco Peregrinus (Peregrine Falcon)

Historically this bird has been bred in captivity and trained to hunt for humans; its head is placed in a hood to prevent it from being overly excited. Imagining what it would be like to be a bird forced into bondage helps us understand what this remedy treats. Falco helps when there is deep anger against anything perceived as a restraint.

A child needing this remedy would be frustrated and angry at routine, school, tests, etc. and does best totally free of expectation. Their ideal is to be travelling the world by impulse with no plans; the reality of life and the expectations of family feels like a terrible burden. There may be deep feelings of being humiliated, undervalued, and misunderstood by the world, as well as an apathetic quality with a detached numbness that everything feels banal and insignificant. When in a state of indifference, they may struggle with memory and concentration. On the flip side, they can be deeply spiritually seeking—they go deep into meditation and into blissed out states—and have both excellent vision and clarity of insight. Compare with Tuberculinum, Carcinosin, and Buteo.

Gallus Domesticus Masculinum (Rooster)

This remedy from the male rooster is for happy, boisterous children who love being chased and fight back when upset. Like all birds, they like to be free and dislike being in closed rooms and new rooms, especially if they see the door is locked. There will be a desire to escape or attempt to climb very high on things, and once they do, they are very proud like they are the king of the world. They may experience intense waves of excitement from the feet on up, making screams and squeals that are loud, like a bottle rocket about to explode. They also may get single minded and fixated on routines, such as regularly checking on rooms of the house, which is a kind of "territorialism."

This remedy is similar to Lycopodium, with a strong feeling of swagger and bravado to cover up a deeply nervous disposition with a fear of looking incompetent and being ridiculed. It may assist with physical symptoms of double vision or issues of focus, as well as issues relating to levels of testosterone.

Gallus Domesticus Penna (Domestic Chicken Feather)

Imagine a backyard chicken—simple-minded, aimless, totally dependent, trapped, and overfeeding to the point of obesity—and you will get a sense of the qualities that this remedy can treat. These creatures of habit will go along with conformity out of fear and see all new ideas as a threat. They are easily taken advantage of, lack substance or character, and have low self-esteem. These kids want to be taken care of and aren't interested in developing independence. Compare with Baryta carb and Calcarea carb.

Haliaeetus Leucophalus (Eagle Blood)

Eagle is a remedy for incarnation, for people who have a yearning desire to be out of the body; this is can be expressed as a feeling of intense spiritual "highness" connected to light and an elation of being "up." They feel like the body is a trap, heavy and perhaps associated with pain and trauma. There may be aggression and anger at the world, with screaming at the top of their lungs out of a kind of existential anguish. They want to rise above difficulty and when they do, life becomes like a dream. People who need this remedy are likely to be perfectionists who understand the importance of precision, such as what it takes to land an ice-skating jump or touchdown a plane. They love the thrill and intensity of being fast and agile, like riding a skateboard. The proving of this remedy had the theme of twins; I once treated a twin boy who had acute immune thrombocytopenic purpura (ITP) and teeth sensitivity who was assisted by Eagle. It may also assist with visual issues, such as tracking and focus issues or lazy eye with a desire to watch lights. Compare with Aurum, Platina, and Canibis indica.

Passer Domesticus (Sparrow)

The ordinary sparrow lives in close proximity to humans, and many children are familiar with them living in their backyards. For this reason, I have often prescribed it for children who have strong themes of the birds without the unique attributes that differentiate higher order birds such as vultures or owls. These children tend to be spirited and boisterous, but also anxious, with an inner restlessness that makes them unstable or ungrounded. There is less yearning for freedom or spirituality compared to other birds and they are likely to feel comfortable within a place of containment, such as a closed yard or some sort of "nest." Like many other birds, they may have separation anxiety with fear of being alone and want to feel safe and cared for. Compare with Carcinosin, Phosphorus, Aconite, Butterfly and Calcarea phos.

Tyto Alba (Barn Owl)

The owl represents understanding and wisdom. A child who needs this remedy will be deeply curious about how things work and ask all kinds of probing questions like "who is God?" and "how does sound travel?" Like many bird remedies they are sociable, talkative, and love travel. Tyto, however, helps with unusual sensory perception issues, especially around vision and hearing. For example, a child needing this remedy may have far-sightedness and depth perception issues, such as crying for a bottle that is right in front of them; or "Superman" hearing, where the child can hear the water travelling through the pipes in the house and will try to discover via their senses where the water travels. They may also be drawn to lights with a desire to look at the sun or watch the moon, especially loving things that glow from within. Physically this remedy will assist with frequent nausea with a need to retch or regurgitate, especially due to sensitivity to smells with pressing pains in the liver and stomach area as if something in the digestive tract needs to come up. This remedy helps those who are spiritually striving tap into their inner wisdom, third eye, connect with the astral world through dreaming, and break through fear of death.

Mollusc Remedies

The evolution of humans started in the Ocean! Seventy percent of our planet is the sea and where we can find the largest number and diversity of animals. There is an evident link between life in the sea, the salinity of our blood, and our life in the uterus. The ocean represents the mother, yin, negativity, our deep dark watery nature, coldness, as well as themes from the remedy Natrum mur (salt) including isolation, loneliness, and over sensitivity.

Ocean animals are generally different from social mammals; busy, high-energy insects and spiders; and high-flying birds. They tend to be more grounded, often times shy, avoiding people and interested in a simple domestic life. In homeopathic terms, they tend to be psoric, or operating from a deficiency mindset, always needing more security and comfort.

Molluscs are animals with a shell including oysters, snails (Helix), and cuttlefish (Sepia). The shell is about containment—they withdraw, close off, shut in, are defensive, and keep the world outside by staying out of reach. These remedies overlap with mineral remedies like Natrum carb and Calcarea mur, who are by nature shy and yielding. The remedy Calcarea carb is actually made from oyster shells and thus can be considered an animal remedy as well as a mineral remedy. These animals build around them a shell for safety and likewise the children who need them will carry around a blankie or item to give them security too. Calcarea carb kids may dislike change so much that, like an oyster, they won't budge from their place. They have a stubborn attitude and can unwaveringly stare you down; it is their way or the highway. Socially these children may also stay on the outskirts of the playground, often too nervous to engage and take center stage. But their mineral nature can make them strong and steady children who, when they practice routinely, build up towards success, becoming a star player on the soccer field or slowly perfecting a piano piece. Words parents may use when talking about kids who need mollusc remedies include in a shell, watery, receding, closed in, out of reach, grounded, closed, and withdrawn.

Confining themselves to a smaller, limited set of experiences and being fearful of trying new things, children who need molluscs can have an immaturity to them. They can be very dependent on their family and anxious about breaking out of their comfort zone, and therefore act younger or like toys and activities meant for younger kids, and they will insist on sticking with them. They prefer to keep a safe distance from people and emotional contact is limited to prevent them from being hurt, but they also want support from others. In this way they may feel negative about their family and hold grudges that keep an emotional distance. A family that needs sea animal remedies will be aloof towards one another and have a hard time giving hugs and saying "I love you," but at the same time they never leave each other due to their insecurities. The remedy Sepia, from the cuttlefish, is known for being "cold" to their family. I once treated an anti-social ASD boy who needed this remedy because he would shun and run away from all family members, push away hugs, and walk away from social gatherings. Sepia is a common women's remedy to balance hormones that can also show up in girls who are detached from their emotions and direct all their energy into a physical activity such as gymnastics.

Kids who need mollusc remedies love being domestic and will spend hours quietly completing puzzles, building with LEGO bricks, playing board games, digging in the sandbox, and prefer no noise or calm music. Molluscs and coral are all about the creation and maintenance of a physical structure for their safety. Likewise, these kids love to build, create rules and routines, and operate within the confines of a safe container.

Sometimes we see that what the animal looks like is what it helps to treat. For example, the remedy Spongia tosta (sea sponge) looks like a lung and treats dry, hard, croupy coughs. Corallium rubrum (red coral) can help treat redness and flushing. Jellyfish can help treat overly sensitive, neurotic people who are ungrounded and spacey. Water is also a fundamental element to sea animals and they may be fearful or have a strong need for the element of water. In general, I have found these cases have a "damp" energy to them, with a lot of tendency to cold clamminess, yeast, and tinea infections.

Natural Mollusc Behaviors

- Stuck in one spot or a small zone
- Need to regulate water
- Defensive

- Have simple, basic needs they expect to be fulfilled—can eat the same thing every day, live comfortably in one small environment, etc.
- Withdrawal; closed, shut in, pulled in
- Keeps the world outside; goes into a shell and out of reach

Notable Mollusc Features in Complex Children

- Afraid to join the group, observers of the group
- Wallflowers, shy, dislikes socializing, loses contact
- Can be flat, apathetic, and unexcitable due to being cut off; neutral tone
- Likes to stay at home, feel safe and contained
- Skin issues, dryness, eczema, birthmarks, moles, hyperpigmentation; dislikes lotions
- Hormonal imbalance, hypothyroidism, water balance issues
- Desires routine, dislikes change, has a small comfort zone
- Attached to a comfort object
- Throws items over themselves and hides away (like going into a shell)
- Interested in calm activities like reading, puzzles, building, knitting, board games, quiet and calm music such as classical
- Loves boats/navy/nautical themes, movies about ocean life (especially *The Little Mermaid*)
- Sensitive to sound, gets overwhelmed and wants to shut everything off
- Does well with structure, likes to set their own rules, likes to take their time to do it right
- Gets stuck, obstinate, immature desires, regressive
- Loves playing in the sandbox, digging in sand, moving water
- May be afraid of water and showers, dislikes water on the head or in the eyes; but may also be ameliorated by bath time or the sound of water running; fear of the beach
- May roll along the floor or walk in contact with the walls
- Compare to Baryta carb, Calcarea mur, Kali carb, Natrum mur, and Silica

Calcarea Carbonica (Oyster Shell)

Like an oyster, a child who needs this remedy will be "in a shell," with their vulnerable soft insides showing up as timidity with a lot of anxiety, and their shell showing up as a rigid stubbornness. They even have a tendency for being "clammy." This is a key remedy for delayed development, weakened immunity with frequent respiratory infections, ear infections, and/or pneumonia. Please refer to pages 209-210 for more information on this common remedy for kids.

Corallium Rubrum (Red Coral)

The shape of this animal resembles an arterial system (think of tubes/pipes branching off in different directions) and this remedy is indicated in cases with active congestion. It can be used for congestion of the nasal passages or lungs, congestion of blood vessels (indicated by red spots/eruptions), congestion of blood to the head, and for hemorrhages. It also may assist very rapid violent coughs, possibly with blood expectoration, preceded by a suffocative feeling and followed by exhaustion, such as in whooping coughs. Compare with Belladonna.

Helix Tosta (Toasted Snail)

This remedy can be useful for hoarseness, difficulty breathing, chronic coughs that are dry, tickling, and worse at night, and blood-tinged coughs. It belongs to the tubercular miasm and can be a good fit for shy children who are too open energetically, similar to Phosphorus.

Murex Purpurea (Sea Snail)

Like many mollusc remedies, the child who needs Murex is antisocial and anxious; they will shy away from attention and want to go and hide, such as crawling into a pile of blankets. At the same time if they are told no or pressured to do something, it will make them very angry and they can explode in anger and defiance. This remedy is especially helpful for healing iron imbalance, dark birthmarks, and hyperpigmentation looking like dark bruising, particularly if this occurred during pregnancy. Compare with Natrum mur, Ferrum met, and Sepia.

Octopus

Octopus states are heavy, dark, and despairing. People who need this remedy may feel trapped in a nightmare or a dark hole, yearning for deliverance. It is possible that they also have hidden talents due to high intelligence, for example a nonverbal child who can write impressive poetry on his letterboard, seeking an outlet for all his angst. These cases are also sensory sensitive and overwhelmed leading particularly to biting, gnawing, or clenching very tightly. This clenching is similar to symptoms of Cuprum met; curiously octopus animals have cuprum/copper based (not iron based) blood. Octopus can also treat digestive disorders, excess stomach acidity, and heavy metals such as mercury or lead. The person who needs this remedy may feel ugly, cold, cut off, hurried, and nervous, with a need to move or travel. Compare with the hiddenness of the lanthanides, the tightness of Cuprum, the heaviness of Aurum, and the restlessness of Tuberculinum.

Sepia Succus (Cuttlefish Ink)

Depressed children with low affect, who are irritated by their family and want to get away from them, may need the Sepia remedy. These kids want to avoid social gatherings; they tend to block out people with indifference and react to demands on them with defiance and negativity. They have difficulty expressing love and affection, and will shirk hugs and avoid emotional communication. In school they have a hard time engaging with teachers and schoolwork due to lack of interest and poor concentration. It is possible there is a history of abuse or neglect from a parent who is, in turn, irritated at them. In this case the parent may also need Sepia. Sepia mothers may have had vomiting during pregnancy (from being oversensitive to smells) and painful back labor, and they may have had some depression from not wanting to be pregnant in the first place. Physically, people who need Sepia are either sluggish and weak from exertion or they desire a lot of activity, sports, and exercise. They can be sensitive to smells, easily nauseated, and have motion sickness. While Sepia can treat both sexes, it is an especially good remedy for girls who are hormonally deficient, have delayed breast development, and are delayed in getting their period. Sepia can also treat recurrent tonsillitis or cystitis, fungal infections, and jaundice.

Spongia Tosta (Sea Sponge)

Spongia is primarily an acute remedy for dry, barking, croupy coughs. The cough is a type of spasm; think of the sea sponge as it quickly retracts in response to any kind of stress. The croup or cough will be worse before midnight and better from warm drinks. There is often extreme dryness of the mucous membranes and there can be a sensation of a plug or foreign body lodged inside. It is also useful for swollen, hardened glands and imbalanced thyroid glands, and is closely related to halogen remedies such as Iodum, Muriaticum, Bromium, and Chlorum.

Venus Mercenaria (American Scallop)

Just like a scallop, the person needing this remedy feels stuck in their house, cut off from excitement. They are looking from the inside out and feel weighed down by the responsibility of caring for their house and family. They may be lonely and depressed, having lost the capacity for expansiveness and connection. A child needing this remedy has so much insecurity and fear that they continually demand security by staying at home. This remedy is for migraines of digestive origin or pains from too much contraction in the body; bones of the head may feel tight and immobile. Compare with Calcarea carb.

Fish Remedies

Fish remedies have thin skins and are one with the water, as opposed to the thick-shelled molluscs. Like birds, kids who need fish remedies also have a desire to be weightless and unbounded and can be constantly moving and busy. They don't have the sophisticated range of interests and self-expression of bird or mammal remedies, and are happy when their simple needs are met (which is often playing in the water). They may show some strong preference for ocean themes and animals—many of my fish cases have had a nonstop obsession with the movie *Finding Nemo*. Words that parents use when describing kids who need fish remedies are buoyant, weightless, water, floating, pool, crashing, swimming, flopping, and dysregulated.

Fish remedies are like a watery Phosphorus, meaning they are friendly, communicative, likeable, and have poor boundaries that can be easily taken advantage of. This lack of a sense of self can lead them to join groups due to a fear of being alone and a great need to feel connected to others. Ultimately this lack of independence leads them to feel resentful and manipulated with moods that swing towards depression. They can cycle back and forth between feeling very happy and "in the flow" to feeling sad and isolated.

Many complex kids in this category are so sensory sensitive and easily dysregulated that they have a hard time staying their natural bubbly self, and will often attack, rage, and crash into things or people. This is not so much out of aggression like reptile, insect, or spider remedies; these kids want love and affection but may awkwardly seek it out by smashing into you. They react more out of sensory overwhelm and internal frustration, as if they are just trying to figure out how their body works in their surroundings. Many fish cases I have seen like to push their heads or bodies into things to calm themselves, or will suddenly bolt out a door.

Kids who need these remedies are generally more physically oriented than they are mental, and love running, jumping, sports, and swimming. However, they can have problems with speaking, memory, dyslexia, focus, fogginess, executive processing, and thinking for long periods. They can be defiant and stubborn when trying to get them to do what everyone else is doing, because they want to be in their own flow. New provings on fish remedies show them to be helpful for organic brain disease such as dementia. Dosing a fish remedy can help a child function better in a classroom and be more verbal.

Natural Fish Behaviors

- Always moving/going—in the flow
- Swimming in schools, moving in circles
- Sticking with a group, operating under group mind
- Thin boundary/skin, one with the environment, unaware of cold
- Buoyancy, floating

Notable Fish Features in Complex Children

- Hyperactive, high energy, physical, always moving
- Hate containment; dislike being strapped into a carseat (like birds), but may love car rides
- Bolting out the door, fearless, seeking adrenaline thrill
- In their element being in the water—can spend all day in the bath or pool, loves the aquarium, may overfill sinks, leave faucets on, or flush things down toilets
- Being in the water drowns out the cacophony of the world, they prefer to live in a muted, blurry space
- Head banging, pressing forehead strongly against other people's heads, hits themselves in the head then falls over
- Crashing into things, awkward, flopping on the floor; not worried about getting hurt, numb to pain
- Love running around stark naked; indifferent to being cold or dirty; cold and clammy skin
- Interest in ocean life and ocean-themed tv shows and movies
- Poor boundaries, helpful, easy, affable, empathic
- Very chemically/environmentally sensitive, allergies, weak lungs
- Low verbal skills, poor memory, dyslexia, low attention span, foggy thinking

- Low ego, low self-identity, very low sense of self
- Floating, buoyancy, spaced out, euphoric, exhilarated, ungrounded
- Going with the group, going with the flow
- Moving in circles
- Fear of being alone and anxious if not connected
- Can be aggressive and confrontational due to poor boundaries; forceful affection (grabs your head and forcefully nuzzles)
- Headaches and pressure in the head, worse pressure
- Easily affected by others; will cry if others cry, can get sad
- Diarrhea, worse milk; watery poop
- Aqua marina and Aqua pura are complementary remedies

Carassius Auratus (Goldfish)

Children who benefit from Goldfish are typically empathic, clairvoyant, and affectionate, often pressing into you. Or instead they may be spacey, ungrounded, and more out of body. They tend to be very sensitive with allergies to pollens, trees, etc., and also sensitivity to pollution, radiation, weather, and sound. They like pressure against their head and often push their head against things. Similar to a goldfish in a bowl, many who need this remedy lead a confined existence (such as in an apartment in a city) and may have a desire to escape. This remedy can be beneficial for headaches with pressure and it can also be indicated for brain tumors or strokes. Compare with Phosphorus, Stramonium, Belladonna, Opium, and Iodum.

Galeocerdo Cuvier Hepar (Tiger Shark Liver)

This remedy helps heal subconscious fears, especially fear of death and a mother's deep instinctual fear for her child's survival. It can treat feelings of urgency, immediacy, and quickness to anger, as well as an attraction to sharp objects such as saws and teeth. Symptoms are left sided and include full body itching and sharp pains. Compare with Belladonna and Stramonium.

Hippocampus Kuda (Seahorse)

Seahorse is similar to Goldfish but has more alternating moods and emotions. These children can be averse to socializing but at the same time don't want to be alone. They tend to be sensitive to noise, odors and tastes and may have frequent nausea or heartburn. There may be ringing in the ears or they may be hearing impaired where sounds are muffled as if they were underwater.

Medusa (Jellyfish)

Children who require this remedy are often highly sensitive, clairvoyant, and empathic beings who distance themselves from others. For them, getting close means getting stung, so these children push away anyone who might get too close. They try to demonstrate their independence from others, but in reality they are yearning for belonging. They tend to be artistic with a unique skill that sets them apart and may also have a strong connection to outer space. Physical symptoms may include electric shock sensations, numbness, burning, pricking heat, and the feeling of pins and needles; it's also helpful for nettle rash and urticaria. Compare with Pulsatilla, Natrum Mur, and Butterfly.

Oleum Jecoris Aselli (Cod Liver Oil)

This remedy is indicated for malnutrition resulting in emaciated, undersized, chilly babies and children, atrophy in muscles, and milk intolerance. It is a liver remedy and useful for pains in the liver and liver region with great soreness. Those needing it may be worse from or unable to take cod liver oil. It can also be helpful for frontal headaches over the right eye and palpitations of the heart with cough and shortness of breath. It is associated with a deficiency of vital heat, coldness (especially in the evening), weakness, and a general lack of energy.

Reptile and Amphibian Remedies

Representing some of the darker aspects of our nature are the reptile remedies. We all have a "reptilian brain" (medulla/hindbrain), which is responsible for our basic survival functions. A more positive way to view the reptilian energy we all have is that it represents our life force; in yoga it is called the kundalini energy, which is coiled at the base of the spine. When we can tap into this energy without suppressing or judging it we have more power, more creativity, and more capacity for healing. Two snakes coiling up a staff is what creates the caduceus, the symbol of medicine and healing.

Snake remedies can heal a wide range of infections, sepsis, constrictions, hormonal disorders, sore throats, coughs, pneumonia, and epilepsy. These remedies are also crucial for healing violent and destructive children who intend to do harm by their actions. Kids who bite, attack, and strangle are often medicated or removed from their home, and knowing this, parents will often isolate their child at home for fear that they will be taken away or harm someone out in the world.

This isolation is an aspect of the destructive, syphilitic miasm (see pages 81-83). Snakes represent destruction on all levels: mental, emotional, and physical. Mentally, snakes can easily lie and manipulate those around them—including the homeopath. Challenging cases that give me the run-around with attempts to hook me into their drama often need snake remedies (particularly Lachesis). People who need snake remedies can also be two sided, wanting only to show off their good side and even come across as "holier than thou," while hiding their hidden, aggressive, controlling, or depressed sides at home. Parents who need snake remedies can have many anxieties and fears that get projected onto their children and they can, in effect, create more issues in their children. I once treated a mother who was afraid that her child would suffocate to death in the middle of the night due to swollen adenoids and she would stay up all night watching him breathe. She also happened to be a respiratory therapist and the remedy Python helped her move through this anxiety. Learning intuitive testing was a turning point in my practice because I realized I couldn't always take the word of my patients as truth—truth is constantly manipulated, even by people who tell you they want to get better!

Those needing snake remedies who are well-compensated can also be outgoing, creative, expressively dramatic, have a big and loving heart, and be generally well-liked. They love to put themselves on stage for attention and get energized by this. I once treated a young singer who needed Lachesis—she would perform on stage and then afterwards lock herself in her home, fearful to emerge because of debilitating anxiety. Snake remedies are well known for bipolar disorder and the remedy Lachesis helped her find a middle ground between these extremes. Many snake people are psychic and empathic. They will warm up to you with their sensitive social skills and they can make very loyal friends (if you go along with them, and if not, watch out!). Snake people are also known for natural intelligence and can easily charm others with talkativeness, quick wits, and knowledge.

Being syphilitic, snake remedies are also blaming and claiming victim-hood, creating drama by projecting their issues onto everyone else around them. They are also prone to all sorts of destructive infections, parasites, blood sepsis, etc. As a result, multiple nosodes are often needed as part of their treatment. Because these cases can have a strong destructive quality, it takes a lot of work to move them in the right direction. I often find some spiritual or even past life healing is required. Many snake remedies have on some subconscious level a sense of violence, murder, and death on their minds and only some deeper levels of spiritual healing through forgiveness and self love can help them move forward. Helping them to recognize and rise above the constant victim/aggressor polarity that they create can be critical.

Physically, these people are of the earth—they can be powerfully strong and sexually oriented, although they may try to hide or suppress this aspect of themselves. Many children who need reptile remedies have strong issues with sexuality; I have often seen a history of pornography addiction in the fathers of these kids. The time of puberty in many children, especially boys, can bring ancestral sexual issues to the surface and snake remedies may help. I always tell parents to be open about discussing sexuality, because when it is judged or dismissed it can create some unhealthy guilt complexes. There are a good handful of PANDAS children I have seen whose triggers were the thoughts they had of sex around the time of puberty that they felt bad about, and remedies like Lachesis, Calcarea brom, Kali brom, Staphysagria, or Anacardium were helpful to release this self-imposed shame. Many reptile children also have massive appetites and literally swallow down food whole, but then have very slow digestion with a tendency towards constipation, especially if they are stagnant and not exercising. There is also a blood and cardiovascular component to snake remedies; they can help with blood clots, heart issues, strokes, and so on. Many mothers who need reptile remedies have a history of hemorrhage during delivery or very traumatic deliveries where their life was at stake. On a hormonal level, snake remedies are of great use to women who have strong mood swings, PMS, endometriosis, hot flashes, or menopausal difficulties.

Not all people who need snake remedies are violent and destructive. Some children who need these remedies instead are very sensual and affectionate and love pressing their bodies into other people (this can be seen in Boa and Python). One boy I treated who needed a snake remedy was obsessed with Valentine's Day and loved hearts and hugging people.

Children who need snakes can often be sedentary and slow, with bursts of speed and intensity coinciding with some rage or inflammation. Many snake cases also overlap with remedies from heavy metals like Mercurius (violence and speed), Aurum (depressive heart effects), Bismuthum, Plumbum, and Polonium (sense of lost power). I also see many snake constitutions need mineral remedies from stage 17 that are negative and blaming (Natrum fluor, Chlorum, Iodum, Bromium), and these can help what appear to be thyroid issues and slow metabolism. Pyrogenium (rotting meat) and Gunpowder (for sepsis) have also been needed regularly in the snake cases I have seen.

Phrases that parents may use when describing a child who needs a snake remedy are "uncomfortable in his own skin," "there is something wrong with the blood," and "I don't trust him."

Natural Reptile and Amphibian Behaviors

- Hiding and deception
- Competition and one-upmanship; competition with the feeling that they are at a disadvantage, requiring cunning to survive
- Themes of superior and inferior
- Planned, conspiracy, calculative and scheming; manipulative
- Jealous, suspicious
- Split in the mind, or antagonism with oneself
- Sexuality, lack of morals
- Clairvoyance, vulnerable
- Show and appearance, loquacity, vivid and descriptive
- Poisonous, venomous
- Sensations of constriction, getting tighter, suffocation, choking
- Sensations of twisting, engulfing, wringing the neck, crushing
- Sudden movement, sudden unpredictable attack
- Concealed, never seen, disguised
- Feeling of being pursued and desire to hide
- Miasm: mainly syphilitic

Notable Reptile and Amphibian Features in Complex Children

- Violent, sudden attacks—scratching, biting, pulling, squeezing
- Fearful that the child actually wants to kill you; child intentionally wants to cause pain or be mean; desire to stab, choke, suffocate
- Writhing, "S" movements of the body
- Double natured, bipolar, extremely happy then depressed
- Sensual, slow and sluggish, slurring speech
- Artistic; desire to color, draw, perform; drama
- Competitive; likes sports, dancing
- Can be very social, naturally manipulative to get what they want
- In their "reptile" brain—tendency to masturbation, violence, eating
- Low executive functioning, low self control
- Family may be religious, but child acts up in church

- Acting up in public followed by desire to escape and isolate oneself; can be antisocial, agoraphobic
- Desire to look attractive, cool, gain attention
- Can be talkative, high energy, hot in the body, energy always needs to flow out
- Hard to sit still; impulsive
- Tendency to sepsis, bacterial, and parasite infections
- Can be very amorous with siblings, or jealous of them
- The reptile aspect of people can be easy to miss, as people are likely to want to hide that aspect of themselves
- Tries to test your limits when you see them, looks at you slyly
- There are many reptile remedies that are fearful, powerless, and simple-minded like Bufo or Natrix natrix
- Flopping onto you—no backbone, wrapping limbs around you
- Dislikes tight clothing
- Hormonal imbalances, easy bruising
- Similar violent remedies: Belladonna, Hyoscyamus, Tarentula, Veratrum album
- Similar sluggish remedies: Pulsatilla, Sepia, Lycopodium

Amphisbaena Alba (Legless White Snake Lizard)

This is an unusual remedy that does not have extensive provings, but I have used it in several cases of deeply entrenched psychosis, such as a strong personality disorder where a person cannot "see" their issues. This lack of "insight" is reflected by the fact that this is a mostly blind snake that lives underground with the appearance of having two heads. Similarly, someone who needs this remedy may seem like they have two personas in one person, like Jekyll and Hyde. Children who can be helped by Amphisbaena may have episodes of insanity, like "blind rage," and then flip a switch into their normal sweet selves. Or it may show up as strange behaviors such as odd vocal tics that the child doesn't pay attention to or even recognize. Ultimately this remedy heals a true dualistic struggle and inner split that is deeper than what is seen in Anacardium and Lachesis.

Bufo Rana (Toad)

Much has been written about Bufo as a remedy for simple-minded children who have developmental delays, brain inflammation, history of brain trauma, and poor impulse control showing up as a preoccupation with masturbation, constant licking of lips or playing with/biting the tongue, seizures, and tics. However, cases do not need to have issues with masturbation or playing with their tongue to be assisted by this remedy. Bufo can also assist a more functional child with a learning disability or a child who is socially delayed but extremely gifted in a particular way. The essence of this remedy is distilled by Paul Herscu, ND, as being helpful for children who are overwhelmed by sensory stimulation making them shut down a part of themselves or seek solitude. In this solitude, they will use a form of communication such as repetitive singing or echolalia as a release of energy. However, they get stuck in this narrow focus of communication and if interrupted in what they are doing, they may have a fit or a seizure leading to more confusion and withdrawal from the world. This remedy may also assist with sepsis and lymphangitis. Compare with Hyoscyamus and Mercurius.

Cenchris Contortrix (Copperhead Snake)

This remedy treats qualities of a personality disorder where the person can't see beyond themselves resulting in extreme jealousy, possessiveness, fear of rejection, and intense control over the parent or caretaker resulting in violence. It is well known for manic depression or insane behaviors particularly around hormonal cycles/PMS and menstrual flow—like a more intense Lachesis.

Chelydra Serpentina (Snapping turtle)

The turtle shares some themes of the reptiles including a tendency to strike out or misbehave creating feelings of guilt, but there is a quality of plodding slowness that sets it apart. There is also a sensation of being contracted in a "shell" with small mindedness such as being engrossed in simple household tasks and black and white rules. They will move very slowly as if drugged and just want their simple needs to be met. There may be a sense of greediness around eating where they assume someone is trying to take their food. They feel trapped inside a heavy body and are irritable at others; there may also be a special interest in shapes. This remedy is like a combination of Calcarea carb, Graphites, and Lachesis.

Crotalus Horridus (Rattlesnake)

This is a useful and important remedy when there are recurrent, deep rooted infectious states occurring with Lyme, bacterial infections, or immunodeficiency. These chronic infections cause jaundice, necrosis, or acute infections that quickly devolve into sepsis, pus, and hemorrhage of dark unclotted blood (such as with gastrointestinal bleeding). It is an important liver remedy with a tendency to right-sided symptoms. Mentally this person is not as intense as Lachesis and is more likely to show depression and despair. Compare with Lachesis and Secale.

Crotalus Cascavella (Brazilian Rattlesnake)

The child who needs this remedy has a desperate fear of being alone and hangs onto their parent for dear life, as if something bad is going to happen or death is just around the corner. There is a weak helplessness and desire to be part of a family in order to survive, such as with a child who is completely abandoned and given up for adoption. These children may be lost in their own worlds and act as if they communicate with spirits. While most snake remedies have a tendency to left-sided symptoms, Crotalus has right-sided symptoms and may also heal aggressive skin disorders such as burning urticaria. Compare with Hyoscyamus and Stramonium.

Dendroaspis Polyepsis (Black Mamba)

This is one of the darkest, heaviest remedies in the reptile family and is useful for deep (possibly suicidal) depression and feeling like a victim, alone and forsaken. There is also a strong selfishness with lack of feeling or care for others resulting in harsh, cruel words, argumentative communication, and an "I am always right" attitude. The body may have a dragging, weak, sluggish feeling with absent mindedness and numbness. Dendroaspis can help when people go into a very dark hole inside themselves that comes periodically causing addictive desires and numbed out feelings.

Elaps Corallinus (Coral Snake)

This is a helpful remedy for digestive complaints, especially if accompanied by a feeling of coldness in the chest or stomach after drinking cold liquids. The child may also crave ice and cold drinks. Digestive symptoms may show up as peptic ulcers, abdominal pains better lying on the stomach, gastritis, esophageal spasms, and the vomiting of blood. It can help children who present with behavioral issues like bullying with competitive desires to prove themselves and a constant fear of failure. Compare with Lachesis, Lycopodium, Veratrum album, and Nux vomica.

Heloderma Horridus (Gila Monster)

This is a truly "cold" remedy with strong internal and physical coldness and also emotional numbness and coldness. It may assist depressed children whose lives are punctuated by episodes of cold-blooded rage, where power/violence/cruelty is exerted with no remorse. A child needing this remedy may complain of boredom with a need to engage the mind, then watch hours of videos alone in their room, and then suddenly attack their parents verbally or physically. The slowness and heaviness in this remedy may be felt as slow digestion, dragging and congestion in the lower pelvic area, and a feeling of lost passion or desire. The coldness of this remedy also creates the tendency for deeply entrenched fungal or yeast infections showing up as destructive nail fungus, loose stools with much gas, spaciness, and scaley, itching, cracked skin. Compare with Bufo and Chelydra serpentina.

Lacerta Agillis (Lizard)

There is not a lot of information on this remedy, however cases I have seen of Lacerta demonstrate an internal feeling of unacceptance, possibly from neglect during childhood, that shows up outwardly as vanity. This vanity expresses itself as strong need for attention, a desire to be the best, materialism, desire for money or someone with money to take care of them, and a strong concern about one's appearance. Still, this person will be sociable and likeable with a desire to please (like Pulsatilla), or have poor impulse control (like Argentum nit). There may be a tendency to numbness and paralysis, sensation of constriction in the throat, bacterial infections, GI irritation, bloating, and skin eruptions.

Lachesis (Bushmaster Snake)

This is the most commonly prescribed snake remedy and it has broad ranging effects that can be useful for many cases. It is a key remedy for children who lash out aggressively, lie, manipulate, or tend to get infections, sepsis, and deep-seated inflammation. Like many reptile remedies, internally there is low self-confidence but externally there is a need to boast, be the best, and be seen as unique and special. Their inner insecurity arises with anger upon losing, taking offense easily, suspicion, jealousy, and criticism of others. There may be internal feelings of guilt felt in the heart that are projected onto others through blame, harsh words, and making others feel guilty. I tend to prescribe Lachesis when there is strong loquacious/talkative energy representing a kind of fullness in the body that needs release. This fullness also shows up in high blood pressure, heat, redness, and heart and circulation issues; likewise these kids cannot stand to wear tight or restrictive clothing. Lachesis cases especially hate constriction around the throat, and it can help treat throat infections, throat constriction, and throat ulcers.

In some cases it becomes apparent that the mother needs Lachesis, which may indicate it for the child as well. These mothers often present with strong mood swings, hormonal hot flashes, menstrual disorders such as endometriosis, history of hemorrhage during delivery, as well as an intense and sometimes overbearing personality with a tendency towards negativity or drama. In these situations, discharges ameliorate the intensity. Discharges can include feeling better upon menstruation, releases of body heat, sexual activity, talkativeness, or expressions of strong emotionality. Lachesis can also assist when there is a family history of alcoholism, stroke, verbal abuse, or manic/bipolar/schizophrenic behaviors. Many complex cases have a Lachesis layer but it can take time, intuition, and deeper investigation to unveil this true inner state, as people are sometimes unwilling to share these tendencies about themselves or their children. Compare with Sulphur, Lycopodium, Medorrhinum, Hyoscyamus, and all other snake remedies.

Naja Tripudians (Cobra)

In ancient times, the cobra was revered as a symbol of royalty, protection, and divine authority. Naja is medicine for the heart and a more refined reptile remedy for people with great sensitivity to others around them. They often have anxiety about the health of their family and fear of failure when doing their job. Their greatest suffering is the guilt that they feel in their heart, which shows up physiologically in issues with the heart valves and neurological tics and twitches. These are generally popular, likeable people and while they perceive the shadow of their reptile nature as a darkness over their heart, they seek out help from alternative healers and find solace in a spiritual path. Compare with Phosphorus and Medorrhinum.

Python Regius

Just imagine a large, thick bodied python who kills by strangling its prey and you will understand the essence of this remedy, which helps with feelings of constriction, oppression, and fear of suffocation. Physical swelling of the ears, throat, glands/adenoids, or respiratory system (asthma) may bring on this survival-based fear of suffocation. Cases of this remedy that I have seen are generally sluggish, thick-bodied people with a large appetite, and in a way they are larger than life. Their fullness isn't quite as threatening or directed as Lachesis, but instead they are controlling of the people around them. A mother who fears for her child's survival and "smothers" that child with attention could be helped by Python. I have also seen this remedy help more affectionate children who enjoy a strong squeeze to settle their systems, but there may still be issues of rage. Python is similar to the remedy Boa constrictor.

T-Rex (Fossilized Dinosaur Bone)

This unique remedy is made from a fossilized dinosaur bone. While it may be challenging to consider treating a child with a remedy from an extinct animal, T-Rex can be very effective. In the cases that I have seen, the child presents with the strong intensity of Lachesis but has the potential for being even more fearless, precocious, and tapped into their primal power. They have a natural desire to be headstrong and dominant to the point of bullying and calling other children names. They may try out bad behaviors just to challenge authority, and if they don't get their way they will throw a fit. The child likely has a strong interest in dinosaurs and enjoys acting them out by behaving downright prehistoric; they love to be wild and free, gleefully stomping in mud puddles or running around naked. Compare with Platina, Veratrum album, and Lachesis.

Vipera Berus (German Viper)

This remedy is similar to Lachesis but has strong keynotes of swelling of the limbs and blood pulsating and throbbing in the extremities, such as would happen if you got your finger smashed in a door. This sensation is relieved by raising the limb up. A child needing this remedy may be cunning, perceptive, and knows how to strike painfully at just the right moment.

Conclusion

The sole driving force in animals is SURVIVAL—through competition, hunting, hiding, aggressing, defending, attracting a mate, and bearing young. As humans we differentiate ourselves as bigger brained and more evolved. But if we intuitively perceive the subconscious undercurrent that creates our behaviors, we see that we really are not that different from animals. There is the unique signature of an animal in each of us. When we dose an animal remedy, we put ourselves in touch with a deeper, subconscious, driving force in our life. We bring balance to the reasons underlying our behaviors, instincts, and even physiology.

In actuality we ARE the animal world. When we dump pesticides on the insect world, we pollute our own nervous system and bodies. When we cage mammals in zoos or corral wild horses, we suppress our own natural passions. When we overdose cows with antibiotics and hormones, we create hormonal imbalances and dysbiosis in our own bodies. In the Native American tradition, when we speak with a "forked tongue" we are lying, like reptiles. Remedies from animals can help integrate parts of ourselves that we have denied or suppressed. When we learn that we are all one and not separated from the natural world we move back to wholeness, back into our life force, and back into the garden of Eden.

Chapter 5

Plant Remedies

According to Cherokee lore, many years ago plants, animals, and humans were able to communicate with one another and they all lived together in harmony. As time passed, mammals complained they were killed only for their fur, and without blessing. Insects complained about being stepped on. Each group of animals held a council to discuss the humans' disrespect. They worried that soon the humans would outnumber them and the animals would be crowded, hunted, and killed to extinction. The animals declared war, and together they devised human diseases. Fortunately, the plants were listening and took pity on the humans. For every disease invented by the animals, the plants designed an antidote. The plants then made a covenant that any sincere plea for help would be answered by the necessary medicinal plant.

True to lore, almost every plant has a level of medicinal value, and homeopathic remedies allow us access to the healing properties of thousands of plants. Homeopathy also allows us to connect to the spirit of each plant by encompassing its full energetic signature, healing us mentally and emotionally, beyond scientifically known pharmacological effects. Native American and other shamanic traditions learned how to use medicinal plants through direct intuitive access, talking directly to the unique spirit of each plant. Deep within us, we all have this capacity. When we get our rational mind out of the way, we can connect to our inner shaman to unite us with specific plants to heal ourselves and our children.

The therapeutic profiles of plants can also be understood by studying their herbal usage, which often matches up with the homeopathic materia medica. For example, herbal artemisia is the same plant as homeopathic Cina, and both treat parasites. If there is a plant medicine you are attracted to for its herbal qualities, or even a plant you are simply drawn to in nature, learn about it homeopathically and you may realize it's a good fit for you in potentized form as well. Likewise, a plant that you find highly problematic or irritating, like poison ivy, or a plant you may have overdosed on, like Cannabis indica, Coffea (coffee), or Thea (tea), may also be a useful remedy to clear the lasting effects these plants may have made on your system.

Plants can treat highly specific complaints in the body. For all the unique mental, emotional, and physical symptoms and sensations that we have, there is often a matching plant medicine to fit that sensory manifestation. These sensations often show polarity between two extremes, such as bending forward versus arching backwards, expansion versus contraction, or heaviness versus lightness. If you can understand the extreme polar states in a patient, you can sometimes find a plant to match it.

Plants can also have organ specificity, so if you need to treat a specific organ system you can find many plants in homeopathic form to help. Sometimes prescribing these remedies in low potency, such as 12X or 6C, taken daily, can help the functionality of these organs.

- Breast: Bellis perennis, Phytolacca
- Eyes: Aconite, Staphysagria, Symphytum
- Genitals: Pulsatilla, Conium, Thuja
- Glands: Phytolacca
- Heart: Aconite, Crataegus, Convolvulus, Digitalis, Cactus, Spigelia, Lycopus, Salix fragilis, Veratrum viride, Tabacum
- Joints/musculoskeletal: Bambusa, Kalmia, Rhododendron, Rhus tox, Ruta, Symphytum
- Kidneys: Berberis, Lycopodium, Uva ursi, Cactus, Equisetum, Sarsaparilla, Staphysagria, Juniperus, Petroselinum
- Liver: Chelidonium, Lycopodium, Carduus marianus, Taraxacum, Leptandra, Juglans cinerea, Myrica, Nux vomica, Podophyllum, Sanguinaria, Ptelea
- Lungs: Sticta, Sambucus nigra, Lobelia, Laurocerasus, Ipecacuanha, Aconite
- Skin: Thuja, Calendula, Iris
- Spleen: Carduus marianus, Helianthus, Ceanothus, Quercus
- Veins: Hamamelis, Aesculus

While there are thousands of plant remedies that could be included here, this chapter focuses on those that I have found to be most useful in complex children. In particular, plant remedies can be critical to help address pain sensations in the body. When a child is in pain and their life revolves around it, this is the main symptom that should be addressed and plants become prime candidates.

Questions to Ask to Help Find a Plant Remedy

Describe the feeling/sensation/pains in the body, go into detail.

If a child is in pain, this is the first thing that needs to be treated. Imagine what that pain/discomfort is like. Is it burning, sharp, dull, aching, cramping, shooting, stabbing, gnawing, twisting, cutting, etc.? Do you see an image like a band, or vice, or an explosion? What do the tissues look like? What makes this pain feel worse? Imagine you have a camera that can go into the body—what would you see? Imagine how your child holds their body when stressed—what does it remind you of? Are they floppy, rigid, scattered, etc.?

What would the opposite feeling of this pain be?

Describe in detail what would make them feel their best and how does that feel? For example: free, euphoric, not in their body, wanting to be in utero, etc.? Close your eyes and image the pain, and then

DRAINAGE, GEMMOTHERAPY, AND FLOWER ESSENCES

Another wonderful way to support specific organ systems is with low potency combination "drainage" formulas, which are sold by companies such as Seroyal or Pekana. UNDA numbered compounds help keep pathways open by draining certain organs and cells in the body, which allow homeopathic remedies to work more effectively. There are also gemmotherapy remedies, which are low potency (usually 1X) plant extractions from buds and other new growth in liquid form. Gemmotherapy remedies help to recalibrate and regenerate the vital force of specific areas of the body—for example stimulating the immune or endocrine system, re-mineralizing bones, calming the central nervous system, or detoxing the liver or kidneys. They are a more energetic form of herbal medicine falling somewhere between herbal tinctures and homeopathy.

Flower essences come from plants as well, and they are similar to homeopathic preparations in that they are subtle dilutions of flowers, however they do not undergo serial dilution and succussion like homeopathic remedies do. Edward Bach, the originator of flower essences, was a well-known homeopath who created flower essences to treat imbalance on the more etheric dimension. This book doesn't list flower essences because there are so many available, but they are a gentle and effective way to treat emotional issues in children. I generally muscle test flower essences and create a formula that has 1 to 5 flowers in it, to be taken daily for 1 to 3 weeks. Although they don't often have significant physical effects, they can help kids with issues such as nervousness in speaking up for themselves, sleeping in their own bed, or helping them be more centered in their heart (and therefore more themselves) when socializing at school.

imagine walking into nature—does a plant show itself to you? Can you picture anything to alleviate the sensations of the body? If there is a polarity between the sensations the child feels when at their best and worse, what is that polarity?

Do you or your child have a specific relationship with a plant already?
Is there a plant in your yard, or one that your child seeks out and enjoys, that could be healing for you or them? Look into it. Often plants that can offer us healing grow very near us!

Plant Families

The remedies in this chapter are organized by their botanical plant family—or in some cases higher classifications—since their biologic similarity creates related physiological effects and healing properties. Contemporary homeopaths such as Rajan Sankaran and Jan Scholten have developed systems that organize key themes and sensations of plant families, and many of these will be listed below. I cannot go into detail on all the plants in each family, but if a given plant family stands out, I suggest you do further research on other remedies within that family. The plant families below are listed alphabetically by their common name or most well-known plant representative and include buttercup, cactus, chocolate, citrus, club moss, coffee, cucumber, daisy, fern, figwort, fungus, gentian, hardwood trees, hemp, heather, latex, lily, magnolia, mint, nightshade, orchid, pea, pine, poison ivy, poppy, rose, spurge, and wild yam. There are many additional plant remedies listed in the charts for specific types of kids in Chapter 10.

Buttercup Family: Emotionally Sensitive and Traumatized

Plants from the buttercup, or Ranunculaceae family, bring balance to states of emotional oversensitivity where reactions are "somatized" or suppressed into the physical, or when oversensitive emotionality has a strong hormonal component. Remedies of this family include Aconite, Ranunculus bulbosus, Cimicifuga, Staphysagria, Actea spicata, Pulsatilla, Helleborus and Clematis. In general, they are important remedies for stuck patterns of emotional trauma that create sensitized emotions in children and adults. When emotions like fear, grief, humiliation, indignation, or anger arise, the body can experience associated overwhelming sensations including tremors, raw nerves, or electrical feelings that radiate or shock. The emotional system gets over-sensitized so the person is easily hurt or triggered, crying over small things like commercials or having outbursts about minor issues. Their emotionality is in a way childish, and there will be desire for comfort and to cling to a parent/teacher/friend for support, acting soft and yielding like a puppy that wants to be taken care of. These emotional events don't easily clear in people needing these remedies; instead they can cause brooding, resentment, and burying of emotion, especially towards the person or event that insulted them. Emotional suppression eventually leads to hysterical outbursts and attention-seeking behavior. If their caregiver/friend/parent doesn't provide this support, they will feel abandoned. Over time, the nervous system can get blunted, slowed, and numbed with low stagnant energy and hormones, causing all types of physical symptoms.

Aconite

Aconite rescues children from panic attacks, the lasting effects of shock, and various anxieties such as claustrophobia, bad dreams, fear of flying, fear of going places, or even fear that their parents may die. The anxiety of Aconite is often felt around the heart with palpitations and restlessness. It can also be a key remedy for the acute onset of colds and flus when dosed at the onset of infection, and can help low-grade, chronic viral infections when the person is on-edge, agoraphobic, easily startled, and restless. Aconite is useful for parents who have had many trips to the emergency room or challenging episodes with their children that leave them in a PTSD state. I have seen several cases of children who had traumatic deliveries with a lot of intervention that left them in a chronic state of shock. These babies will seem highly alert and on edge. Aconite can be similar to Belladonna with acute inflammatory states such as sudden ear infections or sore throat with a high fever. Belladonna will be more delirious and Aconite more fearful and wakeful. See the differential on anxious children (pages 350-352) for remedies similar to Aconite.

Cimicifuga

While classically a remedy for women in menopause, with a feeling of gloom and doom like a black cloud is over them, I have also given Cimicifuga to both boys and girls going through puberty. In these cases, the child has problematic moody emotions, easily breaking into tears. This may seem like Pulsatilla, but in a Cimicifuga case the child is trying to shut down or suppress their emotions and sexuality for fear of growing up, or fear of having their sexuality judged. The person needing Cimicifuga may also have a stiff neck and back, joint pains, and a pressing outward pain in the head.

Helleborus

Helleborus helps heal the sequelae of head injuries, traumatic birth, or chronic inflammation and swelling in the head and represents the more dulled aspect of the buttercup family, differentiating it from Aconite. A child needing Helleborus will be pushing on the head and doing various jaw movements in an attempt to alleviate the pain. There is also likely low vitality and mental slowness—slow speech, memory, and general functioning. I once treated a woman who fell off a horse, hit her head, and had memory loss and slowed mental function; a few doses of Helleborus restored it. Under this dulled stupefaction, there is a deep fear of rejection in love or suppression of emotions. Many complex children are in this state from birth injury, meningitis, vaccine-induced brain inflammation, or other head injuries. They may space out on a regular basis, or push on parts of their heads in an attempt to release a tight feeling in the skull bones. I have seen several children on the spectrum need this remedy who had parents with a history of multiple concussions or other head trauma from sports or motorcycle accidents. See pages 387-390 for more on head trauma remedies.

Pulsatilla

Pulsatilla is a very common remedy for children (more often girls) who are emotionally over-sensitive to their friends and parents. They need too much attention, affection, and approval, which can end up stagnating them. It is a remedy from the "wind flower," and moving with the wind typifies the changeable emotions and symptoms of a Pulsatilla case. They are quick to tears, easily influenced, and indecisive. Their need for love may lead them to seek comfort foods (often fatty or sugary ones). They become overheated and phlegmy with runny noses, and act like spoiled, pouting babies. As an acute remedy it can help with ear infections, colds with thick mucus, hay fever with a lot of mucus and sneezing, clogged ducts and conjunctivitis with green discharge, and UTIs. It can also be a remedy for sadness when there is much weeping, and it plays an important role in women's health by balancing hormonal stagnation. The boys I have seen who need this remedy are underlying Sulphur, Lachesis, or Argentum constitutions—all warm and social kids with a strong allergic tendency.

Staphysagria

Staphysagria can be very similar to Pulsatilla but tends to have greater suppressed emotions including anger, grief, indignation, and resentment, especially towards another person or event from the past. The physical symptoms that can emerge as a result of this suppression of emotions range from UTIs and styes to stomach aches and PMS. Children who are very sensitive and are victimized—such as from being bullied, being bit by an animal, being yelled at excessively, or even sexually abused—can benefit greatly from this remedy. These children tend to be soft and sweet without the capacity to stand up for themselves, so the cycle of victimization can continue. I have often seen children who need Staphysagria because their mothers do; they may have witnessed their parents battling it out and this can become deeply traumatic to the child. Later in life this deep anger may arise through standing up for such causes as animal rights or women's rights, making it similar to the idealistic remedies Causticum and Ignatia. The loss of sense of self in Staphysagria also overlaps with Carcinosin, and they can be used in complementary ways. Physical symptoms that Staphysagria can treat include swollen adenoids, itching anus, eczema, colic, teeth decay, scoliosis, styes and ingrown toenails.

Cactus Family: Contracting and Prickly vs. Expanding and Euphoric

The themes of the Cactaceae (cactus) family can be understood by imagining what it would be like to be a plant surviving in a hot desert, needing to contain all your fluid and resources within a thick, spiny skin that says "don't touch me." It is an extreme environment, and as such, materia medica for these remedies show some extreme polarities, particularly between the sensation of contraction (holding all your water/resources inward, shutting down the heart) and expansion (releasing, opening the heart, dissolving boundaries in a vast environment, euphoric). Deserts are often considered spiritual places, and there can be a spiritually "out-there" quality to people needing these remedies. On the other extreme is survival on bare necessities, feeling isolated in a threatening world, separated, and solitary. Remedies include Anhalonium, Cactina, Carnegie gigantea, Cactus grand, Opuntia and Cereus bonplandii. Children who need these remedies may be silly, euphoric, free spirited, and light (like they aren't in their bodies), alternating with feelings of oppression in the lungs/chest and feeling trapped in the constrictive body. Symptoms tend to congregate around lung/cardiovascular and kidney congestion.

Anhalonium

Also known as peyote or mescal, this hallucinogenic plant is used ceremonially by Native American tribes. Its symptoms include audiovisual hallucinations, hearing disorders, schizophrenia, depersonalization, hysteria, and suicidal tendencies. The expansion side of the polarity of the cactus family, which is the dissolution of self, loss of boundaries, and merging with nature, is truly exemplified by this remedy. However, this loss of identity leads to an inability to function in society, loss of contact with others, loss of sense of time, and existential anguish that can lead to suicide. This extreme state has been found in a few cases of true psychosis where the child had such severe brain inflammation (overlapping with states like Stramonium and Veratrum album) it led them to extreme raging, visual disorders, and hallucinations that, without this remedy, would have landed these children in psych wards. Another case of this remedy was a child whose mother had diabetes and severe kidney disease, was bedbound while pregnant, and had severe edema and immense water weight (she did well with Cactina). Her child had many medical incidents and by the time I treated him she called him her "angel;" he was floating around totally not present in his life, as if drugged. His mother said after the remedy, "It was like he was hovering outside the window of our house looking in, and now it feels like he is in the house." This remedy is comparable to Cannabis indica.

Cactus Grandiflorus

Opposite to an expanded state, people who need cactus remedies can be very contracted and prickly, with a lot of fear. This contraction is seen in the remedy Cactus grand with constricting pains around the heart, sharp pains around the chest (like angina), and spasmodic pains in the body. These sharp pains can be thought of like the spines in the cactus, and this person is often suffering from heartache and fears, similar to Ignatia and Natrum mur. This was the state of one mother I treated who needed this remedy. During her pregnancy, she was in a verbally abusive relationship and felt intense hatred towards her husband, whom she still loved, which created a feeling like her heart was dropping, constriction in the chest, stabbing sensations, and suffocation while breathing. On the flip side, her child, who had an autism diagnosis, was not in touch with people but was always euphoric, happy, light in his heart, and unburdened by life. His survival strategy was to escape into the feeling of space and euphoria. I gave both mother and child Cactus grand and they became more engaged and social; the boy came into his own life and the mother let go of old grievances. This is an interesting example of how polarity in a remedy can span a mother and child.

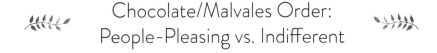

Chocolate/Malvales Order: People-Pleasing vs. Indifferent

Chocolate is a food that is loved by almost everybody, and people who need remedies from its related family of plants can create this loving quality in themselves as well, acting warm, outgoing, wanting to please others, while suppressing/denying aspects of themselves (such as anger, sexuality, etc.) in order to belong to the group. Remedies in the Malvales order include Abroma augusta, Cola nitida, Daphne indica, Gossypium, Hibiscus sabdariffa, Theobroma cacao (chocolate), and Tilia tomentosa. They say that chocolate is a replacement for love, and the sensation of the plants in this family have the desire of falling in love; they are affectionate and communicative creating a merging and loss of self. On the flip side people who experience this kind of merging (like in the first stage of a romantic relationship), will eventually desire to separate, become indifferent to their partners, and gain confidence through independence. The overall polarity is attached and then detached, joined and then separated, in love and then indifferent to those they love.

Daphne Indica

Daphne indica is in the Malvales order in the Thymelaeaceae family, which has a sensation of limbs wringing and twisting to the point of cutting off, or as if feet or head are separated from the body. Their desire to please others causes them to become detached and separated from themselves. This disconnection comes from a feeling of not being appreciated by parents/family, not valued for talents and achievements, and feeling unloved and uncared for. These people will bend themselves into all kinds of positions to be accepted and appreciated. They feel as if they are always being told what to do, causing overwhelm with anxiety, deep anger, blame, and then guilt and repentance. One case of this remedy was the child of a mother who had autoimmune lupus and chronic joint pains while pregnant. She experienced burning, tearing pain in the tissues along the spine as if tissue was being pulled away from the bone, which was better with movement. The pulling of the tissues created a strangulation feeling as if circulation and flow to the extremities were blocked. Her nonverbal child experienced these same physical sensations even more intensely and was deeply uncomfortable; taking this remedy resulted in significantly more ease in his body.

Hibiscus Sabdariffa

While this remedy is not well known in homeopathy, it can be helpful to complex children who feel they have lost contact and are detached from the world of people. They feel as though they have no place in the world or are wrongly positioned in it. They want to experience love, and even romantic love, but cannot speak, or are afraid to speak out and express themselves for fear of being rejected. They are retiring, shy, and afraid of others being angry at them but desire to be more extroverted and connecting. There may be a missing connection with their mother; even though the mom makes herself available to everyone else, she has frustration and anger towards her own child (this remedy may combine well with Natrum mur). The child may be stuck at home, sluggish, without much stimulation, and experience eating problems and indigestion.

Theobroma Cacao

People who need the remedy from chocolate have a strong need for connection but feel sad, alone, and estranged. They desire to be seen, comforted, and cared for. Lack of affection causes them to withdraw into their own creative world, or to become independent and indifferent to relationships. A child needing this remedy demonstrates that they are loveable and affectionate (like Pulsatilla) but also detached and spacey with a weak memory. There may be marital discord between their parents or fighting in the family that creates panic. They want the closeness of a mother, but perhaps never received it; the feeling is like a newborn child requiring the connection and nourishment of breastfeeding, but that close feeling is taken away, causing panic and distress. Children who need this remedy may have separation anxiety, lethargy, eating issues, and difficulty concentrating.

Citrus Family: Compressed Pressure vs. Lassitude

What is it that we all do with fresh lemons and limes? We squeeze the juice from them, and this simple act comprises the general sensation of the Rutaceae plant family: the feeling of connective tissues being crushed, squeezed, then snapped or broken leading to feeling lazy or drained. Remedies in this family include Citrus limon, Ruta graveolens, Ptelea, Angostura trifoliata, and Xanthoxylum. On the mental/emotional level, Jan Scholten describes people needing the Rutaceae family as doing well under pressure. They are hard-working perfectionists who are tough, want to meet high expectations, don't complain, and "overexert themselves, squeezing themselves dry". While this isn't a major family for treating special needs children, I have found a handful of the remedies useful for the children of hardworking parents (particularly moms) who are Type A Ignatia/Nux vomica people who have jobs that require active minds and a lot of focus. Children who need these remedies are likely to be stringy in their body, lively, active, desire sour foods and stimulants, and may have weak liver function and tight tendons, making them want to always stretch.

Ptelea Trifoliata

This remedy assists stomach and liver disorders where there is aching and heaviness in the liver, worse lying on the left side, as well as ravenous hunger (possibly due to worms), empty sensation in the stomach, frontal headaches, or itchy skin due to liver congestion. A child needing this remedy may have a history of jaundice, prefers eating sour/acid things like lemon juice or vinegar, is worse from heavy foods, and will be restless with nightmares at night. The child's mother may feel they are under too much pressure from work, feeling unfairly overburdened and resentful, putting her into a Sepia-like state.

Ruta Graveolens

Ruta, from the plant rue, is well known for the treatment of acute sprains, strains, and joint injuries where there is sore and bruised aching with restlessness. Mentally, the person who needs Ruta is inflexible, factual, frustrated at having to adapt to people, prone to restlessness, and occasionally snaps out of anger or bitter regret (hence the saying "rue the day"). Once a friend of mine gave this remedy to her partner for a ganglion cyst on his wrist. Within minutes of taking the remedy he jumped up, ran out the door, ranted irrationally for ten minutes, came back, apologized, and in that span of time the cyst disappeared!

Xanthoxylum Americanum

The remedy from prickly ash is useful for joint pain and sciatica. It is particularly suited to working moms of nervous temperament who are trying to support the family, perhaps even running a whole business, and are so totally exhausted that their menses are suppressed or they have painful periods. The child who needs this remedy (likely of the aforementioned mother) would prefer sour, juicy foods but have a poor appetite, appearing thin and emaciated with poor absorption. They may have neuralgic issues like shooting pains or numbness in their extremities, and a dry feeling in the mouth.

Club Moss Family/Lycopodium: Napoleonic Complex

Lycopodium, the remedy of club moss, is one that almost all people at some point can benefit from. It has wide ranging effects but is generally a liver-focused remedy that shows up when there are underlying confidence issues that cause a person to try to be something more than they are. Lycopodium can best be understood based on its own natural history. Thousands of years ago it was a large tree, but now it has devolved into a small moss. So it's a little guy that thinks it's a big guy whose importance has been diminished, and it feels vulnerable and threatened. This can also be described as a "Napoleonic complex"—someone who acts confident, strong, bossy, and critical but underneath there is insecurity and the feeling of not being enough.

Lycopodium is often an intercurrent remedy that I give when the particular characteristics described above arise. I am mostly clued into Lycopodium for kids when they have gassiness, bloating, and constipation. This liver backup can show up in the morning, when a child wakes up irritable, with a furrowed brow, acting demanding towards their family. However, once they are amongst peers their insecurities arise. They feel easily vulnerable, fearful of conflicts, fearful of losing, and fearful that they aren't good enough. They may have a lot of anxiety from overthinking (and they can be very intellectual kids), but on the flip side they may have academic issues, such as poor memory and dyslexia. Their insecurities may drive them into becoming bookworms, but sedentary behaviors only tend to exacerbate the liver stagnation. They may also come home from school and release their insecurities by bullying or criticizing a sibling. This remedy can help them get out of their heads, back into their bodies, and be more genuinely self-confident. A Lycopodium parent is typically well-established in an intellectual career, may be dissatisfied with their spouse, seems nice outside the home but is critical of their family at home, and has some obvious physical stagnation. They generally need more exercise (but they already know that).

Not only do Lycopodium kids have a fear of confrontation, they also fear losing and won't play games (or will cheat) simply because they don't want to lose. Their underlying confidence issues result in always feeling like they aren't good enough; they don't like trying new things and they get depressed if they feel they have failed. Lycopodium infants often have well-developed heads and small bodies, were born jaundiced, and have scalp eruptions with yellow discharge. Even as babies they may have a furrowed brow, as though they are anxious from overthinking. Dyslexia, confused thinking, and poor memory are also common Lycopodium features. These children often brag and exaggerate to others as a way of compensating for their low self-esteem.

Coffee Family: Over-Stimulated Raw Nerves and Exhaustion

The Rubiaceae family includes coffee and the key remedies in it are Galium aparine, China officinalis, Yohimbinum, and Coffea. According to Sankaran, the sensation of these plant remedies is overstimulation, which aggravates the nerves. These are people with many ideas and thoughts (think drinking coffee in a café and endless topics of conversation) and a lot of creative pursuits. They tend to be bright, shiny people who are social climbers and like to be seen in the limelight. Eventually this will turn to either an oversensitive, nervous state creating strong irritability or a dull, sleepy state.

China Officinalis

China (the source of quinine which was used to treat malaria) is the most important Rubiaceae remedy and has helped many immune-compromised kids. Interestingly, I did have one case in which a child developed toxic effects after being overdosed on the medication quinine while in Africa, but most cases are children with an underlying parasitic or Lyme-associated infection (similar to malaria). These infections cause a great oversensitivity of the nervous system creating sensitivity to touch, such as a great dislike of having their hair brushed, clothing changed, or taking showers. These children have abundant ideas and can have trouble sleeping from too many excited thoughts. They have contradictory personalities and hate being told no but love screaming "no!" Underlying this intense layer of China these children can be very sensitive cases to begin with, and remedies such as Argentum met, Argentum nit, or Phosphorus are often follow-up remedies.

Coffea Arabica

Most people are aware of the effects of coffee—it makes us mentally active and lucid, and even have rushes of thoughts and ideas. Too much coffee can cause nervous agitation, insomnia, and over-acute senses. Children who respond well to this remedy may have parents who drink a lot of coffee and are overly driven, busy, ambitious, and hurried. It can assist kids with neuralgias, tics, twitches, throbbing headaches, oversensitive senses, dry heat in the face with red cheeks, asthmatic breathing worse from excitement, and sleeplessness. Many people who drink coffee regularly are in a subtle chronic state of the remedy Coffea. If coffee drinkers have worked up nerves and poor sleep, they should ideally quit drinking coffee, but most are loathe to give it up. Classical homeopaths may even say that coffee antidotes homeopathy, although I have not found this to be the case. Instead, caffeine tends to divert energy that the body would use for healing from the interior to the exterior. This pushing towards the exterior and sensitizing the nerves is a key sensation of Rubiaceae.

Cucumber Family: Intense, Sharp Pain, Better Stillness

Cucurbitaceae is the plant family of the bitter cucumber, and indeed, people needing it tend to have deep, bitter feelings of resentment towards life. This may be accompanied by sharp pains in the body (especially the gut), as if they've been stabbed. The deep desire of people who need these remedies is to reach a place of calmness, stillness, and quiet. They don't want to be bothered anymore and interactions with people are generally considered an oppressive annoyance. These remedies include Elaterium, Bryonia alba, Colocynthis, Cucurbita pepo, and Luffa.

According to Sankaran, the sensations of these remedies are "cutting, stabbing, sharp, stitching, pinching." These are typically overworked people who show irritability when questioned and have a deep, antisocial bitterness with aversion to being disturbed, desire for total rest, and avoidance of people. The Bryonia alba keynote of "pain, worse motion" characterizes the feelings of this family well.

The bitter cucumber family remedies are often needed by children of hardworking mothers who are serious about work and investing for the future but feel oppressed and burdened by their jobs. It is always important to understand how a mother felt while pregnant and working—in these cases a lot of anger can arise around work, and there is sometimes an abusive boss in the picture. They can be useful remedies for parasite infections as well, where there is a feeling of being persecuted by their work, which is sucking the life from them.

Bryonia Alba

The core mental state of Bryonia is one of deficiency, to the degree that they have to keep very still so as not to exert any extra effort (which would be painful). For them, movement, talking, and coughing all aggravate because these things use energy that is in short supply. People needing this remedy are generally hard-working and a bit uptight; they are "all business" and hasty in their manner and are easily irritated, much like Nux vomica. They also tend to be homebodies who are conservative and anxious, like Calcarea carb. They have used up all their resources at work and want to come home and sit in front of the TV or hole up in their bedroom. Bryonia is wide-ranging in its action, treating afflictions such as appendicitis, migraine headaches, flu, painful coughing, and painful joints.

Colocynthis

I have seen several strong Colocynthis cases in ASD children whose mothers were bullied while pregnant, usually by a boss or a teacher, and they held it all inside. In one case, the mother had a huge meltdown directed at her boss (who was picking on her) and passed out. The feeling of Colocynthis is that they are stuck in a bad situation and feel insulted or put upon, which makes them angry, impatient, and offended. They hold anger in the stomach, giving them cramps, spasms, and sharp pains, but then it all comes out in a tantrum or through movement, restlessness, or vomiting. The ASD children of these mothers had gut issues, and they too were angry and indignant, especially when something was asked of them. Colocynthis is also a wonderful remedy for sciatica, facial nerve pain, and ovarian and back pain.

Cucurbita Pepo

Pumpkin seeds are known for treating parasites, especially tapeworm, and as such the materia medica of this remedy fits children who are contradictory, demand attention, and are holding in suppressed anger, perhaps from some feeling of being mistreated or abused.

Daisy Family: Beat Up and Wounded

Commonly referred to as the daisy or sunflower family, Compositae (or Asteraceae) is a large and widespread family of flowering plants that includes many edibles and herbal teas. These remedies are all well known for treating a feeling of being beaten, bruised, and wounded resulting in a loss of bodily integrity, with long-lasting fears of accidents or traumas. Most people who need these remedies constitutionally will feel they can't really get comfortable in their bodies and are wary from the touch or approach of others since they on some level still feel traumatized. They tend to be accident prone and may have a history of multiple car or athletic accidents.

According to Jan Scholten, "The Compositae family has a strong drive for individuality, independence, and living their own lives. They have a strong aversion to being interfered with. They want to do things on their own, going their own way. They prefer to say that things are going well rather than being interrupted or intruded upon. This is exemplified by the well known symptom of Arnica when someone is sick but says they are well and sends the doctor away. Even when they are sick, they do not want to be hassled by doctors or others. They hate operations, vaccinations, medications, and any other intervention. They want to keep their integrity, also in their body. Any blow, beating, accident, or hemorrhages in any form is an intrusion of their boundaries, a violation of their integrity. A basic expression of the remedy is a feeling of vulnerability."

There are many daisy family remedies useful for acute conditions:

- Arnica—bruising and swelling from trauma, contusions, surgeries, sore body

- Calendula—wounds/cuts/abrasions/lacerations; easily frightened, tendency to start
- Eupatorium perf—bone pain and chills during flu/fever; chest oppression/cough
- Taraxacum—mapped tongue, gallstones, night sweats, joint pain; impatient and irritable
- Abrotanum—emaciation of limbs, big appetite without weight gain, malnutrition, joint pain
- Bellis perennis—pelvic soreness, deep tissue trauma, childbirth tissue trauma, breast tumors
- Echinacea—sepsis from bites/wounds, gangrene, lymphangitis, appendicitis, sore throat

Arnica is the best-known remedy of this family and is generally the first choice for acute traumas, blows, and injuries in children. I always carry a small vial of Arnica or a tube of Arnica gel in my first aid kit and car. Any surgeries or dental procedures can also be followed by a dose of Arnica to reduce swelling. I generally dose Arnica as an acute remedy for kids and it can be a constitutional remedy for adults in occupationally hazardous professions, such as athletes or construction workers. Bellis perennis, which is called the Arnica of the pelvis, can also be useful for women who had traumatic births or are at risk for breast cancer, but I have not seen this remedy useful for children specifically. Eupatorium perf can be an important flu remedy for deep bone and muscle aches, and I have occasionally used it to help clear deeply suppressed viruses in the body. But by far, the two most useful and important remedies to understand for chronic treatment in children are Cina and Chamomilla. These remedies are quite similar—both are contrarian and will reject things offered to them, and they have a great oversensitivity to pain that makes them whine and tantrum.

Chamomilla

Chamomilla is a top children's remedy that can go hand-in-hand with Cina. If one doesn't work, it can help to try the other. Both can have contrary behaviors such as refusing things right after they ask for them, and show gut discomfort with whining, demanding, impossible behavior. The main difference is that Cina will be more obstinate about the thing they want and Chamomilla will be more changeable and emotionally unstable. Chamomilla is also an excellent remedy for teething and colicky babies where there is deep nerve discomfort, as well as ear infections. A unique keynote of Chamomilla is that a single cheek will be flushed and red while the other is pale, specifically when the child is having a tantrum or crying from pain.

Cina

Cina is an indispensable remedy for the treatment of parasites in children. A reliable behavior on which to prescribe Cina is when a child strikes, hits, or throws toys out of nowhere, coinciding with whining and tantrums. This childish, attacking behavior seems to be an external reflection of the internal parasitic attack. Children with parasites may also have deep neurological inflammation and seizure symptoms. For problematic parasites, I often have parents give Cina 30C two days before, the day of, and two days after the full moon every month, which is a time that parasites replicate in the body. For more information on parasites see pages 281-288. Parents will often notice that their child suddenly develops these behaviors around the new or full moon. Other symptoms include picking the nose and butt, shrieking, and disliking touch including having their hair combed.

Fern Family: Hiding Parasites

There is only one remedy within the fern family, Filix mas, that stands out due to its ability to help with parasites, particularly tapeworms. The mental state of Filix mas and ferns, according to Vermeulen, is a desire to hide or to be invisible or guarded. This fits the energetics of a parasite, which is an organism that hides, tends not to evolve, and seeks to control others around them. People who need this remedy do not want to become an adult with their responsibilities. They may act strongly male on the outside (even backwardly chauvinistic), but in reality they are childish, sensitive to criticism, and averse to change. Symptoms often cycle with the full moon.

Figwort Family: Loose Connections and Detachment vs. Holding On

The figwort/Scrophulariaceae family is useful for people who fear showing the ugly side of themselves or their family, keeping their dirt/discharges, stool/urination/bodily functions hidden. The remedies from this family include Buddleja davidii, Digitalis, Scrophularia nodosa, and Verbascum thapsus. I also include Gratiola below because it has similar themes. They are reserved, mild people who do not open up easily to the point of being secretive, with suppressed anger causing liver, digestive, and elimination problems such as constipation, diarrhea, and enuresis. The underlying sensations and themes are loose connections and bonds leading to fear of separation, disconnection, and detachment causing a desire to reattach, hold on, be stable, and reestablish connection or be tenaciously sticking and adherent. Interestingly, a handful of the complex cases that have done well with these remedies were children conceived via IVF (in vitro fertilization), with some of the pregnancies occurring after many miscarriages. So imagine the feeling a mother has when trying to get pregnant, with a great desire to "hold onto/attach/establish connection" with an embryo and fearful of "separation". Possibly the fertility issues and IVF are kept private, it stays in the family. The children in these cases often have issues with bowel movements, enuresis, and "letting in all out." They can be very attached to their mother as well.

Digitalis

This is the remedy of the flower foxglove and treats disconnection in relationships affecting the heart chakra. A child needing Digitalis may have had difficulty bonding with their mother, or perhaps experienced inconsolable loss after getting attached to a caretaker/nanny who leaves and after that they are never quite the same. The deeper cause of the disconnect may be due to intense familial conflict or rejection in relationships during pregnancy or infancy which caused the mother's heart to almost stop (like a dropping sensation) such as intensely angry arguments with loved ones that created a disconnected feeling in the heart chakra. The child may demonstrate a desire to bond and feel connected with loved ones, but when separated from someone they love it feels like death. This relationship drama eventually leads to an indifferent attitude towards others. The child's state looks a lot like Ignatia or Natrum mur, but they are not as emotionally closed or suppressed. Digitalis is known for treating regulation of the heart beat/pulse, angina, or feelings of the heart stopping. These heart issues may not be experienced acutely in a child, but the children I have seen who need this remedy have a lot of left sided issues, sensory issues around their head with a lot of pushing, neuralgias, numbness and tingling, an intense need to jump hard into the ground (like a frog) as if trying to move energy, and a lot of restlessness in the body with a strong desire to move. They may also have nausea or a congested liver which shows up as a bad temper, irritability, and impatience, similar to Nux vomica.

Gratiola Officinalis

While this remedy is not technically in the figwort family, it is in the same order (Lamiales). In the past it has been considered by homeopaths to have the same themes and is useful for people with a need to hide their negative side in order to preserve their image. It has gastrointestinal tract symptoms including colic, bloody stools, stomach cramps, diarrhea, jaundice, rectal constriction, or diarrhea that is forcibly evacuated making it similar to Podophyllum and useful for diseases such as ulcerative colitis. It can also assist with brain and neurological symptoms such as jerking, tics, hydrocephalus, and a feeling that the brain is contracting. It proved useful in a child (conceived by IVF) who had irritable bowel symptoms; some days he would run to the bathroom for stool many times and other days he would be constipated but not want to push out the stool. Sometimes when he pooped, only little amounts of stool would come out and would remain attached to him. During his birth process he also got stuck halfway, and as an infant he didn't want to progress through his milestones, not due to inability, but from a fear of change. He was so attached to his mother that she always had to push him forward in life. After he took this remedy his bowel movements normalized and he became more open to change.

Scrophularia Nodosa

This is a useful remedy for glandular swellings, particularly if there is a strong history of cancer in the family, breast tumors, or Hodgkin's disease. Children who need this remedy may have eczema around their ears, enuresis, crushing headaches, parasite issues, cutting pains in the abdomen, and pain with bowel movements. Jan Scholten writes that this remedy is useful for families who try to protect/cover up family problems by acting controlling, suspicious, and being careful not to tell too much. There is a feeling of "us against the world." The parents of these children or the children themselves may exert excessive control out of fear of separation or disconnection; fear starts when the connection breaks.

Verbascum Thapsus

The remedy Verbascum (mullein) can be useful for enuresis or bedwetting, especially when there is shame about it and fear that someone outside the family will find out. They will be fearful of sleepovers or going on vacations lest people discover their bedwetting or other things about them that are unacceptable. In general, they are timid and will try to hide all their problems. Is also useful for colic, constipation, mucousy colds with bronchial coughs, deafness, ear pain, neuralgia, and overaccumulation of salty saliva in the mouth.

Fungi Family: Reckless and Reeling

Mushrooms (fungi) are a fascinating family in their own kingdom from which we've derived antibiotics (such as penicillin), psychedelic drugs, and even bioremediation methods. Mushrooms are well-known immune system adaptogens that build our immunity, yet some molds in the fungi family are also responsible for the hidden deterioration behind the walls of our houses that can cause rampant infection and damage in those who are immune-compromised.

Sankaran describes the qualities of fungi as "invading, burrowing, digging, excoriating, gnawing, corrosive, ulcerative, penetrating, spread, superhuman, egotism, courageous, fight, strength." On the flip side, there will be a sense of emptiness, like a hollow void, and then tendency to passive hemorrhage. My sense is that we know a handful of these remedies in homeopathy but that many more need to be understood and explored. It's possible that EMF predisposes people to more fungal infections and the spread of the internet has the qualities of fungal growth.

Children who need fungi remedies tend to be adventurous, reckless, and fearless. They are hot in their bodies and crave sugar, but too much sugar can make them spacey, giggly, reeling, awkward, falling out of chairs, and all over the place. They can have poor boundaries and hemorrhage easily (like Phosphorus), have psychic abilities, and often have an underlying cancer or tubercular miasm with weak immunity and a lot of anxiety. They also tend to have very changeable symptoms—energy moves quickly through them, and they can change in a split second from crying over not getting their way, to laughing, jumping, and screeching. They seek stimulation and excitement, can spread themselves thin doing too many things, and have trouble gaining weight. Their general openness allows them to get quite attached to people and things easily, and if they don't have that thing they so desperately want, they will feel a deep void (like Nux vomica). There is also a great spiritual seeking quality to people who need fungi—they are seeking another world to inhabit, like a portal to a whole other dimension of being. Fungi are associated with the uranium series on the periodic table of elements, which has the themes of the universe, magic, and intuition. For more on fungi remedies, see pages 269-275.

Agaricus Muscarius

This is a red-capped mushroom (also known as amanita) that can cause sensory hallucinations if consumed, and is the mushroom that Alice ate before falling into the rabbit hole of Wonderland. Children who need this remedy are easily influenced, don't have a strong sense of themselves, (like Phosphorus or Carcinosin), and can almost come out of themselves becoming fearless, reckless, over-excited, talkative, and even feel enlarged as if in a drunken state. They don't want to work and can seem lazy, giggly, and spacey. An interesting physical keynote of this remedy is itching of the feet as if frostbit or a general sensation of being frozen or frostbit. Agaricus can also treat family history of alcoholism, spasms and tics of the muscles, twitches, and incredible itching. There may be sharp pains in the back, yet pressing on the spine causes laughter.

Bovista

This is the puff ball fungus and children who need this remedy have alternating moods—(they can go quickly from laughing to crying), are overly sensitive, and easily take offense. Like other fungal remedies they may be uncoordinated and awkward in their body, and even awkward in speech such as stammering. They have a tendency for nosebleeds, acne, eczema, itching, vertigo, and tension headaches. Both the Banerji Protocol from India and Joette Calabrese, CCH, suggest regular dosing of Bovista 200C for chronic food and gluten intolerance in general.

Secale

This is a remedy from a fungus called ergot, which grows on rye plants and when consumed can cause hallucinations. Secale can be useful for passive hemorrhage, such as sudden and intense bloody noses, and for ataxia (stumbling around uncoordinated). Children who need this remedy can be fearless and reckless while climbing over everything, doing flips, and generally rolling around. The child's mother may be very spiritually seeking, such as meditating regularly or wanting to live in an ashram, and she sees her child as a gift from the divine.

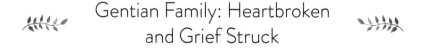

Gentian Family: Heartbroken and Grief Struck

This group of remedies is fundamental in healing the diseases that are a product of the Type A, workaholic, over-thinking culture we live in. The gentian, or Loganiaceae family, includes the remedies Ignatia, Nux vomica, Strychninum, Gelsemium, Upas tieute, and Spigelia. These are ambitious, goal-oriented people who work hard to achieve the perception of a successful life—the perfect house, the perfect marriage, the perfect job—only to realize that they are perpetually wired and tense. These remedies can aid them in opening up to their authentic emotions.

Children are learning to be in their bodies and a healthy immune system requires healthy emotional embodiment, which they learn from their parents. However, if parents are not emotionally connected, which often happens in this culture (such as when we are required to be "professional"), it can disconnect children from their emotional bodies. This results in various manifestations of imbalance, such as meltdowns if they don't get their way, or emotions getting suppressed into the nervous system causing tics or twitches. Professional parents should take off their "work hats" at home and make a conscious effort to be emotionally present for their children, allowing them to openly express their feelings.

The core emotional disconnect that the gentian remedies heal is bringing to the fore suppressed grief that hasn't been properly processed or expressed. Our culture typically suppresses grief because we don't have healthy models of how to process and work through it. For example, children of parents who are divorced often have a deep layer of grief that is suppressed. The emotional energy gets redirected on the neurologic level and may also create patterns of strong workaholism or idealism out of a deep need for recognition and approval. Most of these remedies have neurologic symptoms such as insomnia, trembling, tics, twitches, or irritable bowel syndrome from anxiety.

Many cases, particularly PANDAS (pediatric autoimmune neuropsychiatric disorders associated with streptococcus) cases, have a weakened immunity linked to suppressed grief in the family that can be tracked back to their parents or even further. This unprocessed grief weakens the lungs and boundaries (immunity) of the child, and easily affects the nervous system creating various emotional overreactions. Ideally, emotions flow like a river, but with suppressed emotions we create a dam that will overflow and cause disasters. The disasters will further amplify the desire to dam up the emotions again, creating a cycle of unhealthy emotional release followed by withholding of emotions. Unfortunately, this pattern of emotional cycling is almost a new norm in our culture.

The homeopathic sensations listed by Sankaran that characterize the gentian remedies are "heartbroken, shattered, disappointed, unresolved grief from broken relationships, shock so sudden as to paralyze, difficulty weeping." A death of someone close or a series of challenging breakups can lead to this state. Being raised by a parent who didn't love unconditionally, but rather based on performance, can also create this state. Or there is a heartbreak that does not find resolution and shuts down the full and open functioning of the heart chakra. The disappointed person then redirects their energy into ambitious motives, thinking that if they only made more money, or were more successful, or if their children received straight A's, then it would make up for this loss, this hole in the heart.

While there is a slight tendency for Nux vomica to be prescribed to males and Ignatia to females, often people who need one can also benefit from the other. The remedy Strychninum is made from an alkaloid present in the gentian plants, and when the energy of heartbreak and disappointment is extreme, I will prescribe this remedy instead. Or, if Ignatia or Nux vomica have been useful but haven't fully cleared the picture of a keyed-up nervous system I will dose Strychninum.

Ignatia

A great majority of people who withhold emotions, especially grief, can benefit from Ignatia. They often have an ideal life or partner in mind with an actual life that never meets their ideal, setting them up for continuous disappointment after which they will set an even higher bar. This cycle can only be broken when this person realizes that true love is an act of giving and not reliant on performance that you can fail at. People who need Ignatia often feel heaviness around their breathing or chest and a lump in their throat. The feelings around their heart can feel closed off or broken.

Ignatia is a common remedy given to parents with special needs children who have a sense of sadness and disappointment. It is also a key remedy for children who have suppressed streptococcus infections and tend to be perfectionistic, and it can be useful given alongside one of the strep nosodes (see page 248-252), especially for feelings of stuckness and aching around the throat. These tend to be contradictory children with strong desires and keyed up nervous systems, who only find release when they have an emotional blowout. Similar to a baby that needs to have a good cry before falling asleep, kids with an Ignatia constitution need emotional release to help their body relax. However, if they attempt to control and hold in emotions, they will have insomnia and various neurological symptoms. Other physical symptoms that can be helped by Ignatia include anorexia and other body image issues, colic, constipation, croup and coughs, spasms and general oversensitivity, sore throat, and tics and twitches. All the other remedies in this plant family can be complementary to Ignatia.

Gelsemium

Gelsemium is the most anxious of the gentian family with a lot of floating anxiety and fear of being put on the spot, or anticipatory anxiety. They fear being let down by some bad news and may have a history of emotional shock. I once treated a mother who needed this remedy constitutionally with a history of grief stemming from her estranged father who always disappointed her by not showing up for his weekends with her. Gelsemium is also a big influenza remedy with weakness and trembling as major keynote symptoms. It seems that many flu epidemics also have a connection to media scares and this itself feeds into the Gelsemium state. Likewise, Gelsemium can be a common remedy for immunodeficiency and chronic fatigue cases that have a suppressed viral component, or an etiology of successive annual flu vaccines. These kids are in a perpetual state of anxiety which shows up as weakness, nausea, trembling, tics and twitches, and many fears.

Nux Vomica

Nux vomica is the most workaholic remedy of the group and people who need it are often driven by a deep emptiness that they have a hard time putting their finger on. Sometimes this workaholism is just an energy reinforced by our culture of making more and more money and a need to keep busy. People who respond well to Nux vomica may rely on stimulants like coffee to keep them going and alcohol to calm them down, which ultimately creates a wired nervous system causing all sorts of physical issues such as poor digestion, gas, irritable bowel syndrome, diarrhea, and sensitivity to cold. Children of these parents easily fall into this pattern as well, being competitive in school and sports and making to-do lists like their parents. When they get worn down, they can yell and be irritable to friends and family; those around them walk on eggshells. This remedy is very common in many diagnoses and is often used for PANDAS. Nux vomica also helps to treat addictions, colds and flus, liver and stomach issues, headaches, nausea and vomiting, and insomnia.

Spigelia

Spigelia is similar to Ignatia, but more anxious and agitated. This person can't stand thinking about pain and may have a particular fear of sharp or pointed objects like pins, which correlates with a type of pain they get that is sticking, pinching, or sharp. They may suffer from pains around the chest like angina, stitches around the diaphragm, migraines, neuralgias, and shortness of breath. It is also a useful remedy for worms.

Hardwood Trees: Heavy, Dull, Dragged Down vs. Light and Free

Place a mental image of a tree in your mind. Imagine its roots anchoring its weight in the earth, the sheer massiveness of it. And then imagine its branches reaching upwards towards the sky, leaves lightly blowing in the wind. These are the two sensations that make up tree remedies—the polarity of feeling heavy, contained, dragged down like roots versus a feeling of being in open air, light, free, imaginative, and moving, like the top of the tree. As humans, we mirror trees, we need to be rooted and grounded to the earth and also connected to the sky and our spiritual selves, and we move between these two polarities. Tree remedies span many plant families such as Fagaceae, Sapindaceae, and conifers (see pine/Thuja). They include remedies such as Myrica, Fagus sylvatica, Castanea, Betula alba, Quercus robur, Carp bet, Ostrya virginiana, Alnus rubra, Acer saccharum, and Hornbeam, and they help the body equilibrate its connection between earth and sky.

Hardwood tree remedies are often for sturdy, dependable types, who may be the strong and silent people we rely on for trustworthy, service-oriented jobs. They can be so grounded that they tend to get a sense of heaviness, compression, or sadness with dulled senses. Often when someone who needs a tree remedy is describing their sensations, they will speak of their body like a wooden box or crate, and usually there is a corresponding physical rigidity. To escape this, they may have a desire for freedom that is different from animal remedies. It is a freedom of the mind—creativity, openness, poetry, music—as well as the openness of fresh air, sun, and nature that brings them true joy.

Acer Saccharum

Animals aren't the only category that children can imitate, some kids will show love and imitation of plants! While Acer saccharum, the remedy of sugar maple, is not well known in homeopathy, I gave the remedy to a child who had a deep love of this particular tree. Maple is in the Sapindaceae family of trees, which according to Scholten are for people where rules have become too strict and immovable; their need for comfort and safety leads to excessive rigidity. They can be overly intellectual or separated from their body, leading to feelings of vertigo. Other remedies in this family include Aesculus and Acer campestre. In the case of this child, he would posture his body or other people's bodies to be like trees and create bridges out of his body with his arms and legs. His favorite activity was to go on long walks looking for leaves, particularly red maple leaves. He would find and distinguish different leaves by calling some of them mommy, some daddy, and some baby leaves, and identified various tree types by leaf shape. He loved deep red colors so much he would go into the store "Victoria's Secret" so he could be surrounded by it, and would also keep and collect red produce stickers or price tags. Physically he had an itching, oozing red eczema that flared easily. This remedy helped not only the eczema but shifted all of the stuck behaviors that gave him an ASD diagnosis.

Betula Alba

The remedy Betula alba from the silver birch tree has a heavy tiredness in the body while mentally there is a desire for lightness, serenity, clarity, and bringing order to chaos. This person is self-sacrificial, wanting to serve others with generosity and compassion, but toughened by working in a hard life, almost like a pioneer in the Wild West would have felt. A child needing this remedy would feel heavy and fatigued in the body, possibly rejected, isolated, and misunderstood. Instead of being bossy like Quercus robur, they are more mild-mannered, shut down, closed, and anxious, especially when around chaos. Physically they may have eczema, shooting pains in the urethra, stiffness in the body, and hypoglycemia.

Quercus Robur

This is the remedy from the English oak tree in the Fagaceae family, and this family is known for treating people who are responsible, reliable, and duty oriented with strong will power that can make them almost dominant. People rely on them for their wisdom and leadership, making them good at running organizations, being in the military, or taking positions of authority. Because of this inner strength they can have high expectations of themselves, take on too many burdens, get overstrained, and become fearful of letting others down. Adults needing this remedy may become depressed, alcoholic, and/or develop liver disorders. Children needing this remedy may be bossy to the point of barking orders at their mother, requiring routine/schedules for their predictability, and want to do every-thing on their terms. They are likely to have a large appetite and act irrita-ble and bossy (with livery qualities like Lycopodium), and very much want to prove to others that they are capable. Sensation wise, this child will feel that all the chaos of the world makes them want to hunker down, making them feel heavy in the body, angry, and frustrated. On the flip side, a child needing this remedy can also daydream a lot and seem light/spacey and even feel their head is spinning when they are checked out. While they like the sun, they may also be sensitive to sun and light, giving them headaches or fatigue. It is also useful for eczema, gassiness, and vertigo.

Heather Family: Stiff and Restless

Another group of plants to treat restlessness are the heather, or Eri-caceae family, which includes the remedies Kalmia, Rhododendron, and Ledum. The sensation these plants treat is stiffness leading to a need for wandering movement. According to Jan Scholten, "In general these people are not very marked. They avoid standing in the center of attention and feel better doing their job in a quiet and practical way. But they long for recognition and compliment." These remedies are well known for treating the aching musculoskeletal symptoms of Lyme disease including wander-ing joint pains that are worse damp weather. Ledum has been known to prevent Lyme disease if taken after a tick bite. This family also treats eye and kidney disorders. I include them here because of the Lyme etiology common in chronic immune disorders, but see chapter 10 for more Lyme-related remedies.

Kalmia

This is a great remedy for chronic Lyme pain, especially if migrating from joint to joint or moving down the limb. The pain can come on sud-denly and severely and be paralytic, with neuralgia or cracking joints. Stiff-ness may also be around the eyes, with pain on moving the eyes. Pain in general is worse with motion or cold and better with heat. Kalmia may also help with facial neuralgia that is right sided, such as in post-shingles neuralgia. People who need this remedy are generally mild in disposition.

Ledum

Ledum is known as a remedy to take after all puncture wounds, such as bites or injections, and may prevent tetanus, Lyme disease, and side effects of vaccinations. It is also helpful for black eyes and hard swellings. The site of the wound may be cold to the touch but feels better when cold or ice is applied; drinking cold water is also desired. Ledum can be useful for arthritis that begins in the feet and moves upwards, or stiff joints that are better with cold applications. Emotionally, the person who needs Ledum may prefer solitude.

Rhododendron

Rhododendron's well-known keynote is that symptoms are worse on the approach of a storm or wet weather, with sensitivity to electrical changes such as lightning and thunder. It is a useful remedy for vertigo when lying down, better with movement. People who need this remedy may also have intense tinnitus, loss of memory, or sudden disappearance of thought.

Hemp Family/Cannabis Indica—Bright and Creative vs. Dull and Lethargic

Like trees, the cannabis state has a strong separation in sensation between the upper, imaginative realm and the heavier, dragging down energies. It's typical for people to sit on their couch not moving much and then get lost in their imagination when they smoke pot. The middle chakra, responsible for will power, gets weakened. Parents who use it a lot can also pass on a miasmatic cannabis pattern to the kids. These kids, if overly exposed to pot, will be spacey and have a hard time incarnating—just BEING in their bodies—which creates a lot of anxiety, and they will be too open on sensory levels making it hard to engage in the real world. However, there does not need to be a history of exposure to cannabis. Cannabis indica can be useful for overly sensitive, absent-minded children who become anxious because they are not well-grounded. Paul Herscu, ND, often uses this remedy for ASD children who are really into sensory stimulation, like looking at colors. Strong hallucinations and imagination, lost sense of time and space, clairvoyance, blissful states, being exhausted after a short walk due to weak lower limbs, an involuntary shaking of the head, as well as loss of memory and fear of insanity can all occur with people who need this remedy.

Lily Family: Belonging and Holding On vs. Forced Out and Excluded

The lily (Liliaceae/Melanthiaceae) plant family includes the remedies Veratrum album, Veratrum viride, Lilium tigrinum, and Paris quadrifolia. Scholten states of this family, "They have an outgoing quality, behaving as if the world belongs to them. But there is also a fear that they are not accepted and easily neglected. So they have to make themselves bigger, boasting of what they are and can do in order to be really accepted. It is a difficult state as they want to preserve their position of being great and good and on the other hand feel they are losing it and will be treated easily at any moment as a beggar." This desire, to not only belong to a group but to be elevated in status by the group, creates the sensation of needing to be attractive to others and hold onto their status, versus a fear of being excluded or forced out of the group. Physically this forcing out fear shows up as pressure headaches, nausea, vomiting, diarrhea, and even a feeling that the pelvic floor will be pushed out.

Paris Quadrifolia

This remedy is for talkative, loud, rude, self-satisfied children who are attention seeking. Perhaps they are "only" children, overly complimented and adored, while at the same time not taken seriously. With their friends they may feel they are more mature, but they act too hyper or impulsively without caring about the reactions of others, always speaking about themselves in an egotistical way. They view themselves as the center of the world and feel worse from being excluded. Physically they can get swollen sensations, one side of the body hot and the other side cold, and headaches where their head feels enlarged or constricted. Pressure is also felt in the eyes where the eyeballs feel enlarged or protruding, as if the lids would not close, and there is a drawing sensation in the eyeballs.

Veratrum Album

The main remedy of significance for complex children in this plant family is Veratrum album. The child has a need to belong to a group and to be seen, often as a leader, but there is also a great fear of being disliked, pushed out, or not included. This can show up in gifted adolescents who fear being rejected and have a strong need to be perceived as smart and special. These tend to be intelligent, precocious kids with disconnected emotions that can result in cruel, unfeeling behaviors that they have little remorse for. They can have manic states where they are dominant and haughty, VERY restless, verbally abusive, or cutting or tearing into things. This manic state can alternate with a weak or collapsed state where they are afraid of being abandoned or left alone and become needy. The over-mentalized state in Veratrum album tends to create paranoid delusions that people are out to get them or that there is a mass conspiracy, making it a useful remedy in schizophrenia. I have seen two Veratrum album cases where there was a family history of cruelty, murder, or crime, and it is not beyond a child needing Veratrum album to commit serious crime.

Veratrum Viride

This remedy is similar to Veratrum album with its destructive restlessness, but it is more effective in cases where children are having strong central nervous system inflammation symptoms showing up as convulsions, occipital pressure/pain/congestion, or meningitis. They will feel hot in the head and faint with a rapid or irregular pounding pulse, bloodshot eyes, and dilated pupils. It's comparable to Belladonna and can be considered as an alternative to it. The child may have pneumonia, violent stomach pain with nausea/vomiting, acute joint pain, and a keynote of a red streak down the center of the tongue.

Water Lily/Nuphar Luteum

The water lily is in the Nymphaeales family and actually doesn't have much to do with Veratrum album/viride or Paris quadrifolia, but is a useful remedy for children at the opposite end of the spectrum—those who have very little identity and have suffered abuse. The water lily is a symbol of purity because it looks clean despite growing out of mud. Similarly, the remedy Nuphar luteum (yellow pond lily) helps to restore the purity that was lost in children who were victims of abuse, incest, exploitation, or torture, especially if this was at a young age when there was total powerlessness. This abuse creates confusion of identity, lack of will power, loss of root chakra, sexual imbalance (lack of desire or hypersexual) and a sympathetic love of animals. This remedy can clear "potty mouth" behavior with inappropriate focus on genitalia, much like Hyoscyamus, in children as well. Physically it may help colitis, diarrhea, and fatigue.

Magnolia/Lauraceae Family: Confused, Withdrawn, and Adaptable

This group of plants includes some well-known spices such as nutmeg, and contains the homeopathic remedies Nux moschata, Magnolia grandiflora, Myristica, and Asarum. The sensation of the Magnoliidae group according to Sankaran is, "The world is a place of confusion—I am bewildered or beclouded, everything is strange; and because the world outside is so bewildering and confusing, I feel isolated and not part of it, and I withdraw, and create my own world, which is familiar. The shutting out of the strange world can cause a sense of being sleepy, blankness, floating, unconscious, and I might even pass out. And the reaction to this state is becoming easily adjustable, adaptable to a strange/new/confusing situation." Scholten also describes this plant family as, "They have a child quality... giving them a duality of stability and instability. They have a feeling that they belong somewhere in the world, but the place they belong is dangerous or falling apart, so they feel unsafe."

The Lauraceae family is related to the magnolia family, and also feel as if they are losing everything in a strange world; they are lost and confused and do not know where to go to survive. They may attempt to be more expansive, enthusiastic, and ambitious in order to overcome their underlying fears. Camphora and Cinnamomum are in the Lauraceae family.

This picture seems to fit the thematic state of many autism cases where the world is a confusing place, resulting in a withdrawal. It is similar to Carcinosin, in which the world is felt to be chaotic, so they become co-dependent. However, this group of plants is not a panacea for autism; there is a very specific quality that needs to be met to prescribe these. Imagine your house is intruded on, you are abducted, and then taken to an alien planet and everything is so new and strange. You walk around like every day is a new day and you are so overwhelmed that you just pass out—that is the feeling of this group of remedies.

Camphora

Camphora has shown up in two of my cases where there was a traumatic birth experience with multiple epidurals and problems with anesthesia, after which the mother felt strange and cold, then lost sensation, and then passed out during birth. This beclouded state is then transmitted to the infant. There is a sensation that you feel as if you are going to die and are relieved to find yourself alive. Camphora can negate the effects of anesthesia or other shocks to the system that cause a state of collapse. There is a coldness to the body, sometimes with violent convulsions.

Cinnamomum Verum

Children who need the remedy made of cinnamon feel overwhelmed, like a child lost in a strange world who desires to be in a safe, small world. Parents may be absent or going through a divorce and overall their world has been turned upside down. It's possible that the mother has a symbiotic relationship with the child to avoid having a relationship with their spouse, and there is general confusion about the nature of relationships and how to make contact with the world. The child may be hysterical, dissatisfied, discontented, and crying loudly especially at night. Physically there may be nosebleeds (or history of hemorrhage in the mother), constipation, diarrhea, nausea, vomiting, and stomach cramps.

Magnolia Grandiflorus

This remedy is useful for children who have an absent parent. The parent may have left the family or may just be working so much that the child barely sees them. Either way, the child lacks attention, feels disoriented and lost, and becomes attached to other parental figures such as grandparents. Physically they may have difficulty breathing/lung complaints, erratic heart disorders, joint pains, and stiffness.

Nux Moschata

This is the most "lost" of all the remedies in this group, as if a child has lost his family and is living in a strange place and does not know how to get home or find safety. This situation could occur with an orphan or in a family of immigrants who do not speak the language of the country they are living in. The child is likely nervous with a changeable temperament, oversensitive to light/sounds/smell/touch, overwrought, confused with loss of memory, depressed, uncoordinated, and possibly even narcoleptic. The mother may have felt confused during her pregnancy and her child is therefore dreamy and bewildered.

Mint Family: Overexcited Pleasure vs. Lack of Reaction

There is a natural urge when you are around herbs from the mint family, such as basil, mint, lavender, and rosemary, to pick their leaves, crush them in your hand, pleasurably inhale their aromas and experience a kind of joie de vivre. When this kind of sensory pleasure to touch or smell is overdone, it creates an overexcitability in the nervous system that remedies from the mint family can treat. Children who need these remedies are sensually oriented, highly strung and overstimulated, and wanting to do everything in life at the same time. They are vivacious children who want to do well in school, have a lot of friends, and be physically active with a lot of stimulation to the body. This looks a lot like the Phosphorus constitution, however it can be overdone and result in burnout or lack of reaction. With a burned-out nervous system, symptoms such as tics, twitches, and neuralgias can also arise. There are many remedies in the mint (or Lamiaceae) family including Mentha, Lamium album, Lycopus, Agnus castus, Clerodendrum inerme, Collinsonia, Teucrium, and Origanum, and I have only used a small fraction of them. Many deserve more exploration, especially for children these days who tend to be overwrought from excessive stimulation.

Clerodendrum Inerme

Clerodendrum inerme is wild jasmine from Southeast Asia. A mother of a child with frequent tics and twitches once brought this plant to my attention because she heard that as a tea it treats neurological tics. I bought the plant, made a remedy out of it, and gave it to the child of this mother, and it did in fact reduce her tics and twitches. It seems to be specifically helpful for children who are too open neurologically, with big open eyes and who get easily overexcited. They are often into dance, gymnastics, and being with friends. This remedy brings a sense of calm and almost a yin essence to the child. Similarly, Gelsemium, known commonly as yellow jasmine (but from a different plant family)—also heals the polarity of nervous excitability versus collapsed states. White jasmine (also in a different plant family of Oleaceae) is known in toxic overdose to produce nervous system overreaction/twitches followed by coma. As an aside, I find it curious that all these forms of jasmine come from different plant families all over the world, but carry the same name and similar nerve calming effects.

Origanum Majorana

The remedy from sweet marjoram, Origanum is known for sexual desire that has increased to the point of being tormenting creating masturbation and nymphomania, particularly in girls who are longing for love and contact. This may also show up as nervous unrest, despairing with fear of one's own sexual impulses, or dullness caused by excessive masturbation.

Teucrium Marum

This is the remedy of catnip and most of us know what happens when a cat gets hold of some of this stuff—they get super excited and stimulated and almost act drunken with pleasure. Like a cat, children who do well with this remedy like to stretch and may also have worms, an itching anus, a large appetite, and ingrown toenails. These children tend to have open, sympathetic, and over-excitable personalities and also do well with remedies like Phosphorus, Argentum nit, and Lac Felinum.

Nightshade Family: Central Nervous System Inflammation

The Solanaceae family, also known as the nightshades, include the homeopathic remedies Hyoscyamus and Stramonium, which are well known for treating central nervous system conditions and are fundamental to many complex cases. Belladonna, one of the more important of all acute remedies, is used extensively for inflammatory conditions, particularly those accompanied by very high fevers. Other nightshade remedies are more rarely used but important for various inflammatory conditions, including Capsicum, Atropinum, and Mandragora. The nightshade family includes many commonly eaten foods such as potatoes, tomatoes, eggplants, and peppers, which can cause flares in some people with autoimmune or arthritic conditions.

While there are many other remedies that treat an inflamed central nervous system, such as Helleborus and Zincum, children needing nightshade remedies are distinct in the intensity of the manifestation of their acute fight or flight response and attacks of rage.

Sankaran states in his book *An Insight Into Plants, Volume 2,* "A well understood theme of the nightshade family is fear, especially fear of death, fear of sudden death." This fear of death can be rationalized by the fact that the child's central nervous system is truly under attack. The sensory nervous system of these children will often be acutely sensitive; the approach of a large dog, a slight whiff of an allergen, or the noise of the blender turning on can lead to a sudden, explosive, violent, spasmodic rage with kicking, screaming, and a great desire to escape. The child cannot be blamed for bad behavior; these rage attacks are triggered by a deep survival-driven response.

Some children are in a chronic nightshade state; perpetually in fight or flight mode touched off by the slightest of triggers. Parents of a child needing these remedies stated, "His aggression comes on out of nowhere. He will switch moods and is SCARED—like he's a different person, and then he comes out of it. When he is like that he gets red, rashy, and hot to the touch from the chest up. You're almost afraid he could kill you. He goes after us, bites, clawing, everything in the house is destroyed. Rages vary—last week it was 4 days, sometimes 3-15 minutes. We don't know what brings it on, it can come any time of day out of the blue. He gets more anxious around the time he is about to have a rage. He'll keep wanting to know what is happening next: when he will eat, when we will go home, when the next car ride will be. When he has his fits, his hands are moving up and down, twitching, pulsing, and his eyes get dilated during a rage."

In these chronic cases there is often a history of many trips to the emergency room for various infections. There can also be a history of intense traumas during pregnancy and delivery where there is hemorrhaging, or intense pain states with fear of death (similar to the poppy family). The child often has a history of intense fevers during infancy, and perhaps has been chronically ill for most of their life, with many suppressive treatments and toxic accumulations leading to a gradual decline towards the more severe inflammatory states. Such a case, however, will involve many layers of other remedies to bring the system back into balance. I had one ASD case where Belladonna reduced her rages, but she still had extremely high levels of adrenaline on lab tests and was incredibly hyperactive. She responded fantastically to the sarcode Adrenalinum (see Chapter 8).

Other healthier and neurotypical children may have a more standard constitutional state like Calcarea carb or Ignatia and move into acute inflammatory states where they need a nightshade remedy, such as an ear infection with high fever requiring Belladonna. Belladonna 30C, dosed when a fever reaches higher levels (above 103.5), and/or if the child is delirious, will naturally support a necessary and healthy immune response.

It's important for parents to learn how to dose these remedies and give them in the moment when they are seeing the onset of a flare. Properly timed, a dose can prevent the entire episode. Some parents have even given these remedies to teachers and aids to administer to the child if a flare is taking place while at school. High potencies up to 1M and 10M may be needed, depending on the intensity of the reactions, but very sensitive children may also react successfully to low potencies when they have rages.

Many children who exhibit these states regularly are on suppressive medications including corticosteroids, antipsychotics, antiepileptics, or mood stabilizers. While these medications may be deemed necessary for the child to function, they can certainly make homeopathic treatment more difficult since the drugs may be suppressing or altering normal immune or other physiological responses. Even with these medications, homeopathic treatment is a worthwhile pursuit and different dosing strategies can be used.

Many cases have ongoing inflammatory triggers that need to be addressed to make progress. If inflammation is continually triggered by environmental toxins, molds, allergens, a standard American diet high in sugar, or even harmful EMFs, these maintaining causes need to also be recognized and reduced as much as possible to assist in healing the child.

General Mental Symptoms for All Nightshade Remedies

- Immense fears—especially fear of death, but also fear of the dark, fears after watching a scary movie, fear of water, fear of sudden noises, fear of abandonment, etc.
- Night terrors
- Fear of death combined with reactionary violence (as opposed to pre-meditated violence which is characteristic of other remedies)
- Aggression directed at themselves or others
- Ritualism to calm their fears
- Depressed and on guard
- Poor impulse control, lack of inhibition, cursing, Tourette's, or inappropriate sexual behaviors
- Jealousy
- Hyperactivity

General Physical Symptoms for All Nightshade Remedies

- Seizures
- Migraines of a bursting, throbbing nature with strong sensory sensitivity
- Dilated pupils

- High adrenaline
- Abnormal EEGs
- Strong light and sound sensitivity
- Superhuman strength during rages/tantrums/flares
- High fevers with delirium
- Tics, twitches, and jerking motions
- History of head injury, encephalitis, meningitis
- Acute infections with sudden onset and high fever (such as ear infections, bronchitis, pneumonia, sore throats)
- Great thirst, especially for electrolyte fluids like lemonade
- Worse heat
- Hallucinations
- Deep-seated viral, bacterial, and parasitic infections
- History of suppression, worse after vaccinations

Belladonna

Belladonna is the most commonly used of all the nightshade remedies. Many children, particularly those who are strongly built, can swing into an intense inflammatory or fever state, or congested throbbing migraines, that is eased by Belladonna. Kids who need it constitutionally do well with routine, or being told ahead of time what is next, as they can react poorly to unpredictability.

Belladonna is often given as an acute remedy for high spiking fevers and is indicated when there are sudden inflammations, but children who need Belladonna constitutionally will likely be in a perpetually intense state, with bodies that are strongly built, loud, talkative, and warm. They are commanding kids who will easily rage and strike out, reacting strongly to little stressors in their environment. This over-reactivity finds some resolve when these children have a sense of control or know what is happening. This can look a lot like Ignatia, and both can be reactive to situations of injustice with anger. I often find Belladonna cases that later do well with doses of Ignatia. Other remedies that often overlap can be Apis for high inflammatory states and Medorrhinum or Lachesis for chronic infectious states.

Atropinum is an alkaloid of Belladonna that is also available as a remedy. Sad, morose, and keeping to themselves with sudden attacks of rage, these children present as very thirsty with dilated pupils. Try this remedy if Belladonna worked well and stopped working. Sankaran categorizes it as tubercular, and the one time I used it successfully was in a tubercular child whose rages were triggered by the inhalation of dust (she also had asthma that improved with the remedy Blatta orientalis). Mandragora (from the mandrake root) is also a very similar plant to Belladonna; try this remedy if Belladonna worked well but stopped working. It has keynotes of constipation and eye disorders.

Capsicum

Capsicum is the most irritable, easily offended nightshade remedy. These children can scream and be oppositional for no good reason but are not as intensely rageful and fearful. They tend to be flabby or obese and may have swellings or inflammation behind the ears (mastoid region) and burning sensations but are chilly in their body and worse from cold. Capsicum is a good remedy for parasite infections (in herbal form as well) and looks similar to Natrum sulph, Calcarea carb, Cina, or Belladonna.

Hyoscyamus

The Hyoscyamus mental picture can get quite intense, with rage, obscene behaviors, Tourette's, swearing, schizophrenia, nymphomania, and so on. In an extreme state, a Hyoscyamus person may have perverted sexual thoughts, a desire to exhibit their genitals inappropriately, or will abuse those they seek to control out of jealousy. However, there are Hyoscyamus cases that present in a more subtle way. An example is a girl with strong chorea who gets very emotionally upset when her friends don't prioritize her. Or it may present as silly, annoying behaviors in an overactive child without a filter. I have also seen this picture arise when a younger sibling is born and on a subconscious level the older sibling experiences rage, jealousy, and feelings of abandonment. These reactions cannot be rationalized with the person since they are arising from the deep subconscious. This remedy is the most intense in its need for attention and underlying this is a deep, primal fear of being abandoned. Hyoscyamus is also a powerful remedy for chorea, tics, twitches, seizures, and nosebleeds. It helps with the lower intestine/colon, plus issues around elimination such an encopresis, fecal impaction, and excessive masturbation.

Stramonium

Stramonium is the most intensely fearful, and darkest, of all the nightshade remedies. Deep unconscious fears, lashing out, fight or flight reactions, seizures, and nightmares or night terrors are all symptoms that may be aided by Stramonium. In most cases these children are like deeply frightened animals, with big eyes and dark, dilated pupils, soft-spoken and innocent. Stramonium is also a remedy that can be used in a wide range of kids—from average children who develop night terrors to severely autistic children who have seizures or rages in response to sensory over-reactivity. It is similar to Aconite, with an underlying fear of death or injury, but Stramonium is darker than Aconite, prone to images of horror and talk of zombies, witches, jokers, clowns, fear of the dark, etc. These kids may get ritualistic or have secret behaviors to help manage their fears. It is also possible that a Stramonium case has been exposed to extreme fear and violence. I have taken the cases of several adult women who witnessed extreme crimes and afterward their personality became like soft-spoken children with big eyes brimming with fear, and always on guard. In children these deep fears correlate with brain inflammation, and reactions may range from repetitive behaviors when stressed, to self-abuse, to chorea. Stramonium cases are not as loud and outgoing as Belladonna or as animalistic as Hyoscyamus. The tendency is that the fears and their reactions to those fears drive them inwards, and they will become shy and receding, possibly even stammering in speech. These children may be very sensitive to light and sound, grind their teeth, complain of headaches, suffer from throat spasms and constrictions, and have vision issues and disorders.

Orchid Family: Overly Cerebral and Sensual

Remedies in the orchid family include Vanilla planifolia, Cypripedium pubescens, and Phalaenopsis gigantea, with many new orchid family provings conducted by homeopath Lou Klein. In his book, Orchids in Homeopathy, he elucidates this family as useful for the "modern child" who is overly adapted to technology and affected by it, where there are heightened senses, extreme sensitivity, excessive cerebral activity, and engrossment in electronics (especially with strong interest in gaming), leading to overwhelmed senses, a need to block out, exhaustion, and need for sleep. While they are likely intelligent, they can experience ADHD, dysgraphia, and dyslexia. They will compensate their overwhelm through OCD, need for control, and desire for perfection. Balance is a challenge for them; they can be extremely shy alternating with total lack of social inhibition or have very high energy and then complete exhaustion. Their mood may be happy one day and depressed the next.

These plants have weak root systems; likewise a child needing orchid remedies may literally have issues at their "root," manifesting as foot pains/injuries and poor circulation to the feet, or as ungroundedness that leads to an over-impulsive, silly, exuberant, and even narcissistic/hedonistic nature (into sex/parties/drugs). Their behaviors may attract people, but they feel like an outsider with fear of rejection leading to shallow and artificial relationships. They may even tend to deceive or mislead others to get what they want.

Orchids are used to make a space beautiful, and people who need orchid remedies will have a strong aesthetic sensibility with a desire to be surrounded by beautiful and even luxurious possessions. A materialistic teenager, for example, who must wear the finest most stylish clothing and maintains fastidious surroundings. Symptoms may also include seizures, neuralgias, numbness and tingling, insomnia, hormonal imbalances, food and environmental allergies, or EMF sensitivity. Lou Klein also states they are useful for the effects of vaccines and post viral infections. Orchids compare to fungal remedies like Agaricus, stimulant remedies such as Coca, Coffea, and Thea, nervine remedies such as Scutellaria and Valeriana, as well as animal remedies ranging from Butterfly to Lachesis.

Cypripedium Pubescens

This remedy is known for treating the keynote symptom of when children wake up in the middle of the night, very exhilarated, playing and giggling. They may have excessive cerebral activity or brain disorders showing up as chorea, twitching of limbs, sleeplessness, or epilepsy. Emotionally this is a child who loves to retreat into a fantasy world while in the real world the need to obey and adapt to rules creates internal anger and irritability. Overstimulation of the child may cause fever with restlessness and they may have irritability from worms. Cypripedium also treats joint pains following infections such as strep, as well as enlarged lymph nodes.

Phalaenopsis Gigantea

This orchid remedy is particularly suited for issues with memory and comprehension. There may be problems with writing and clarity of communication, dysgraphia, an overall state of confusion, or ADHD. Emotionally there may be feelings of frustration, anger, and blaming others for communication problems, which cause social embarrassment. The person needing this remedy may feel hopelessly lost or stuck with a desire for escape. This whole situation is parasitic in nature, where a person who needs to be taken care of could begin to feel resentment and self-pity. Physically there may be clumsiness, issues with depth perception, swelling and numbness of hands and feet, allergies, acid reflux, spasmodic pains in the stomach and abdomen, dizziness, parasites, and herpes infections.

Pea/Legume Family: Scattered, Weak, and Coming Apart

Most people have seen pea vines growing up a trellis. They wind, twist, and shoot out in all directions. The central stalk is skinny and needs support and all energy is pushed outwards, into the creation of the pea and seeds. Interposing the image of a pea plant on a child, we can understand that this plant family treats children with a weak core/central nervous system whose energies are excessively pushed outward, making them scattered and fragmented. This shows up as a child who is apathetic, low energy, lacking in ambition, and absentminded, wandering around confused and stimming or picking at useless things. Somehow, they can't "get it together" and these remedies can help their systems feel more unified, determined, and useful. Being a source of food/energy, legume remedies (the adaptogens Astragalus and Glycyrrhiza glabra included) can also be used to treat low energy and chronic fatigue. There are also themes in the family, identified by Jan Scholten, of fear of poverty or of resources becoming exhausted, creating an over-serious dry personality with conflict between duty versus pleasure. There are many remedies in the Leguminosae/Fabaceae family, including Medicago, Melilotus, Baptisia, Robinia, Physostigma, Caesalpinia, Lathyrus, Astragalus, and Trifolium pratense. Baptisia has keynotes of confusion of identity during illness and the feeling that the body is scattered in the bed, which taps into the quality of this plant family.

Interestingly, pea plants were at the origin of modern genetic studies and some of the cases I've treated with these plants had genetic issues, including a family history of degenerative diseases such as Alzheimer's and multiple sclerosis. Children needing these remedies also seem to have issues of insufficient mineralization with pica/mouthing behaviors, locomotor ataxia, sensory oversensitivity, motor planning issues, and sensory processing issues where senses seem out of synch or they can't seem to "get it together" to perform basic tasks.

Caesalpinia Bonducella

This is a nut native to India called nata which is used homeopathically to treat asthma, leprosy, and tuberculosis; however, I tend to use it more for treating hot, restless children with poor concentration. Children who need this remedy may, like many other remedies in this family, have poor digestion, picky eating, and what seems like poor mineralization. They may have high or low energy but are neurotic and wired with weak lungs, stringy bodies, and a "tubercular" constitution showing up as allergies, breathing issues, and poor ability to "contain" themselves. Their energy and even sense of self feels scattered, fragmented, and "out there," as if all internal resources to hold it together have been exhausted. It's possible that this is the child of a family with burned out working parents who travel a lot and what this child really needs is a lot of quiet down time with nutritive, mineral rich foods to ground and cool their bodies.

Lathyrus Sativa

Lathyrus is the remedy of wild vetch that, in homeopathic form, is used for locomotive issues where there is progressive weakening and emaciation of limbs, a set of symptoms also common to many neurodegenerative diseases such as multiple sclerosis, poliomyelitis, amyotrophic lateral sclerosis (ALS, or Lou Gehrig's disease), and Parkinson's disease. If these conditions are present in a family, and a child presents with motor deficits, this is a remedy to consider. Lathyrus can be a miracle for children in a truly destructive situation where their nervous system is ceasing to function at all leading them to feel depressed and trapped by life's circumstances. In an ASD case successfully treated with this remedy, the child was sitting in a bed all day, picking at the sheets or hiding under them, and he would occasionally hit his limbs as if to try to feel them or awaken some feeling of numbness, and when waking up he would kick his legs to get feeling into them. He also experienced easy sensory overload from noises and sunlight, as well as poor digestion with pain in his stomach. Treatment with this remedy over a period of time took him from being bed bound to running in the park, and he became much more at ease and joyful being in his body. Also consider this remedy for infantile paralysis, issues of reflexes, paraplegias, and emaciation of limbs. It can complement the action of Alumina, Kali, and Natrum remedies.

Robinia

This is a digestive-oriented remedy within the pea family and is good for people who tend to have excess acidity, heartburn and stomach disorders, and colitis. It's also useful for infants with colic or who have a sour smell to their body, stools, or vomit. These issues contribute to an overall irritable, uncomfortable, restless child, who, like other remedies in the pea family, is easily overstimulated and scattered. Their senses are not synched and they can't focus their attention. A child needing this remedy may be hungry all the time, have poor impulse control, and always be looking for something to put into their mouth to ease feelings in the stomach (such as pica, a disorder where people eat non-food items like dirt or chalk).

Trifolium Pratense

Red clover is a plant that draws minerals from deep in the earth, making it an effective cover-crop that helps mineralize soil. Taken as an herb, it can support our own body's mineralization and hormone balance. The materia medica on this remedy is limited; it has only been proven to treat dry cough, asthma, blood disorders, and confusion of ideas. However, it has a broader use for sensory processing in children. One such case effectively treated with this remedy was a boy who had sensory processing issues such that he could not read nonverbal gestures and facial expressions (he would see a kid cry and say she is happy). There were also motor planning issues where he couldn't visualize what do to with his body—for example when going down stairs he would get paralyzed and say "my body doesn't know what to do." Overall this child couldn't "put the pieces together." He also had anaphylactic reactions to peanuts (in the legume family) and eating hummus caused him to vomit and break out in hives. He had various midline defects and bad tooth decay. The mother's pelvis during pregnancy also oversoftened, so mineralization was a problem at that point. His mother said that he would get frustrated with toys that were supposed to stand on their own but couldn't and needed a stand to help them be upright. The strength of the remedy Trifolium pratense brought this child wonderful gains in speech and understanding, and even helped him develop a sense of self.

Pine Family: Weak and Hollow on the Inside vs. Strong on the Outside

The conifer (or pine) tree family includes the remedies Terebinthina, Abies nigra, Thuja, Pix liquida, Pseudotsuga, and Sabina. This is a key family of plants, with Thuja being the most commonly used, and the main sensation is a core weakness that could be described as fragile, vulnerable, and fearful. Often there is a weakness in a person's self-identity and ability to project their true self authentically, and this is mirrored by immune weakness because they can't effectively push out foreign influences. In order to compensate for this weakness, the person takes on an outer persona that is "put on;" an appearance that they are tough, hard, strong, and can handle anything or even protect others. This outer personality takes over and the person eventually becomes disconnected from their true self. These remedies can help them connect to their own life force more deeply, so they can push out any harmful external influences, whether diseases or ideas.

Thuja

Thuja is one of the most common remedies for complex, layered children because it works deeply to help push out foreign influences and infections, particularly viral ones. It is best known as the remedy that can be given at the time of vaccination to help prevent vaccine damage, and also for its ability to get rid of warts on the skin. I often dose this remedy intercurrently with a viral or vaccine nosode to help clear a viral layer.

Kids who need Thuja often have a sweet, people-pleasing disposition, especially when younger, and in a way are overly sensitive to the needs of others. They will sacrifice their own self-expression in order to fit in. This is similar to (and can support) Silica, and both have skin conditions reflecting their issue with "outer appearances." Kids needing Thuja easily absorb outer influences such as trends and media, as well as viruses and infections, and eventually these children will get so bogged down by these outer influences that they lose touch with themselves and get depressed.

Thuja can be a great remedy for children addicted to social media or video games. This makes it similar to Medorrhinum, which can also complement Thuja. Both of them have a tendency to keep secrets, however Thuja is more internally weak and insecure than Medorrhinum. The secret-keeping of these remedies is due to a desire to seem perfect on the outside while hiding something "unacceptable" from the rest of the world, who would reject them if they knew. These similarities to Medorrhinum are characteristics of the sycotic miasm in general (see pages 78-81).

Poison Ivy Family: Trapped, Stiff, and Restless

Anacardiaceae, the poison ivy family of plants, includes the remedies Rhus tox, Rhus radicans, Rhus venenata, Rhus glabra, Mangifera indica, and Anacardium. The two most commonly used are Rhus tox (poison ivy) and Anacardium. Homeopath Tinus Smits, who focused on special needs cases, listed these as two of his top ten remedies which heal on the universal level—meaning most people can need them at some point. This plant family has a feeling of being stiff, rigid, and tight in the body, which then creates a kind of trapped feeling resulting in restlessness and always being on the move. The rigidity in the tissues comes from a deeply suppressed anger held in the body, and taking the remedy helps to release this anger, irritability, and stiffness. All of the remedies in this family are worse from damp and cold, better when they get moving and from continued motion, and also better from hot showers.

In complex children I have also found this plant family helps to heal deeply suppressed viruses, especially herpes infections and other skin disorders that have been suppressed into the nervous system. Taking a remedy from this family may result in an itching rash, eczema, or a herpes flare as the body is healing these viral infections. They are also key remedies for healing joint manifestations of Lyme disease.

The bodily sensations of tension, tightness, and restlessness common to the ivy-family remedies share some similarity with spider remedies and the spurge plant family. The internal psychological split and the sensation of being "trapped" can also look like Lachesis or other animal remedies. The self-loathing and lack of self-esteem of Anacardium can resemble that found in the remedies Staphysagria, Thuja, or Carcinosin, and the deep guilt is similar to Kali brom. The tightly wound irritability and anger of Rhus tox can look like Nux vomica or Ruta.

Anacardium Orientale

Anacardium is a key remedy for psychiatric and behavioral disorders. Anacardium kids can be varied in appearance—some are sweet and people-pleasing with mild depression while others may come across as oppositional, violent, depressed, and disturbed. What is common in them is a deep suppression of the self, with low self-esteem and an inner dialogue of self-hatred, which can arise in a child directly following medical suppression of strep or other infections.

A keynote of Anacardium is "angel on one shoulder, devil on the other," and this speaks to an inner battle in which one voice encourages right action while the deeply suppressed and angry part pushes them to act out in destructive ways. This inner conflict can create a split in the personality where they actually start to hear voices and have auditory and visual hallucinations, although this aspect isn't necessary in all Anacardium cases. The inner "demon" in the child may act out cruelly towards animals or younger children, or even become self-abusive. The archetype of the bullied outsider who is so deeply angry he brings a weapon to school (and possibly even uses it) fits Anacardium. These children may also have dreams of violence, or mental images of violence that disturb them, similar to Stramonium. Anacardium will help heal depression, suppressed anger, bipolar states, Tourette's, delusions, hallucinations, and violent anger, especially when there is a history of abuse or alcoholism in the family. It can also treat constrictive headaches, constriction in the chest, a sensation of a band in the extremities, or a feeling of something stuck in a part of the body.

Rhus Tox

Rhus tox is an excellent remedy for angry and oppositional states when paired with musculoskeletal pains and joint stiffness. I have seen this quite often in teenage boys who are irritable and restless in their bodies. They may have back or joint problems that are worse damp weather, with some sort of skeletal weakness underneath. People who need Rhus tox tend not to be very social people and can even be verbally cruel or attack someone out of rage, but have a stronger sense of self confidence than Anacardium.

Remedies with weak skeletal structures, such as Calcarea phos and Staphysagria, have an inner restlessness that overlaps with Rhus tox. Ruta is a remedy similar to Rhus tox (tightness in the body and joints with some repressed anger), but Ruta has a feeling of "snapping out" rage, or parts of the body "snapping."

Rhus tox is often an acute remedy for injury to the joints where the tissues stiffen up to compensate and require stretching/motion to loosen up. Symptoms are generally worse on beginning motion and better with continued motion and walking, while prolonged motion or exertion of any kind leads to exhaustion. It can also be a great remedy for flus where the entire body hurts with aching pains that feel like bruises, and they toss and turn to get comfortable. Skin infections and acne are also helped by Rhus tox, especially if there's an eruption on top of another eruption such as an abscess on top of a rash.

Poppy Family: Sensitive to Great Pain, Suffering, and Numbing Out

The poppy (or Papaveraceae) family of plants, all of which are highly medicinal plants with pain-killing alkaloids, provides the remedies Morphinum, Chelidonium, Sanguinaria, Opium, Succinum purum, and Codeinum.

There is a strong polarity present in these cases, with a great sensitivity to pain and suffering on one hand and a tendency to numbness and desire for escape on the other. Often when these people witness pain and suffering they feel it acutely in themselves, and in this sense they can be deeply empathetic with others. However, they can also be numb to their own pain. A child may burn himself on the stove and it isn't discovered until later, or an adult buries himself in addictions to escape pain. Sankaran describes some themes present in this family as "torture, intense suffering, as in war, murder, violence," and indeed it was the violence of war that brought these plant families into pharmacological use for pain relief. The opium dens of China flourished during a time where war was rampant and people would escape into a refuge of drug addiction. In today's world people still rely heavily on opiate drugs from heroin to oxycodone to avoid the pain of their own lives. These can also be remedies for intense rage and seizures, or intensely painful GI disorders and colic. While all remedies in this family have issues with pain alternating with numbness, how it manifests in each one is different.

Chelidonium

Chelidonium is a common remedy for immune-compromised kids when there is a history of jaundice and digestive symptoms such as floating stools, poor appetite, and abdominal pains. These kids may even have high liver inflammation markers. They have strong and dominant personalities. They want to help people but can be bossy and want their advice followed, getting irritated and offended if it's not. These kids may feel guilty and take the blame if something goes wrong, which makes them insecure and feel disliked or disrespected, so they get worried and want to help people again. Think of army generals and coaches—these are people who have responsibility for others and feel great guilt if something goes wrong. This remedy is a lot like Nux vomica or Lycopodium. I have also seen it needed in families where there is a history of alcoholism.

Chelidonium can sometimes be useful in low potency, such as 6C, for liver support.

Morphinum

Morphine is an alkaloid of opium. It is still used in painkillers and sleep inducers in modern times. This remedy is useful in treating drug addictions with profound depression and includes keynotes of forgetfulness, indifference, and apathy. The two Morphinum cases I treated both had traumatic, emergency room C-section deliveries—although it was unclear if the mother was given morphine specifically. The children had a low pain sensation but would tantrum very easily, similar to Belladonna. Morphinum can also treat heart palpitations, intense itching as if from a drug reaction, constipation, and nausea and vomiting.

Opium

Opium is closer to the unconscious, unfeeling side of the poppy family polarity. People who need this remedy have a desire to escape situations of intense pain and violence, going into a "den" where they can't feel their body and numbing out. Whereas Morphinum is the most intense and reactive in acute rages, similar to Belladonna, Opium is more of a chronically suppressed state where the world is overwhelming and chaotic, similar to Carcinosin. Sankaran includes Opium within the cancer miasm, and Opium is worse from strong emotions. At the same time, Opium can be a remedy for issues originating from fright—it contains the keynote "epilepsy in children from the approach of strangers, or spasms in children after mother has been severely frightened." Other physical symptoms that Opium can treat include constipation, intestinal obstruction, head injuries, and loss of pain sensation with great sensitivity to sound, light, and smells.

Sanguinaria

These people are empathic, sensitive to pain and suffering, and want to help others. Sanguinaria is a strong liver and gall bladder remedy that helps with right-sided, sharp, liver-associated migraines, and right-sided shoulder pain. People who need Sanguinaria are extremely light and smell sensitive, are easily nauseated, and have burning pains.

Rose Family: Generous and Overflowing vs. Oppressed

The rose (Rosaceae) family not only provides us with beautiful smelling roses, it also provides us with an abundance of fruit, as most fruit (apples, pears, cherries, peaches, plums and many berries), as well as almonds, are in this family. The fruit and flowers are nature's gifts of love and this generosity exemplifies those needing remedies from the rose family, who tend to be generous people who give their all to make their loved ones happy, and desire romantic love. But a person needing these remedies can give too much of themselves, creating resentments that become like thorns.

Or, imagine being a fruit tree and you are pushing water and mineral resources outward to create fruit—it is this sensation of outward pressure, with pinching, pressing, pushing, shooting out sensations, that is thematic for rose plant remedies. Symptomatically, this shows up as respiratory trouble and allergies, where fluid floods the lungs and sinuses creating a feeling of oppression/suffocation/stuffiness. Remedies in the rose family include Amygdalus amara aqua, Prunus spinosa, Rosa damascena, Laurocerasus, and Crataegus.

Laurocerasus

The remedy of cherry laurel is known in the treatment of newborns who have difficulty breathing, low oxygen, blueness of the skin, and coldness (aka "blue babies"). The person who needs this remedy may feel that no one loves them, has been abused, has parents who are fighting, or has experienced a deep fright or shock. Invariably the trauma leads to a shut down feeling in the chest/heart region, leading to clutching and palpitations, as well as possible loss of sensation, epilepsy, chorea, tics, and twitches. This may also show up in cases with respiratory challenges, asthma, or allergies when so much fluid rises up that it leads to congestion and swelling of the tissues; there may be a feeling of suffocation and even brain compression. The child may pinch or press into an adult out of their discomfort from internal pressure.

Rosa Damascena

The remedy from the damask rose is useful for hay fever allergies to flower pollen (itching nose and eyes with frequent sneezing and shortness of breath), and fluid in the ears causing hearing problems or tinnitus. Compare to other hay fever remedies such as Arsenicum album, Allium cepa, Euphrasia, Natrum mur, Nux vomica, Pulsatilla, Sabadilla, Agaricus, Ambrosia, Apis, Arundo, and Wyethia.

Spurge Family: Bound Up, Stretched, and Inflamed

This unique group of plants from the spurge (or Euphorbiaceae) family includes Hevea brasiliensis (the rubber tree) and many others that produce latex—a milky poisonous sap, that when processed, is known for its tensile strength and elasticity. The particular sensation common in this family of plants is a feeling that the tissues, skin, or intestines are bound up, tied up, gripping, or stretched like a balloon (hidebound). A case needing this remedy may feel like the intestines are tied up by a large rubber band, the head (or even brain) is bound tightly, or the skin feels stiff, tight, and stretched, making the person feel "held in" like a prisoner, creating a desire to break free. Remedies in the spurge family include Croton tig, Hura brasil, Stillingia sylvatica, Mancinella, Cascarilla, Euphorbium perf, and Ricinus communis.

Euphorbium

I often prescribe Euphorbium in cases with a lot of dysbiosis and deep inflammatory pain. During the sensation process parents will say that the child's intestines feel like a tight ball of rubber bands with a burning sensation, which leads me to this remedy. These burning sensations may also be felt in the bones and throughout the GI tract, and the skin may be hot and dry. Stagnation in the body can result in headaches, mood swings, or even manic behaviors. There may also be a history of cancer in the family, particularly GI cancer.

Hura Brasil

Hura is an interesting remedy for the feeling of being despised and disgusting, as if you were a leper. I have seen a small handful of ASD children, lost in their own world of stimming, who feel that they are alone in the world and have lost the affection of friends. It also assists with gastrointestinal and skin issues. There may even be a stretchy, rubbery sensation notable in the case. I once treated an autistic girl who was absorbed with playing with the stretchy stickiness of her saliva and snot, and this remedy shifted these behaviors.

Mancinella

Mancinella is an interesting remedy for the fear that one is possessed by evil (or the devil) and there are repetitive thoughts that drive them crazy, as if the brain itself is bound up by tormenting thoughts. Skin disorders such as intense itching, vesicles, blisters, or growths may also be present.

Wild Yam Family/Dioscorea: Twisting Colic

A key remedy for colic in children is Dioscorea (wild yam) from the Dioscoreaceae family, which has the sense that the intestines are being wrung out and twisted with a desire to twist and arch the back to find relief. Stretching and pulling makes the pain feel better. This is often seen in infants who, after nursing, arch and twist their backs in discomfort. Vermeulen also shares that this remedy can arise when "one's individual ambitions encounter the drudgery of domestic life such as when a wife/mom becomes the willing slave of her family." Indeed, I have seen Dioscorea cases of mothers who felt just this way. It overlaps nicely with Pulsatilla (for PMS and women's health issues).

Conclusion

Get curious about plants! If there is a plant that you have an intuitive hit about, investigate it! A family I once treated from India excitedly told me about the use of a plant known as Vacha, or Acorus calamus, which in their native country is placed on the tongue of children to help them speak. Vacha actually means speech in Sanskrit. I gave it in homeopathic form to the children of this family, and it did assist their sense of self-identity which led to gains in speech. While this remedy is not a panacea for speech in all children, for this family we found a resonant plant that helped them progress. The best prescriptions for plants come from deep understanding of the full expression of sensations and feelings in the body. Close your eyes and describe in detail, with your imaginative mind, what you sense in the body, or imagine your child sensing. Picture the body tissues, what are they experiencing? Ask your heart-led intuition to guide you to a plant that matches this sensation. The plant kingdom is always listening, and every plant has a solution.

Chapter 6

Mineral and Periodic Table Remedies

Mineral remedies assist with issues of structure, function, and deficiency in the body and they will be given to almost all those receiving homeopathic treatment at some point. For children who are building up their bodies, their sense of self, and their ability to process information, mineral remedies are key to helping them develop in a solid, stable way. For example, the remedy Calcarea phos helps when children have growing pains and physical restlessness, while the remedy Silica helps children correct malabsorption of minerals so they can build a stronger physical structure. Calcarea carb is wonderful when children are first starting school and have anxiety about following the rules and doing the right thing. Phosphorus helps children who have poor boundaries and are too open to have a stronger sense of self. All of these are examples of classic polychrest mineral remedies that can fit the overall constitutional makeup of the child.

In addition to well-known mineral remedies, this chapter includes remedies that are new to homeopathy. Many of these have only been elucidated in the last few decades, primarily via the work of Dutch homeopath Jan Scholten's Element Theory, which sheds light on the overall thematic patterns present in the periodic table of elements. For example, remedies from radioactive elements are helpful for deep, destructive processes like cancer, and those from gaseous elements like hydrogen and helium are for out-of-body states. According to Element Theory, people who need mineral remedies are more likely to be structured, linear people who are less variable and more fixed in their reactions to situations. In contrast, people who need animal remedies will be more animated and multifaceted, and those who need plant remedies are more sensitive and emotional in the way they speak and present themselves.

Understanding the complexities of Jan Scholten's Element Theory is beyond the scope of this book. However, for the sake of grouping remedies via thematic similarities, I am listing mineral remedies in the order they take place on the periodic table of elements, and according to the "series" (or row) they are on. One aspect of Element Theory is that elements on the left side of the table are building up towards stability, while the elements on the right side of the table are moving towards deterioration, which is somewhat reflected in the materia medica of these elements. To explore this concept in more detail, I highly recommend reading Jan Scholten's book, *Homeopathy and the Elements.*

In addition to elements from the periodic table, other mineral substances such as gunpowder, sugar, and petroleum are covered in this chapter. The range of action of these remedies is broad. Many remedies from organic chemicals like benzolum or formaldehyde help with environmental toxicity and alleviate certain chemical depressant effects on the body. There are also remedies made from gemstones such as diamond or Clear quartz, as well as types of water such as ocean and spring water (see page 193).

Hydrogen Series

The two elements in the hydrogen series are hydrogen and helium. Both are gases found in outer space; 74 percent of the universe is hydrogen and 24 percent is helium. Children who need these two remedies are still connected to the stage of the unborn fetus, floating through space and time, not well-grounded in their bodies. These cosmic kids may actually feel as if they are floating, like a gas, outside of their bodies. A parent of a child who needed Hydrogenium said, "He feels light, drifting around, not grounded, can't hang onto anything. His drawings never had ground planes, they were light and airy like a balloon."

A child who needs Hydrogenium is more intense and potentially explosive, while a child who needs Helium is more angelic and in their own bubble. The matridonal remedies (made from breast milk, placenta, etc.) are important to consider for this theme of supporting the incarnational process as well (see Chapter 8).

Hydrogenium (Hydrogen)

Hydrogenium helps with incarnation. The Hydrogenium state can sometimes be felt in the explosive scream of a newborn baby, as if saying "I don't want to be here on this planet!" Hydrogenium can be useful for adopted children or in situations where the mother may not have wanted the baby and considered abortion, contributing to the child's state of not "being here," and giving the remedy will ground them. Hydrogenium may also assist with children who experienced the death of a loved one (especially a parent) which created a kind of heavenly longing or desire for spiritual unity and are generally challenged by being incarnated.

With Hydrogenium, there is a desire in their activity on some level for having the experience of unity/oneness. They do this by pouring all of themselves into what they do, in an intense way, without boundaries. They may taste, smell, and visualize things more intensely, and feel more empathy than average. Excess energy may be an issue; sometimes these children can feel as if their body is so full of energy they can't get rid of it fast enough; energy or frustration can come out of them like an explosion. Or they may seem out of body and have personality dissociation. They may be very creative and interested in space travel, astronauts, fantasy, sci-fi, etc. Physical symptoms include uneven energy and temperature regulation, numbness, skin formication (crawling sensation), nerve pain, and deep-seated migraines with nausea and vomiting. Compare with Phosphorus, Coffea, Medorrhinum, Causticum, Platina, Palladium, Canibis indica, and other drug remedies.

Also associated with Hydrogenium are the acid remedies (Phosphoric acid, Sulphuric acid, etc.), which are substances that donate hydrogen ions. Acid remedies are needed when someone has burned themselves out by pouring too much of their energy into an experience, relationship, or even an infection. They are useful for post-viral burnout. Too much enthusiasm, fanaticism, or intensity has created a burned-out state that an acid remedy can assist.

Helium

Children who are angelic, as though they have one foot on earth and the other foot in heaven, can benefit from Helium. Sometimes this remedy shows up in premature babies who remain like innocent newborns as they grow up and prefer to be in a safe "cocoon" space, not socializing, sleeping a lot or day dreaming. The parents of one Helium case said, "he was a premie and the perfect baby, never crying, but he was too quiet. Even today he is easy going and compliant. He is not all here, trying to figure it out—not comfortable, awkward, insecure, with a high tolerance for pain. He doesn't feel like he is completely in his body." It is a more internalized state than Hydrogenium and is akin to the state of the fetus in utero, floating in amniotic fluid. Jan Scholten associates this remedy with autism stating, "they don't feel like entering this world, they prefer to stay in themselves to experience their own being." This remedy can also assist children who are born prematurely or in cases of Down syndrome. One child I treated who needed this remedy had Down syndrome and assisted others by communicating with the spirit world. Giving the remedy will help the child ground and engage more on the human level rather than the etheric.

Carbon Series

The carbon series includes lithium, beryllium, boron, carbon, nitrogen, oxygen, fluorine, and neon. These elements represent the development or rejection of core values, what is real versus not real, materialism, and the development of a healthy body and ego or sense of self. This series fits with the stage of the toddler who learns to master the physical dimension by learning to walk and talk, give and take toys, eat, and potty train. Having a strong sense of self can translate into the child taking a toy and stating loudly, "mine!" This taking can be a healthy part of the development of the egoic self. The earlier stage elements, lithium, beryllium, and boron find it harder to take and are more inclined to easily give due to an inner weakness and inability to stand up for themselves. The remedies made from these elements are all helpful for naivety; for example, a child who believes that if he puts on a diaper he becomes a baby, or believes scarecrows are real people. The elements nitrogen, oxygen, and fluorine are

WATER REMEDIES

Remedies from different types of water have a universal cleansing quality and can be given intercurrently to support detoxification.

- Aqua marina: Made from sea water, this can be considered a universal remedy for cleansing the nervous system, lymphatic system, and revitalizing the blood. Similar to the supplement isotonic ocean water, I use Aqua marina in a more generalized way for detoxification support, especially for children who do well with Natrum mur or need remedies from molluscs or fish with a strong draw or aversion to the ocean.

- Sanicula aqua: Made from a famous spring water source in Illinois, this remedy cleanses the gut and settles irritability. There may be poor digestion resulting in a pot belly and behaviors similar to Chamomilla/Cina/Tuberculinum including being easily angered, averse to touch, and irritable with restlessness and shrieking. It's also similar to Silica where there is emaciation with ravenous appetite, foot sweat, and hangnails. There may be a sense of neglect and lack of support and nurturing, either of the child (such as in a foster situation), or of the mother while pregnant. Also helps with stool that must be mechanically removed, such as via enema.

more inclined to take from a feeling that it is their right, stemming from a more arrogant sense of self. For example, the feeling of "I deserve this toy so I am going to steal it." There is also a thematic relationship in these elements to stages of emerging from the birth canal: boron (fear of falling and not wanting to emerge), carbon (stuck in birth canal), nitrogen (coming out into life), and oxygen (taking what you need from life, breath, and taking attention). The carbon series include wonderful remedies to assist children in developing a balanced sense of self.[1]

Lithium Muriaticum or Lithium Carbonicum

Remedies made from lithium salts help those who have a very poor sense of self identity, which leads to mood swings or manic depression. For example, a child who needed this remedy would go from yelling to laughing, then bored, then crying, all in the span of fifteen minutes. His mother said, "He will be sobbing over miniscule details from reading a book; there are three days in his life where he has not cried." These kids may have a high level of separation anxiety or some sense of insecurity about their parental relationships. Lithium mur will particularly help with issues of insecurity around the mothering relationship, while Lithium carb may help with issues of insecurity about the fathering relationship. I have seen cases of people who are on the medication lithium for a mood disorder who did well with the lithium homeopathic remedy in its place. These also treat rheumatic soreness in the heart region and whole-body soreness in the bones, joints, and muscles.

Beryllium

Uncertain children with a poor sense of themselves who yield to others can benefit from Beryllium. They are extremely timid and fearful of being observed. While a child might be able to expertly copy the behavior of others, he doesn't know how to act himself. These children are always adapting due to a deep lack of self-identity. It's also beneficial for children who seem helpless and who lack a sense of what is real and what is pretend, giving them a naiveté that could be taken advantage of.

Borax Venata

One of the strongest keynotes of Borax is a baby who has an incredible fear of falling or being dropped; you lean over to place the baby gently in a crib and she startles with fear, sticks her arms out, and tenses up. They are also afraid of any noises that startle them, and need their mother to hold them. They may have colic and will cry until their nerves wear down and they fall asleep. As the child grows older, she becomes discontented, emotional, nervous, and continues to be easily startled. These children also have a poor sense of identity but with a childish, sweet naiveté. They talk to dolls like they are real, believe completely in Santa Claus, and won't question anything you tell them. Also useful for canker sores, unhealthy skin/complexion and hair, cracked and mapped tongue, eczema, crusty scabs on the nose, painful urination, and vomiting after breakfast. Compare with Baryta carb, Calcarea carb, Chamomilla, and Pulsatilla.

Carbon

Carbon shows up in homeopathy in many forms, usually combined with another element such as Calcarea carb and Kali carb. Carbon also exists in different chemical compositions such as graphite, diamond, coal, and carbon dioxide—there are seemingly countless forms of carbon that could be made into remedies. Carbon is the essential central building block of life, and we all have aspects of carbon central to our make-up, however we may need a carbon remedy when certain themes show up strongly in a case. Rigid, fixed thinking and a strong view of what is right and wrong are strong keynotes for carbon remedies. These people may get angry because they feel so strongly that this is the way it should be. They are solid, well built, "like a block," with self-confidence and a balanced, stable personality, although this rigidity may show up in their bodies. Carbon represents the role of the father/central figure/core/God, and Carb kids really look up to their fathers or take on the role of the father. These kids are interested in material things such as clothes and cars. They may have tons of energy and then suffer from issues of depleted energy; interestingly, carbon makes up sugar, petroleum, and alcohol, all forms of fuels. All of these themes show up in mineral remedies containing carbon, such as Calcarea carb, Natrum carb, Magnesia carb, and Kali carb.

Graphites (Graphite)

The remedy made of graphite is the most common carbon remedy given to kids. Graphites cases tend to relate to physical conditions of the skin and mucous membranes. The skin may have issues like moist, crusty scaling and itching, cradle cap, eczema in folds of the skin, fissures around the mouth, or rashes with sticky discharges. They also often have stubborn constipation and distended bellies. Parents will say they have a strong will and attitude, sometimes defiant, although sometimes they can feel irresolute about decisions. These kids may be sluggish and lazy in the morning but have high energy around bedtime, possibly causing tantrums. A long bedtime routine may be required to wind them down. Like all the carbon remedies, there is rigidity in the body such as stiff muscles or they get rigidly stuck in their ways, such as expecting the same exact traditions every holiday. Many ASD children who are happy at home, stuck in their ways, can't see outside the box, and don't want the introduction of anything "new" can benefit from this remedy. Graphites also carries the theme of the father, and children who need these remedies either look up greatly to their fathers and/or have the feeling of an absent father.

Other Carbon-based Remedies	
Adamas (diamond)	For a strong personality who is deeply perfectionistic and wants things done a certain way. Gets depressed if things are not "just right." Can feel boxed inside themselves and easily block people out with feelings of anger. Similar to Ignatia, with strong rigidity and deep feelings; can complement the prescribing of Ignatia.
Carbon dioxide and Carbon monoxide	Helpful for kids living next to highways or in heavy smog. It can treat disoriented, spaced-out, irritable states and other issues of mental dullness.
Alcoholus (alcohol)	Helps those who are uncentered, sensory sensitive, restless, anxious, and overly emotional get more centered and focused. Also treats impaired memory and mania with excessive irritability. Useful for history of alcoholism; similar to Cannabis indica and Agaricus. Sometimes sold under the name Ethylicum.
Carbo veg and Carbo animalis (wood charcoal and ox hide charcoal)	These remedies are important for a weak vital force and burned-out states due to cancer, pneumonia, bronchitis, and long-term viral infections such as mononucleosis. Helps to revitalize a person who feels cold, sluggish, weak, and unreactive. The weakness may develop slowly due to organic pathology in the liver, heart, or lungs or as a consequence of a serious infection. Can give concurrently with viral clears. Also useful for gas, bloating, and indigestion. Desires fresh air.

Other Carbon-based Remedies	
Carboneum chlor	Insatiable hunger for material things; compulsive shopping. Wants something out of a situation or to take from the partner/parent and then runs away and rejects them for not giving enough of whatever was initially wanted. New moon aggravation felt in midback. Desires carbs. Assists with parasite infections.
Saccharum officinalis (white sugar)	A universally useful carbon-based remedy as our culture has been inundated by refined sugar. Assists with issues of blood sugar, hypoglycemia, and diabetes. For strong sugar cravings, worse after eating sweets, with an empty, weak, hungry feeling. Sugar can compensate for lack of attention, love, or affection and those needing the remedy may have ailments from lack of attention or physical contact in early childhood. Physical symptoms include thrush, putting items or fingers into the mouth, and kicking and hitting after eating sugar. Helps children limit their own sugar intake and behave more sweetly. Often prescribed as an intercurrent remedy while clearing yeast or parasites.

Nitrogenium

These children have enthusiastic, expansive personas and are a flurry of movement and activity. They have rapid speech and are happiest when going places and being social. Because of their larger than life personalities they will have poor boundaries and impulsivity, such as touching everything and talking to anyone. They crave fat and sugar to power themselves. In the one case I had where Nitrogenium deeply healed the child, the mother had been on blood vessel relaxants for high blood pressure while pregnant, which may have contributed to a Nitrogenium state in the child. This child loved posing for the camera making silly faces. His parents said his constant feeling was, "I need to go, I can't wait, why are you staying here, I want to play with you, interact with you, I want you to feel my excitement, my need to move, I will push you and maybe you'll play with me, maybe you'll be laughing, be as excited as me." These kids like to open their mouths wide and will stim with a lot of movement. Nitrogenium is similar to Sulphur and Phosphorus; it can overlap with bird and spider remedies and the tubercular miasm. Themes of nitrogen are also found in

Argentum nit (Silver nitrate), which is helpful for overly impulsive and neurotic children.

Nitricum Acidum

This remedy assists with red, swollen, and cracked sores at the corners of the mouth or around the anus. These people have a tendency to develop warts and get cold sores when sick. There may also be a history of sore throats with a stitching or splintering sensation, herpes or genital warts, rectal malignancy, vaginitis, or swelling of foreskin. Emotionally this child may be peevish and nasty, screwing his face at you, although I have seen sweet and sensitive people, who typically need Carcinosin, needing this remedy for acute splintering or sharp pains around the anus or mouth.

Oxygenium

Oxygenium is a very important remedy for pulling people out of an attention-seeking, victim mentality and I prescribe it often. Children who need this remedy consume all the energy and attention of the household through their demands, tantrums, and neediness but they feel neglected, believe they deserve more, and end up acting selfish. For example, a mother said, "She has the worst tantrums especially when she is in the back seat and her brother is in the front seat, she will just scream and scream. She is like, 'Let me out of this car seat and let me come to you, back here I feel you don't see me!'" It can also show up in a sibling of a complex child who has the sense that they are neglected, feel sorry for themselves, and demand that their needs be met. The mother may have also lacked emotional support during pregnancy or delivery. Oftentimes in Oxygenium cases the father is not present or abandoned the family, which eventually transforms into a deep feeling of neglect and need for attention. Overall this remedy can really help family dynamics and heal the member of the family who feels they aren't getting their fair share. Oxygenium may also be useful for children who were put on oxygen at birth and other low-oxygen situations such as iron deficiency, anemia, or asthma. As an acute remedy it supports the common cold and respiratory tract issues with a feeling of oppression in the chest, cold sores, and raw sore throats. It can even support the healing of cancerous tumors. Compare with Sulphur, Cina, and Chamomilla.

Fluoricum Acidum

Fluoricum acidum helps kids who are emotionally hardened and naughty with no fear of consequences, as if their life and body have no value to them. These kids may have been rejected or are not valued by the family. They may have bad teeth, cavities, or many broken teeth and have been negatively affected by fluoride treatments or fluoride water. They may also have an interest in hard core music, gambling, or criminal behaviors.

Silica Series

This series includes the elements sodium (known as natrum in homeopathy), magnesium (known as magnesia in homeopathy), aluminum, silica, phosphorus, sulphur, and chlorine (known as muriaticum in homeopathy). These elements are fundamentally about how we relate with others and the roles we assume within our family unit. The remedies from these elements all have archetypal relationship themes: Natrum for loneliness, Magnesia for passivity, Silica for standing up for oneself, Phosphorus for friendship and boundaries, Sulphur for deep love and selfishness, and Chlorum for rejection of relationships. These are also minerals fundamental to our physiological makeup; various imbalances we may have with these minerals may be corrected by taking them homeopathically. For example, people challenged with muscle cramping due to magnesium deficiency may do well with a Magnesia remedy; while those who have strong salt cravings may do well with the remedy Natrum mur (sodium chloride/salt).

For many children it is a daily challenge to learn how to create and maintain relationships, and often special needs children are stuck in their capacity to socialize. The right remedies can help them move past these limitations and are key in helping them build a sense of confidence in socializing with peers, adults, and even their own parents. To ascertain whether a mineral remedy will help, think about how your child acts on the playground, while socializing, or when meeting a new friend. Shy children may do well with Natrum, Calcarea, Magnesium, or Silica remedies, while an extroverted child may do well with Sulphur. Phosphorus tends to be too open and wanting to connect, and this may show up as either shy or extroverted.

It's also important to remember that children learn how to relate to others based on how they see their parents socialize; children also gain their sense of confidence based on the unconditional love they get from their mom and dad. Therefore, helping children relate successfully may require helping parents move through stuck patterns as well.

Natrum Muriaticum (Sodium Chloride or Common Salt)

This is a very common remedy and in many of my cases it has been the only remedy that an ASD/Asperger's kid needed. Often these children will have poor eye contact, hide their face to avoid your gaze, and are very sensitive to touch. They are natural loners and may idealize making more friends but don't know how. Natrum mur is a powerful remedy for kids who are in their own world. It can be a remedy for chorea, low energy, lethargy, desire to be alone, viral infections, and poor immunity. These kids may learn to socialize better at some point through therapy but deep down inside have a great fear of being rejected and have poor self-love.

The Natrum mur child is sad and weepy but doesn't want any consolation. Innermost feelings are hidden, and they can be aloof with hugs and affection or push a parent away but will be loving to their stuffed animals. There is an extreme sensitivity and deep, profound emotions. They are generally well-behaved and want to please others but can be irritable or passive aggressive due to feelings of low self-worth. If they make mistakes, they feel bad about it and they are very concerned about the opinions of others, which results in them avoiding the company of people. Fears abound, especially during sleep, and they often fear that something bad will happen to the person they love most.

This is a great remedy for kids who get dropped off at daycare and are grief-stricken. It's also good for separation anxiety and for children whose moms work a lot outside of the home. Likewise, it can be great for a sad child who has been stuck at home and not allowed to socialize. The Natrum mur child may do well academically or can do very poorly in school and not care. Natrum mur kids can have a lot of trouble with concentration and may say they hate math. Also look for feeding problems, such as a capricious appetite, because the child may avoid food in parallel to the way they subconsciously avoid nurturing.

Natrum mur is often the deepest layer under many other layers rooted in disconnection. For example, a child needing Natrum mur who has poor eye contact as an infant may go on to receive many vaccinations, develop neurologic behaviors, and act out putting them into a spider remedy state. This child may then get medicated for their behaviors, leading to more disconnection and needing a remedy like Opium.

On the physical side, children needing Natrum mur may have delayed development and dentition; closed tear ducts; dryness of the skin, mucous membranes, and stool; watery and very itchy allergies; physical over-sensitivities to many things; an emaciated body despite eating well; headaches and poor vision; and they may be pale and anemic-looking. A strong craving for salty foods is also a keynote of Natrum mur.

The key theme of a Natrum remedy is the feeling of being ALONE and wanting something to fill that sense of loneliness. Below are commonly prescribed Natrum remedies for lonely, sensitive, longing children.

Other Natrum Remedies	
Natrum ars	Lonely, closed off. Extremely fastidious about germs and health. Suffers from asthma and headaches. Can be a helpful remedy for moms who are overly concerned about germs.
Natrum brom	Lonely and shut down because of strong guilty or passionate feelings, such as from "sinning" or doing the wrong thing. The guilty feelings sometimes relate to sexual behaviors. May have bad cystic acne.
Natrum carb	Mild and timid, wanting only one friend at a time, all they need is their one best friend. Prefer calm, gentle, quiet environments and soft, soothing music. Very sensitive stomach and milk allergies.
Natrum fluor	Closed off and introverted, not warm and friendly. A bit mean and hard. Loners, but actually like being at parties and feeling glamorous. Wants to befriend only the bad kids at school. Long, lean, sharp, bony body with hardened tissues.
Natrum phos	Lonely unless in the company of parents or friends, which they always need to be around. Very emotionally sensitive, worried that people won't like them. Has easy emotional breakdowns and sobs easily. There are often issues with parasites/worms and noise sensitivity.
Natrum sulph	Desires deep love of a parent or partner. Depression from a breakup or the death of a loved one leading to possible thoughts of suicide. Asthma worse at 4am or after grief. Head trauma causing confusion or mental dullness. Diabetes. Feels better after stool.

Magnesia Carbonicum

Magnesia remedies are for children who become passive in the family due to fear of conflict. An example of a common situation that leads to needing these remedies was aptly described by one of my clients: "His dad and I were divorcing at the time. I would start to cry and his dad would yell, 'Shut up!' Then my son went through a personality change, just withdrawn in general. He shifted from 'the world is a safe place' to 'the world is a dangerous place.' Nobody protected him. He took the divorce so hard, but still has a fantasy we will get back together and won't release it." Other situations when Magnesia remedies are helpful are when kids become passive because their siblings take all the attention, or there are too many children in the household. This can create a general passive aggressive quality and the child may assert himself through whining.

Magnesia carb is a major GI and liver remedy for those who are aggravated by dairy. These children are stressed and anxious when their parents or others are arguing. They are fearful of conflict and attack but can be passive aggressive or have meltdowns due to feeling uncared for. All Magnesia remedies can have some form of cramping such as headaches, stomachaches, foot cramps, and a sense of feeling orphaned or unloved. A child needing this remedy whines about everything and feels like life is unfair to them. They are anxious about all sorts of little things and act infantile. Some keynotes of Magnesia carb include sour odors from discharges, constipation and slow digestion, sleepless from 3-4 am, low muscle tone, lack of strength, and failure to thrive in babies.

Other Magnesia Remedies	
Magnesia mur	Passivity on the emotional level and cramping on the physical level. Whining and worried, feels rejected and judged by mother but needs her attention and wants to be babied. Allergies, liver issues, constipation, worse milk.
Magnesia phos	Passivity on the emotional level and cramping on the physical level that is better with heat and pressure (also a well-known remedy for menstrual cramps). Whining and wanting to be taken care of, picked up, and babied. Squealing, baby talk.
Magnesia sulph	Passivity on the emotional level and cramping on the physical level. Whining and suppressed anger due to unresolved confrontation. High blood pressure and migraines. Feels orphaned/abandoned by those they love most.

Alumina/Aluminum

Many complex children have high levels of aluminum on heavy metal tests, possibly due to vaccines and environmental toxins, and taking Alumina 12C a few times a week can help detox aluminum from their system. Symptoms of Alumina (and likewise aluminum toxicity) may include slowness in answering questions, slow reflexes, and mental fogginess. They dislike being hurried and are easily disoriented, like someone who has Alzheimer's. Parents may say that the child seems uncertain, like lost in a fog, not realizing their surroundings. They may also suffer from constipation, dry skin, dry mucous membranes, and yeast infections.

Silica

Silica children want everyone to be happy and harmonious so they can forgo expressing their own wants and needs. They tend to be refined, mild mannered, and shy, but will still want to socialize. A parent of a Silica child may say, "he is a good student and would never get in trouble. He likes to be presentable and in general will obey rules. While he is a quiet kid, he loves it if a group of kids come up to him. He likes people and enjoys company but can be hard to get to know because he doesn't express his feelings. Sometimes he looks awkward with people, but people still love talking to him."

While they seem sweet and adaptable to others, they can surprise you with their need for success or their strong sense of injustice which can trigger an emotional outburst. Giving the remedy Silica can boost a child's sense of self, bring hidden emotions to the surface, and help them absorb minerals and grow better. Silica also helps when something needs to be "pushed out" of the body, like a splinter, or pus from acne, and especially with ear, nose, throat, and sinus infections or congestions. Some keynotes of Silica include delayed development or failure to thrive in infants; blocked or infected tear ducts; weak, ingrown, and fragile nails; white spots on nails; ingrown hairs; enlarged and hardened glands; acne that leaves small pits in the face; spinal curvatures or scoliosis; constipation where the stool comes out and then recedes; dental abscesses and infections of the gums; sweating feet and scalp; and sour sweat. Silica is a common remedy that many children can need at some point for a physical acute, a stage of growth, or for shy kids who need a boost in their sense of self.

I also sometimes prescribe the remedy Clear quartz, which is made of Silica. Gemstone remedies like this one assist in stabilizing the core structure and spine to help a person feel grounded. Clear quartz, and especially the gemstone remedy Emerald, have a powerful effect on cleansing EMF toxicity and mental fog through keeping the body energetically aligned and connected to the crown chakra. For more information on gemstone remedies, refer to the work of homeopath Peter Tumminello.

Phosphorus

A Phosphorus child is happy and open with poor energetic and interpersonal boundaries. They desire friends and may be quite social and bubbly but can also be shy due to being empathic and sensitive (this sensitivity can be environmental as well, especially to chemicals). They dislike being alone and may be reticent at first, but when they warm up to a person will become like their best friend. They can even carry on wonderful conversations with strangers. They may have moments of sadness and fear people being angry at them. Or they may have floating anxiety or hypochondria or various phobias such as fear of thunder. Parents of a Phosphorus child will say, "she is quite effusive and doesn't want to be alone, wanting to be around people a lot. She loves riding the bus with her friends. She was crying because she was afraid that her teacher would yell at her."

This open contact with the world can result in frequent infections, particularly respiratory ones. Phosphorus falls under the tubercular miasm with coughs, allergies, and respiratory infections. Bloody noses, hoarse throats, and losing one's voice during an illness are also helped by this remedy. The Phosphorus child may have a growth spurt that comes all at once; they also have bursts of high energy followed by exhaustion and the need for naps.

While Phosphorus is a well-known constitutional remedy, it is usually not a remedy I start with in complex cases. Most kids who have this underlying constitution have suffered from suppression due to their poor defensive mechanisms and as a result need remedies that release suppression, such as Carcinosin, Anacardium, or an animal remedy first.

Phosphoricum Acidum

Like Phosphorus, a child who needs Phosphoric acid craves connection with others but they get more burned out from connecting and become flat and lifeless. They need naps in the middle of the day and they crave juice and fizzy drinks. People can enter a flat and depressed Phosphoric acid state after a loved one dies or after an infection that leaves them exhausted with no energy.

Sulphur

Sulphur helps with poor detoxification and symptoms of heat, inflammation, and the tendency to be messy and collect things, which is generally a reflection of their inner toxicity. The mental state of Sulphur is prone to philosophical, imaginative thinking and they can generally be very bright and passionate about their hobbies. These are warm, generous, lazy, messy, funny children who are social but comfortable being on their own. They are very loving to their parents but can selfishly want someone to cater to them so they can have fun playing with their toys, numerous collections, or video games. Often their mother is the one who caters to them, and in return, they have a deeply affectionate relationship with their mother and fear that she will someday not be there for them (this is the classic mama's boy/girl).

While Sulphur is well described in classical homeopathic literature, I have not seen many true Sulphur cases, and if I do, they are generally healthy children. Most complex kids need many other layers cleared before needing Sulphur as a constitutional remedy. On the other hand, Sulphur and Sulphur-containing remedies (such as Zincum sulph, Hepar sulph, Natrum sulph, Calcarea sulph, etc.), dosed in low potency (6C or 12C), can be great intercurrent detoxification support for kids who are poor detoxers and prone to infections with excessive inflammation. Almost everyone who tests positive for the MTHFR gene dysfunction may do well with some variant of Sulphur. Other kids who have digestive problems from high sulphur foods, such as eggs and broccoli, can also benefit from doses of Sulphur. Keep in mind that dosing Sulphur homeopathically can often bring about physical detox symptoms (rashes, diarrhea, mucus). A strong keynote of Sulphur is being hot in the body; classically they run so hot they will stick their feet out from under the covers, although I have also seen Sulphur cases that are cold. They may sweat excessively, dislike heat, and also have burning pains. This heat can be matched with an eruptive, hot temper and easy irritation. Sulphur kids usually look a bit dirty with greasy, tangled hair and have bedrooms cluttered with things they have collected but refuse to throw away. Yet they are easily disgusted by smells and foul substances. They may suffer from itching red rashes, eczema, a weak back, and poor posture.

Other Sulphur Remedies	
Hepar sulph	Chilly, irritable, and sensitive to pain. Useful for swollen glands, pharyngitis, croup, and otitis media. Similar to Psorinum, Graphites, and Calcarea carb.
Sulfanilamide	This remedy was made from the Sulfa drug (Para-amino-phenyl sulfomonide). Useful for a Sulphur constitution who has mental discombobulation/confusion. Helps with detox and better cognitive function. May have a history of bad reaction to Sulfa-based drugs.
Sulphuric acid	A burned-out Sulphur state. Child used to be highly energetic but now sits on the couch and likes to get a rise out of people. Intensely burning stools, burning sensations in the nervous and GI systems.
Ferrum sulph	Has the warm, loving nature of Sulphur but can be more dictatorial, domineering, and forceful due to the Ferrum aspect. Has an eruptive temper and loves to boss people around. Red rashes around the mouth.
Zincum sulph	Wired and nervous constitution, overly fast thinking, repetitive thinking with looping thoughts in the head. Helps clear viral infections from the body.

Chlorum (Chlorine)

Chlorum is not a classic constitutional remedy, but I have found it crucial in treating complex children and chronic conditions like Lyme disease and I prescribe it often. It helps treat a state of strong negativity and the archetype of the self-martyr. I also give it frequently to parents who pour all their energy into their kids and have lost their center, forgetting what nourishes them. A parent who needed this remedy once told me, "I blame myself—I am not loving myself enough. I don't need the extra blame I put on myself. I want to be by myself and just veg…or eat sugar; but I don't get joy from food. I can't eat what I want to eat. I hate everything I eat. Nothing is nourishing. I just want to get away from it all." It is similar to Oxygenium in that they are both negative and victim-oriented, however Chlorum rejects relationships and avoids drama while Oxygenium feels more deeply deserving from others and claims attention.

These children can be quite depressed and feel disconnected from people due to an internal state of negativity. They are contradictory and may be loners who desire to run away while also becoming more depressed from being alone. Parents will say of this child, "He has self-defeating behavior and is hard on himself. He will say, 'I have no friends, nobody likes me, I am bad at sports.'" On the flip side, they can commit all of themselves to a relationship, losing themselves in the process. They don't feel that they are loved as much as their siblings and suffer from any rejection, although they will usually reject others before they experience rejection themselves. Chlorum can follow Natrum mur, especially if there is chlorine sensitivity or thyroid issues. Chronic cases of Chlorum may have either high or low stomach acid and reflux issues worse from sugar. Also, low potencies of Chlorum can improve the appetite of an overly picky eater who rejects food. Other physical keynotes include acidic saliva, GERD, stomach acid issues, teeth that have been corroded by acid and are falling out, and spasms and convulsions.

Muriaticum Acidum

Children who can benefit from the remedy Muriaticum acidum, which is made from hydrochloric acid, are irritable and sad but apathetic. They feel physically weak and may be in a collapsed state but are restless from the soreness in their body. Sometimes there are issues with hydrochloric acid production in the body resulting in difficulty digesting food. There may also be stomach disorders, ulcers, acidity, and nosebleeds.

Ferrum/Iron Series

Remedies in the ferrum series primarily address themes of work and duty, such as how children handle relationships, schoolwork, and work in general. There are 18 elements in the ferrum series: potassium (known as Kali in homeopathy), calcium, scandium, titanium, vanadium, chromium, manganum, ferrum, cobaltum, niccolum, cuprum, zincum, gallium, germanium, arsenicum, selenium, bromium, and krypton. The most common ferrum series remedies that I use are Kali carb, Calcarea carb, Ferrum met, Cuprum met, Zincum met, Arsenicum, Selenium, and Causticum.

These children are comfortable with routine, order, and the rules of society—they may have a fear of breaking the rules or a strong desire to follow them. Their performance or sense of duty is enforced by a certain social conscientiousness and the guilt of doing something the wrong way or being chastised for breaking a rule. Their thinking may be rigid, and they can sometimes be less emotional than others. Quite often, the children who need ferrum series remedies have hardworking, duty-oriented parents who have technical professions such as engineers, computer programmers, and lawyers. Often these parents give me meticulous, detailed intake forms. If a mom was working while pregnant it is always helpful to know the emotional state they were in while working—if they felt pressured, oppressed, or enjoyed their work—as these pregnancy states all have an impact on the child and their attitude towards future schoolwork.

Kali Carbonicum

Kali carb is a key remedy for kids with weak immunity who, after a series of infections and coughs, feel most comfortable just staying at home in their bedrooms reading or playing video games. Their internal weakness is also reflected in an adherence to rules for a sense of security and they tend to be obedient, "play it safe" types of kids. This adherence to rules lends them a certain bossiness. For example, one mother shared about her child that, "sometimes she thinks things have to be done a certain way, like if I give her a bath she gives lots of instructions. Even the teacher said she acted like my boss." They can also be rigid and want to do things in a specific order or will require that you drive a specific route.

Kali children are black and white, rule-bound thinkers who do better at technical thinking than creative exposition. In this aspect, they may have trouble understanding nuance or jokes and tend to be either overly serious or irritable. They may repeat the same phrase or question over and over and lack the reasoning skills needed to hold a conversation. Another parent shared that "he completely lacks creative thinking. He can do some pretend play if we show him to do it, and will consistently do the same thing every time. If I show him how to play the doctor, he will memorize it and do it the same way. If I teach him something step by step it sticks; anything new he won't do." While they fear doing anything new, they will enjoy puzzles, kitchen sets, or blocks and can easily learn math or reading if it is taught step by step. Their main challenge is often issues with social skills and they tend to avoid hyperactive groups of kids. As another parent of a child I prescribed Kali carb to explained, "He is way behind on his social skills. He doesn't understand the concept of games like catch. He likes other kids, he will introduce himself and shake hands but it stops there, he cannot transition. He cannot sustain a conversation. He initiates, says hello, and then doesn't know what to do."

People who need Kali carb may suffer from frequent colds, coughs, and low back pain. They often have weak motor skills and coordination and delayed milestones. As an acute remedy, Kali carb can treat pneumonia with sharp and stitching pains, difficult respiration that's worse when lying flat and better when sitting upright, and coughs that wake you up at night and are worse between 2 and 4 am. I sometimes alternate between Kali carb and Calcarea carb (see below) for kids like this since they are similar remedies and both will boost weak immunity.

Other Kali Remedies	
Kali ars	Very ritualistic and OCD about cleanliness. Has to do something perfectly, like folding clothes or putting something away. Anxious about health and infections.
Kali bich	Conformist who rigidly sticks to things. Important remedy for stuck sinusitis or coughs with thick, gluey discharges. Stomach symptoms alternating with joint pain or asthma.
Kali fluor	Highly rigid and tense in the body tissues. Yelling and contradicting if people don't do things the right way. Deep lack of confidence. May align themselves with the naughty child of the class and become their sidekick.
Kali mur	Similar to Kali carb but sadder, more closed off and shut down. Wants to go by the rules but shuts others out due to a lack of ability to relate. Feels rejected by the mother.
Kali phos	Doesn't have the rigidity of other Kali remedies. More specific for poor memory, mental exhaustion, and depleted states. Helps children who can't remember their lessons, settles the nervous system, and promotes sleep.
Kali sulph	Child is cautious and wants to obey the rules. Once they get comfortable, they are sociable. Craves salty/spicy snacks; warm-blooded. Often described as an "irritable Pulsatilla."

Calcarea Carbonica

This fundamental remedy is one that many children need. There is a fearful anxiety at the core of Calcarea carb, and they cling to something secure which slows them down and can hold them back. The anxiety shows up as timid, shielding behaviors in new places or with new people, and they are especially uncomfortable when being observed. It is most useful when children are stuck or slowed in their development. For example, it can help large, flabby babies who are slow to sit, crawl, or walk. They may have large heads that smell sour. It helps with weakened immunity leading to colds or ear infections and allows children to recover faster. It also helps when children are first dropped off in a classroom and feel deeply scared and timid of the rules, other kids, and teacher. A major fear of Calcarea carb is doing something wrong and being chastised for it. They follow rules like Kali carb but are not as black and white in their thinking. It is also similar to Silica—both are mild and shy yet stubborn. However, Calcarea carb tends to have a larger build and will hide behind others while Silica tends to have a smaller build and stays contained within themselves. A mom once told me of her Calcarea carb child, "He is slow to warm up, he feels that he is unsure, he will stand around and stall, wait, hold back. Once he connects with the kid, he can integrate. He knows he'll have fun. He does seek that. He wants to play with other kids but won't initiate. He's timid. He does what he is supposed to do, by the book and the rules."

Calcarea carb kids do best learning by rote, or systematically, and can truly master a subject when they put the work and practice in. It's best to give them space and time to work through their routines and a heads up on the plan of the day. Once they know what is expected of them and have a routine, they will do quite well. Their response to stress is to get organized or stick to what they know. Physically, Calcarea carb kids tend to be plump and have low stamina, they have sweaty heads especially when sleeping, clammy hands, and must wear socks because their feet are always cold. They may also have delayed dentition, issues with indigestion and constipation, and poor immunity with recurrent ear infections, tonsillitis, and pharyngitis.

Calcarea Phosphorica

This is a common remedy at the core of many immune deficient cases with a weak or unstable physical structure, or growing pains that cause the child to be physically restless or uncomfortable in their bodies and thus irritable and whiny. This child wants to be social and connect but is still cautious and insecure about making friends. It is possible to need this remedy with the flabbiness and poor muscle tone of Calcarea carb but be less stubborn and desire travel and stimulation; likewise they are easily bored and have a hard time sticking with one activity long. A typical Calcarea phos child will sigh loudly, flop onto the couch and say "I'm bored!" But they may be motivated by planning a trip or exciting activity outside of the house. This is a good acute remedy for growing pains, leg cramps, and dentition. It can also be an underlying remedy in immunodeficiency cases, especially tubercular cases, where there are pains and imbalances in the spine or joints such as arthritis or scoliosis.

Other Calcarea Remedies	
Calcarea mur	Can be used to treat children with immunodeficiency states and is an important remedy to consider if your child has done well with Calcarea carb. Looks like Calcarea carb but instead of asserting themselves with stubbornness they instead retreat to their bedrooms and are more closed off and sad. May vomit all food and drink with stomach pain or have ringworm. Kids often move on to Calcarea carb after treatment with Calcarea mur.
Calcarea sil	Less common than the remedies above but may occasionally arise for anxious kids who are chilly all the time due to a lack of vital heat and have a hard time gaining weight. The child is like Calcarea carb but may be a bit more refined like Silica. Cautious and observing, keeps to themselves. Timid but not aloof.
Calcarea sulph	Outgoing, warm, community oriented. Eruptive tendencies of skin, diarrhea, or even emotions. They are anxious about their eruptions, whether skin or emotional. Tendency to sinus infections and abscesses with unhealthy skin and yellow discharges. Can be sensual, disorganized, jealous, and selfish...but funny.

Vanadium Metallicum

Children who need this remedy may feel tortured by fear of failure and perfectionism so they procrastinate and have a hard time getting the task finished. This remedy may help with issues of anorexia and bulimia with an inability to control their appetite as well as a great amount of doubt and insecurity around what to eat, causing vacillating eating tendencies.

Chromium Metallicum

A child needing Chromium may feel observed when trying something new and then gets very embarrassed when they fail. They only have the courage to do something when they know other people aren't looking. They feel that they must do something to prove themselves, but do so carefully for fear of failing. Other mental symptoms include confusion, spacy thinking, and a weak memory. Chromium is good for colds with sticky, stringy mucus; anemia; and pancreatic issues like diabetes or problems with blood sugar metabolism. Kali bich, a remedy well known for moving stuck discharges, is a version of the remedy Chromium.

Manganum Metallicum

The main feature of this remedy is a desire to help and receive acknowledgement for the work they do. They are sensitive, kind, loving, and adapting, and know intuitively how to help. They like to teach and be taught, giving and taking a lot of feedback. However, criticism gives them a feeling of failure and can cause deep resentment. All symptoms, including vertigo, are better from lying down. Desires tomatoes and also worse from tomatoes. May also have ear or throat problems, like the sensation of ears being plugged, pain, tinnitus, etc.

Ferrum Metallicum (Iron)

Ferrum is a common remedy in complex cases where children are oppositional because they are very sensitive to any pressure put on them. They hate the feeling of being forced to do anything and will put up incredible resistance. A parent may describe their child as highly contradictory to the point of never agreeing with them and always wanting the opposite of whatever is offered. There is little ease and cooperation between the child and parent; often the parents feel they must force the child to do things, which is what the child hates most. They also hate criticism and correction and will talk back. A parent of a Ferrum met case once told me, "If he is corrected, he has a problem with it. He might growl at me and say, 'I know how to do it' or 'I never get this right.' He will correct it but is embarrassed if he makes a mistake, he doesn't take correction well. He will try to bargain with us or try to pressure and convince us to get what he wants. If we tell him no, he'll get a cross look and say something mean and walk off."

Often there is anemia or weakness underlying this defiant behavior, which makes everything they do feel like too much effort. Physical symptoms include red lips, flushed cheeks, hot flashes, and dyspnea from going up stairs due to anemia. Children needing this remedy can be bossy, emotional, and domineering; they push through hard work, refusing to rest until the job is done. They can be bossy and mean to other children when trying to get them to do what they want. Alternately they may be the children of dominant, disciplining parents who push them to do their work and the child stubbornly opposes in equal force. Force from either side of the equation is the main issue and taking the remedy will create more ease and flexibility in the situation. If anemia is discovered in cases with this presentation, giving Ferrum phos cell salts should help.

Niccolum Metallicum (Nickel)

Children needing Niccolum are high achievers who need to control everything with absolute perfection. A mother of a Niccolum case will say, "He tries to be perfect. He loves praise, loves doing a great job. We both have that need to be in control." They generally suppress their emotions but can sometimes have outbursts like Ignatia. They may have parents who are unemotional and intellectual or are in professions that require suppression of emotion (like a lawyer); these parents, out of habit, don't connect emotionally with their kids. These kids find love through being successful at school and may be leaders in their class, like a "little mayor." Niccolum is also a helpful remedy for headaches and coughs and can heal impeded speech due to the sensation of a stiff tongue and tightness inside the mouth.

Cuprum Metallicum (Copper)

Children needing Cuprum are tight, clenched in, and closed with the need for occasional neurologic release. They may seem introverted, disliking socializing unless they are around people they know well. Responsible, detail oriented, and independent, these kids can persevere to the point of being overly headstrong about getting their way. An example is a child who is like his father, a dutiful and perfectionistic military man, and the child gets upset at himself if he didn't do things just perfectly.

These children have a tendency towards spasms, cramps, and even seizures, which can be a physical release of all they are holding inside their tightly wound personalities. They may have had spasms or seizures as infants, or epilepsy after vaccination, and be on antiseizure medications. They also find release through a teasing nature, repetitive stimming, or outbursts of immoderate laughter. This remedy is similar to Zincum; cases may alternate between needing Zincum and Cuprum with both having some level of suppression of the nervous system causing neurological complaints. Also consider Carcinosin cum Cuprum, which is a combination remedy created by Tinus Smits that addresses the controlling nature of both Cuprum and Carcinosin along with the oversensitivity of Carcinosin.

Zincum Metallicum (Zinc) and Zincum Phosphoricum

Zincum is an important remedy for healing overstimulation of the nervous system and is useful for children who take in information too quickly. These children can be oversensitive, talkative, hurried, and very quick learners. However, information gets stuck in loops leading to repetitive behaviors, making it a useful remedy for stimming and scripting, behaviors which tend to calm them. One mother of a child who needed Zincum told me that "Watching things over and over again, repeating words over and over again, or talking to himself makes him calm. What makes him anxious are sudden loud noises or fear about emergencies, stuff happening that he can't control or make stop." These kids may want to play with other kids but get too detailed in the play and lose their audience, getting stuck in repeat. Because they can get particularly stuck on tv shows or video games, weaning them off media can be an important step in allowing their nervous system to heal. It can also be a useful remedy for children who have over-studied or been under too much academic stress, resulting in headaches.

A typical Zincum child will also be restless in their bodies, contorting into strange positions and making silly faces or wrinkling their forehead. It's a great remedy for tics and twitches or other involuntary movements. They flop around, push their heads into things and kick, jerk in their sleep, bang their heads, and grind their teeth. Their sensitive nervous system will make them extra ticklish or sensitive to sounds and drafts. They also eat quickly leading to hiccoughs and vomiting after drinking. Even if they eat well, they often don't put on weight. There might be a history of meningitis, encephalitis, or rashes treated with steroids. Eventually dullness can also develop with poor memory, slow speech, and slow response time, making Zincum a useful remedy for mental slowness. Compare with Nux vomica, Cuprum, and Rhus tox, and look at variants below.

Other Zincum Remedies	
Zincum mur	Sense of smell and taste strange/off. Twitching of face and hands. Spasms of hands. Vomits all food but milk.

Other Zincum Remedies	
Zincum oxydatum	Constant impulse to laugh. Sudden vomiting. Diarrhea. Sadness from masturbation. Undulating of muscles.
Zincum phos	Herpes neuralgia, especially of head and face. Locomotor ataxia. Brain fog. Formication all over the body.
Zincum picricum	Facial paralysis. Brain fog. Loss of energy and memory. Cerebral paralysis. Nervous exhaustion.

Gallium Metallicum

When kids become very withdrawn and are stuck in the dull routine of life they may be in a Gallium state; this is likely connected to a parent who is depressed by their work. The child is shut down to the point where they don't even respond when people ask them something, as if they can't hear the question, and you have to yell to get them to listen. May assist with deafness or hardness of hearing. Sometimes the root cause is a systemic fungal infection that can lead to this level of dullness.

Germanium Metallicum

Germanium has similarities to Gallium in that they are going through the motions of work in a robotic way, feeling vacuous and drained of all life. This is generally a remedy that I have given to parents who work in dull, routine-oriented jobs. With Germanium there are also strong keynotes of fatigue, anemia, and suppressed anger with small outbursts and no remorse. Giving the remedy will result in a renewed sense of purpose in life and may lead one to change jobs or career.

Arsenicum Album

Arsenicum kids tend to be high-strung, busy, and anxious with a kind of organized fastidiousness that helps them be top performers in school. They will keep their bedroom, toys, schoolwork, and even clothes and hair looking very tidy. They like having people around and will have an intelligent conversation with you while their mother is sitting next to them; mostly they don't like being alone. Many Arsenicum children will have fears about disease, infection, or someone dying, possibly with obsessive compulsive disorders around their fears such as obsessive hand washing. One Aspergers child I treated with Arsenicum was obsessed with the ways different famous people died. Most cases of Arsenicum are children who have allergies and/or asthma, most often with allergies to cats, dust, and grass. Asthma will alternate with skin eruptions like rashes or eczema and will be worse late at night, better sitting up. Insomnia due to anxiety is a common ailment treated by Arsenicum.

I give this remedy even more often, however, to parents who are very fearful of germs and infection to the point of hypochondria. It can help those who have a strong reliance on their doctor or the medical system, or who have incredible anxiety around their child's health problems resulting in a desire for control and perfectionism. One mother who needed Arsenicum said, "We have had one chronic health problem after another. I always had the feeling like my son's very life was in my hands because none of the doctors ever really knew what to do with him. I felt like there was more for me to manage than I could handle, nothing seemed to be going right with either of my kids. One aspect after another of my life was being robbed. I panic in a hospital or doctor's office situation, I feel like I'm going to lose something. These situations make me feel angry, fearful, and completely drained, and it takes me a few days to pick myself back up." People who do well with Arsenicum also have a fear of being robbed or losing a job or income.

Arsenicum is also one of the best acute remedies to have on hand for food poisoning where there is vomiting and diarrhea with anxious restlessness. It is often given for epidemic influenza when there is great fear of contagion. Arsenicum patients are chilly and desire heat; they have dehydrated, cracked, dry lips and a strong thirst for water.

Selenium

This remedy can result in a wonderful turn-around for kids who show capacity to do well in school but can't be bothered to do the work. In other words, they are lazy and avoid any demands or responsibilities placed on them. They are drained and have little drive; they feel like it's not worth putting forth any more energy into schoolwork because they may fail anyway. They would much rather slump on the couch and watch tv or play video games. Their laziness may show up as simple forgetfulness, messiness, and disorganization; for example, they may do their school assignment but will forget it and leave it at home. They feel mental work is harder for them than for others so they procrastinate, hoping an assignment will go away. They also can get angry and will want to put the blame on their siblings, claiming injustice or unfair treatment. Other common remedies for children who avoid demands (sometimes labelled as "Pathological Demand

Avoidance") are Ferrum met, Sulphur, Chlorum, Agaricus, Bryonia, and Colocynthis.

I've often seen this remedy show up in kids whose mothers are burned out from working in their profession and want to quit, or in mothers who have quit a profession and feel too unmotivated to work anymore. Physical symptoms include excess saliva that may collect and actually dribble from the mouth, scalp eczema, skin disorders, psoriasis, constipation, and acne.

Bromium

Bromium is for a feeling of being exiled, like all effort is worthless and there is no motivation at all. The person is just tired and wants to lay down. There will be zero focus and flat affect in a child who needs this remedy and a desire to be left alone. They won't even care if their parents are around or not. There may be a strong feeling of having escaped from doing something that one feels guilty for, or of being blamed or scapegoated. It can also help with general feelings of guilt, for example when a parent feels guilty that they aren't working hard enough to help their child, or guilty for failing at school, or a child feels guilty about sexuality or sexual thoughts. This guilt leads to negativity about oneself, which results in a shut down state. Physically there may be low metabolism; thyroid issues; left sided tonsillitis; large, stony, hard glands; and a hoarse cough, all worse from heat or being overheated. Compare with Iodum, Chlorum, and Spongia.

Krypton

These children are capable and may even have unique talents or gifts (savant-level) but don't socialize and act as if they don't have a care in the world; they are free of all responsibility. This state of being separated from the world is characteristic of the noble gases in general, including remedies such as Helium, Neon, Argon, Krypton, and Xenon. They are withdrawn but happy living in their own bubble and are not affected by negativity or the people around them. Krypton can be a good remedy for deep seated brain inflammation or deaf-mute children.

Argentum/Silver Series

Like the "silver screen," these remedies pertain to issues of creativity, performance, and self-expression. Overall these children show interest in fashion, art, music, film, and the admiration of others; they are media savvy and enjoy popular culture. Or they may be skilled in scientific exploration, writing, the healing arts, or sports, and will seek out a way to make their unique stamp upon the world. Their talents are supported by a generally high degree of social sensitivity and empathy. While there are eighteen elements in this group, I am focusing on the remedies I most commonly prescribe. The metal remedies Palladium, Argentum, Cadmium, and Indium are warm, open, empathetic, neurotic, impulsive, socially anxious, and have a tendency towards tics and twitches. Stannum, Antimonium, Tellurium, and Iodum may experience loss of voice, cynicism, contrariness, and breakdown.

Often children who need a silver series remedy have parents who encourage their pursuits and even push them to be the best and win recognition or awards. Many of these remedies have an impact on issues surrounding the voice such as stuttering (Argentum), loss of voice (Stannum), or raspy voice (Antimonium tart). They also have an impact on electrical conductivity, the eyes, ears, throat, and genitals. Many kids who do well with these remedies have multiple motor tics such as head jerking, throat clearing, jumping, sighing, clicking the fingers, etc.

Palladium Metallicum

Palladium children are comfortable being the center of attention, performing on stage, and getting recognition; they love drama, theater, singing, and dancing. Ultimately, they desire being liked by everyone more than anything else and are most stressed if they feel someone doesn't like them. They need to be perfect and will cover up any mistakes. For example, in a Palladium case a mom said, "She needs to always be seen as doing things right, she can never do something wrong. She will lie to cover up something instead of getting in trouble." After basking in the rays of attention from everyone they will be exhausted and crash, secretly fretting about how other people perceive them. Being very empathic and socially aware, they can see through other people's problems and compliment people on their best qualities. They are emotionally needy with their parents as well, needing one hundred percent of their attention. They can have right-sided issues in the genital region such as hernias, ovarian cysts, and varicoceles; this is primarily a female remedy like Platina.

Argentum Nitricum (Silver Nitrate)

Children who need Argentum nit are very open and sensitive and can be nervous about how others perceive them or react to what they say. These children are likely to have many friends, are diplomatic and well-liked, and may have a strong social media presence. Argentum is the element that represents the voice, and many Argentum people will have strong voices, large vocabularies, and rehearse what they say before saying it. It can also be a remedy for stuttering. As this mother said of her child who needed Argentum, "At three years old he stuttered fairly significantly—it was like his brain was working faster than how he could speak. But he grew out of it once we started therapies. He is very visual, very expressive, very drawn to art and building…lots of visual things. But I can see that scatterbrained part too. He is silly, always wanting attention, wanting people to play with him. He is just sweet, silly, and fun. The teachers love him. But he is so sensitive to the other kids and that makes him more anxious."

Oftentimes their easy connectivity and creativity makes them apt comedians and performers. Their openness, however, leads them to have impulsive thoughts, such as "what if I jumped off this bridge," or an easy suggestibility that makes them convinced of other people's opinions. Big-hearted, they can also be quite sympathetic and want to be in serving or healing professions. Their neurotic tendency leads to anticipatory fears, hypochondria, claustrophobia, and desire for company, much like Phosphorus or Arsenicum. Occasionally I have prescribed Argentum met instead of Argentum nit when there is the anxious neuroticism of Argentum nit but the person is more contained and less impulsive. Keynotes include tics and twitches, ataxia or staggering, being warm-blooded (but not all Argentum people are "hot"), a hoarse throat, a splinter-like pain in the throat, desiring sweets and sugar, belching, and gassiness.

Cadmium Metallicum

Similar to Argentum nit, people who need this remedy can be gregarious, social, and loud but also overwhelmed by social situations where they tend to be dramatic and overreact. They are very expressive and open, often fearless, and their excitability can escalate into fights. One case that did well with Cadmium as a remedy had very high cadmium levels on a heavy metals test. His mother said that "He loves to talk and almost has a constant need to be making noise. He used to quote movies and TV constantly. When he is excited around friends or the baby he will often make up a silly song. He has a lot of social desire but does get fearful when meeting new people. He is stressed when meeting new people or in a busy situation when he gets into sensory overload. He will be silly and out of control in his body when he is nervous. Birthday parties are hard for him especially if there is a trampoline, bounce house, or loud music. He will have meltdowns if there is a confrontation with a child and it escalates and he doesn't have an adult to help bring him back down. Overall, I would say he has poor emotional regulation and little things make him very upset. He is drawn to people, he just needs a lot of down time too. I think he gets frustrated with himself because he has such a hard time keeping his hands to himself and being quiet. He gets frustrated with his impulsivity." Cadmium is a carcinogenic element and may assist when there is a history of cancer in addition to treating headaches, voice issues, lung complaints, and problems with genitalia.

Indium Metallicum

These kids are also outgoing and easy with friends, enjoying hugs, cuddles, and positive feedback about their skills. They are quite excited about events, holidays, and social situations, but will be anxious and worried about feeling let down afterwards. There may also be nostalgia for past events with much conversation focusing on the past. Often the parent is creative or an artist of some kind and the child has grown up in a home surrounded by vintage art and antiques. Physically these kids have sensitive nervous systems, mold sensitivity, and may complain of a pins and needles feeling in the body, aching legs, tics and twitches, and fatigue.

Stannum Metallicum

Primarily a cough remedy, this person has a weak and hollow feeling in the chest and overall weakness in the body from prolonged respiratory infections. There will be an empty feeling in the chest, especially after coughing, and there may be copious expectoration. Sometimes the depletion and weakness is so strong that the person can't even speak or exert themselves. Likewise, this person may feel "unheard" or depressed that people don't want to hear what they have to say, or when they talk the other person has a hard time paying attention to what they are saying. These kids may be preachy with a true desire that their message be heard, courteous, and well meaning. But they suffer when they feel people ignore their message.

Antimonium Crudum

Primarily a gastrointestinal remedy, Antimonium crud is similar to Chamomilla with irritability, aversion to touch, and aversion to having attention put on them. Gloomy and sad, they whine and moan with all sorts of stomach issues. The crudum component is the inclusion of sulphur in the remedy, which creates a more sentimental, lazy, easily offended person. While children who need Antimonium crud tend to be challenging, adults who need it are milder, sulkier people who keep to themselves. Keynotes include a thick white coating on the tongue; cracks in the skin, mouth corners, and nostrils; and brittle, distorted fingernails.

Antimonium Tartaricum

Antimonium tart is primarily known as a remedy for clearing out the mucus of a wet cough, from serious bronchitis to mild colds. A child who needs this remedy has a rattling cough with difficulty bringing the mucus out. This can cause a feeling of suffocation, cyanosis, and a cough that's worse at night. The cough is so challenging that the child feels tired and weakened after coughing, perhaps even with nausea and vomiting after the cough. This can also be a useful remedy for chronic asthma with rattling in the chest but little expectoration, better being carried upright.

Similar to Chamomilla, the child who needs this remedy is also likely to be irritable and averse to touch. They may not even want to be looked at, are very discontented, and make contrary comments. Although they want to be with you, they stubbornly do the opposite of what they are asked to do (this is also a tubercular trait). Other important cough/phlegm/pneumonia remedies to compare are Justicia, Spongia, Phosphorus, Squilla, Lobelia, Ipecacuana, and Carbo veg.

Tellurium Metallicum

Consider this remedy when there is laziness, poor posture, and offensive discharges such as fish odor from the ears or very stinky gas or stools. This child will be physically weak and may drool or collect spit in the mouth (similar to Selenium). There may be limping from back pain or pain anywhere in the body, worse from straining at stool or cough. This remedy is similar to Sulphur and Selenium and helps strengthen the body's detoxification and clear out smelly, gassy gut bacteria. Like Sulphur, this child wants to please and be social but can tantrum and act spoiled. Like Selenium, there is mental weakness such as poor memory and focus. I've seen cases with poor detoxification do well with this whole group—Tellurium, Selenium, Sulphur, and Oxygenium—all remedies that have to do with laziness, foul discharges, and issues with stool.

Iodum (Iodine)

In cases where it feels like a child may be hyper or hypo thyroid, consider this remedy, even in low potency, to help balance the thyroid. Many children are in metabolic overdrive creating a state of nonstop, obsessive activity. I often see this in tubercular children who eat ravenously and are hot, thin, and wiry. Sometimes children who need fish, bird, or insect remedies—who are constantly on the go or can even get aggressive— can use Iodum to help them calm down. They don't have a stop button and can be obsessive or agitated about an activity or person. They can also get overwhelmed, want to run and hide, escape, or bolt. These kids may have enlarged glands or a goiter and have a hard time gaining weight despite eating voraciously. They can also have allergies/hay fever, asthma, dry cough, palpitations, or a history of lung infections.

On the flip side, Iodum can show up in children whose metabolism is burned out and they are hypothyroid, always cold, and have no energy or motivation. Often there is a history of low thyroid function in the mother. I will see in these families a tendency to expressing negative statements such as, "I would never do that" or "I hate this or that" that keeps them in a depressed state. This negativity is characteristic of the halogens (fluorine, chlorine, bromine, iodine) and in such cases, they can all be useful to dose at some point in chronic negative cases.

Baryta/Barium Remedies

While technically at the beginning of the gold series (discussed below), the baryta remedies can be considered a category of their own and are especially important for the treatment of complex kids. Their profile is very much like that of Calcarea carb, but being heavier elements, they are more deeply stubborn with greater potential for physical degeneration. Baryta carb and Calcarea carb are similar in that both are deeply timid with a fear of being made fun of or doing something the wrong way. But with Baryta carb, this fear is so deep that they regress backwards into immature, childish behaviors and seek the parent to compensate for their inabilities. They don't want to put themselves out there, they'd rather do what is familiar to them. They prefer staying at home and are fearful of busy, noisy places or rooms full of people. Baryta cases can also have problematic physical delays such as swollen glands, abdomen, and tonsils and delayed growth. Some of these may be children who were developing faster than normal and then totally stalled out and regressed. Symptoms may have developed after the birth of a sibling, starting school, or any major change in their life that makes them want to be taken care of like a baby again. Consider the baryta remedies if your child is stubbornly stuck in their maturation, acting younger than they should be out of a refusal to grow up, and forcing their caretakers to do things for them that they should know how to do themselves. When you do give the remedy, make sure to back away from doing things for the child and push them to do things more on their own. While these remedies are known for mental slowness, they can also show up in intellectually capable people who are emotionally immature and stubbornly avoid life challenges due to low self-confidence and timidity, similar to Calcarea carb, Pulsatilla, and Lycopodium.

Baryta Carbonica

These kids have regressive, childish behavior and are very stubborn about not changing. An example is a post pubertal boy who insists on his mother still tying his shoes or an older girl who talks in baby voice. There can be a stuckness with learning new things or grasping concepts, looking vacant despite repeating a simple lesson over and over. They will have meltdowns about not getting their way, are very shy around new people, fear doing new things, and are especially anxious about being laughed at. They may bite their nails or pick their nose when anxious and prefer standing near the door to a room rather than fully enter it. They will need regular reassurance and help with making decisions or doing academic work. Physically, they may have immaturity or atrophy of body parts (dwarfism) such as hands or sexual organs. This remedy is especially helpful for tonsil and gland inflammations and they are chilly and easily fatigued.

Other Baryta Remedies	
Baryta mur	Regressive behavior and focused on hiding, running away. Sadness. Dull and inattentive. Enlarged tonsil, cervical, or parotid glands. Sensation of lump in the throat. Anxiety and pressure in the stomach, sensitive stomach, indigestion, bending double, nausea, and retching. Increased sexual desire.
Baryta phos	Regressive, babyish behavior but friendly, reaching out to others; wants friends but acts too childish/naive. Feels ridiculed, bullied or laughed at by friends. Inability to concentrate. Shy, sympathetic, and yielding.

Other Baryta Remedies	
Baryta sulph	Regressive behavior with baby talk, particularly clingy with mom and wanting to be mom's baby all the time. May be irritable, hurried, itchy, and hot.

Lanthanide Series

These are self-contained and often advanced children who teach themselves how to do things starting from an early age, mastering complex subjects like mathematics, programming, or self-oriented activities such as rock climbing or martial arts. School is a bore since they aren't so much into the social aspect and they can teach themselves what they need to know. They strongly dislike being told what to do or being forced to follow social conventions. When they teach themselves a skill, such as playing a musical instrument, it is primarily for their own self-development, not to perform for others. In fact, they do not care what others think and are entirely self-driven. The lanthanides also have an association with autoimmune conditions, a medical "self-attack" which is mirrored by their self-critical attitude. Many cases with autoimmune conditions, especially people who are self-reflective and desire autonomy, could benefit from these remedies as well.

There are many lanthanide elements; I prescribe them more often to adults and one doesn't stand out more than any other. Occasionally I give these remedies to children who are in their own mental universe and who resist traditional schooling. In some cases, it's important to suggest to the parent that traditional schooling may not be ideal for this child and they may prefer homeschooling. The concept of unschooling may suit these children well.

These remedies are also worth considering for an autistic child with impressive capacities for writing or thinking that they can't easily deliver to the world, possibly because they are nonverbal. For example, they may write beautiful poetry on their device, or draw uniquely expressive cartoons that demonstrate their capacity for deep thought that they cannot easily express otherwise. The lanthanide remedies include Lanthanum, Cerium, Praseodymium, Neodymium, Promethium, Samarium, Europium, Gadolinium, Terbium, Dysprosium, Holmium, Erbium, Thulium, Ytterbium, and Lutetium. A few are described below.

Lanthanum Carbonicum

The name lanthanum means hidden, and these kids are fairly shy and hide away their talents. To cover their vulnerability and fear of observation they have a tendency to tease others. Lanthanum carb seems like Calcarea carb plus Natrum mur, but the child is entirely self-driven and has given up on doing something for the appreciation of others. They love developing skill sets on their own for the sake of learning but will not share their skills openly for fear of being made fun of. I have seen a few lanthanum cases overlap with the mollusc remedies where there is a shelling off from the world.

Holmium

This remedy state is best described as withdrawn, sarcastic, cynical, and bitter about themselves and their situation. These are experts who know everything but instead of sharing, they scoff. People who need Holmium are self-analytical and caught up in their own negative self-reflection.

Thulium

This remedy helps pull people out of a dark, hellish state akin to being trapped in a pit with no way out. There is a sense of being annihilated but also a desire for salvation. I have seen this remedy show up in cases of precocious ASD kids who will express a heavy feeling of being trapped in their bodies and experiencing great anguish but are deeply, spiritually seeking a way out.

Aurum/Gold Series

These are heavy metal elements and include the remedies Hafnium, Tantalum, Tungsten, Rhenium, Osmium, Iridium, Platinum, Aurum, Mercurius, Thallium, Plumbum, Bismuthum, Polonium, Astatinum, and Radon. The remedies explained below are the ones that I encounter most frequently. People who need them possess a certain heaviness in the body or exhibit an emotional gravitas. Some can be prone to depression and isolation to the point of suicidal tendencies, but others have great potential for being powerful, passionate, and impressive.

Children who need aurum remedies often have parents who need them. These parents are invested in power and influence or the accumulation of wealth, often in the high-level corporate world or military, and generally show great confidence. To obtain this influence they will take on a lot of responsibility and can be greatly affected by any loss of power or status (as seen with Osmium, Iridium, Platina, Aurum, Mercurius, and Plumbum). There may also be cases of people who have been deeply disempowered to the core, perhaps through childhood trauma or sexual abuse, who need remedies such as Bismuthum or Polonium. This loss of power can be felt as an energetic weakness in the "dantian," or lower abdomen.

Like their parents, these children are also serious about their pursuits and hobbies and talk about them like an adult would. They often do not consider their parents to be authority figures. They have a strong leadership capacity and like to take charge of group projects or become the coach of their team, easily attracting other children. They may have adult tastes such as classical music or may even try to discuss world politics with you. Children who need remedies like Aurum may get quite depressed by social and political issues in the world and feel personally connected to them.

Sometimes hair or urine testing may reveal high levels of a particular metal but the child doesn't fit the mental or emotional profile of that metal. In these cases it can still be worth clearing the metal using that remedy dosed in a lower potency (such as 6C or 12C) a few times a week (see Chapter 9).

Platina (Platinum)

For the true divas there is Platina. These children love attention, dressing up, fancy jewelry, checking themselves out in front of a mirror, and performing on stage. They are prone to drama, haughtiness, and can act hysterical. The mother of a four-year-old Platina princess once told me that, "She craves attention from her parents and nanny but she's afraid of strangers, snobby with other people, and people have to work hard to get her to smile. She's a bit of a diva. She will eventually warm up to kids, she has a boyfriend who is four years old. Her tantrums are horrible, she's so demanding and impatient. If she doesn't get what she wants that second, she stomps and screams 'I wants it NOW!' She loves to look at herself in the mirror and when she hears music she transforms and stops paying attention to everyone. When the music plays she'll start dancing in the middle of the room."

Platina tends to be a female remedy, but I have seen boys who need it as well. In these cases they tend to act arrogantly towards adults, need to be the best with performance anxiety and/or have strong sexual urges, sometimes towards the same sex. Platina children may have many neurologic complaints such as tics and twitches, numbness, and neuralgias.

Aurum (Gold)

These tend to be serious children with gravitas who connect better with adults than other children. They may watch the news with great focus and feel depressed about the world or state of politics. They may come off as particular and haughty showing great ambition to become a businessman, politician, or leader of some sort. They can also be deeply emotional and feel misunderstood; they're just waiting to get through childhood so they can have the full responsibility and range of experience of an adult.

Children who need Aurum have some association with deep grief, possibly from the death of a parent or grandparent, or there may be a history of suicidal depression in the family. It may also be a useful remedy for children who are depressed due to their own major illness such as cancer or congenital heart disease. In a handful of cases this remedy has shown up in children whose mothers experienced the death of their own father during the time of their pregnancy, which they deeply grieved. Physical keynotes of this remedy include issues of the bones such as stunted growth or deformations, growing pains, coldness felt in the bones, atrophy, undescended testes, and induration of glands.

Mercurius Sol (Mercury)

Mercurius is an interesting remedy because mercury toxicity can show up on many levels. For some children with high mercury levels on lab tests, I have seen only physical symptoms with increased salivation, swollen glands, chronic ear or throat infections, high yeast levels, and terrible eczema, while on the mental/emotional level the child remains average. For others with high mercury, the toxicity will manifest as a violent child who will engage in premeditated attacks; however this outwardly aggressive manifestation is less common in my experience. What I generally see in kids is a more subtle presentation of Mercurius—a closed off, introverted child who is talented, highly independent, and contradicts all authority. The destructive aspect of Mercurius in this case is subverted into a strong interest in shockingly violent movies or video games. On an emotional level these kids can seem quite shut down, often ignoring others and interested only in their own pursuits. When they do connect, they do so earnestly with full attention.

Almost like a human thermometer, these kids are very sensitive to temperatures and easily become too hot or too cold. They may have chronic ear infections, bad breath, excessive salivation, and a tongue that's imprinted on the sides by their teeth. Look for gastrointestinal issues such as ulcerative colitis and a strong urging for stool with a "never done" sensation. Mercurious can seem a lot like spider remedies—reactive and fast in the body.

Thimerosal is an ethylmercury sodium salt that acts as a preservative in vaccines. It was removed from most (but not all) vaccines in 1997. People with mercury symptoms from vaccines (increased salivation, swollen glands, closed behavior, paranoia, interest in violence) should consider this remedy.

Plumbum Metallicum (Lead)

The symptoms of lead toxicity are well understood and congregate around toxification of the nervous system causing lack of reaction and loss of power. This shows up in many symptoms, including slow cognition, slow speaking, slow reflexes, loss of urge to urinate, loss of sensitivity to pain, trembling of hands when holding objects or from slight exertion, emaciation of muscles in limbs, convulsions with flexed limbs, contracture of tendons, ataxia and headache with stiffness and pain in the nape of the neck, and vomiting. There will also be digestive symptoms including profuse salivation, extreme thirst, constipation with impacted stool, pebble-like stools, and a large distended abdomen.

On the mental level there is slowness and/or dullness with the child hiding or evading eye contact. One child I treated who needed this remedy didn't have the energy to stand up due to emaciated limbs, so he stayed hiding under his bedcovers, chewing the sheets and hitting his forearms and legs because they were tingling. Plumbum and the remedy Lathyrus, which are also known for treating the symptoms of polio, restored power to this child and he was running in the park within months of treatment. With Plumbum, there is a general feeling of being forsaken, so the child will want to make silly faces, act out, strike, moan, or whimper for attention. Likewise, a mother who could need Plumbum may exaggerate or make up health complaints for her child, excessively seeking the attention of the doctor (like Munchausen's).

The symptoms of Plumbum are very similar to Alumina with the slowed nervous system, dryness, constipation, induration of glands, and depression. In most cases with these symptoms I would ask for a heavy metals test, if there isn't one already. If these metals show up high on tests, I will give them the metal in the potency 12C a few times a week if not daily, along with chlorella for chelation. Compare with Baryta carb, Silica, Natrum mur, and Kali remedies.

Bismuthum (Bismuth)

Bismuthum is known as a remedy for gastritis when there is abdominal pain along with great fear, like fear of death or being alone, causing anxious restlessness; this is similar to Phosphorus or Arsenicum. With Bismuthum there will be great thirst for cold water but vomiting when water hits the stomach.

This remedy has shown up on a chronic level in cases when there is dark, heavy depression in the family and a sense of loss of power. The elements Bismuthum, Plumbum, and Polonium feel as if power has been taken from them resulting in a deep vacuum, as if a part of their soul is missing. In one pediatric case that did well with both Bismuthum and Polonium, there was a family history of incest that left a deep scar on the parent. On top of this, while pregnant, the mother was told by doctors that the child would die after delivery due to a cyst found on an ultrasound. While she did not die, this imprinted a feeling of loss/death onto the child. As a baby, the child had a lot of diarrhea and vomiting and a constant serious expression. Nothing made her happy, but she needed to be constantly held. As this child grew up, she had back and bone pain and would cause herself to dramatically fall as if someone pulled a rug out from under her. Bismuthum was a key remedy in helping this child reclaim her power and become a strong, creative young woman.

Uranium/Actinide Series

Uranium remedies are useful for cancer, extreme sensitivity, and also deep ancestral anger that needs release. The impressive, advanced, "old souls" who need uranium series remedies communicate better with adults than children and may teach themselves advanced skill sets. They can be empathetic or psychic with an interest in religion, world events, magic, angels, the occult, life after death, or meditation. Some of these children may have experienced serious and complex medical conditions, such as cancer or operations at an early age. I have also seen the children of mothers who are medical professionals and who work with serious health conditions (like in a cancer ward), especially while pregnant, need these remedies.

Other children who need these remedies may suffer from genetic conditions that are severe and may be nonverbal. They tend to have very big, open crown chakras with an ability to go "out of body," partly because being in the body is heavy and challenging. Physically they may be exploding with energy or very exhausted and debilitated. They tend to crave eating meat. These children may seem to have a halo of light around their head and look older than they are. Sometimes they actually test high for radioactive elements like uranium or thorium on heavy metals testing.

Below are three uranium series remedies, but the list of available radioactive remedies includes Radium, Thorium, Protactinium, Uranium, Plutonium, Curium, and Californium. The theme of explosions, glass, broken glass, and melting glass also showed up frequently in the proving of these remedies. Uranium series cases often move to needing aurum series remedies afterwards.

Radium Bromatum

People who need this remedy are overwhelmed by the thought of death, God, heaven, and the afterlife. In their body they feel tired and irritable and desire to have someone near. It may be useful for children undergoing cancer treatment or X-rays causing exhaustion, deep aching pains, radiation ulcers, or severe headaches. I have also given it to children who have a parent undergoing cancer treatment.

Uranium Nitricum

Uranium levels can show up high on heavy metals tests in children, particularly those in the western United States. In the cases of high uranium levels that I have seen, these children tend to have high parasite loads, although this may not be a direct correlation with Uranium. They also have a tendency to rage/attack—like a volcano bursting—which is correlated with deep nervous system inflammation due to oversensitivity, toxicity, and parasites. However, when they are calm, they are capable of being very advanced in academics or some skill which gives them a strong sense of self confidence that draws people to them. This is also a remedy for malnutrition, fluid buildup in the abdomen (ascites), diabetes, and nighttime bedwetting.

Plutonium Muriaticum

This remedy can clear the weight of a deeply traumatic ancestral history of oppression, genocide of whole groups of people, and deep depression or internal rage due to the trauma or sins of the ancestors that has been passed from one generation to the next. Plutonium may also show up when there is a rare genetic disorder in the child. These children tend to have very open crown chakras and show difficulty on the physical plane.

Other Minerals and Substances

The remedies detailed in this section don't fall into the categories above but are worth mentioning as I have found them useful for complex kids. Many are carbon-based and can help with the effects of chemical exposures such as kidney toxicity and metabolic and blood disorders.

Ammonium Carbonicum

Often used for chronic fatigue in the elderly, Ammonium carb can help some debilitated ASD cases where there is an oppressed sensation in the chest. It also treats stagnancy states such as sluggish circulation, heart conditions, and being overweight. These kids may be closed off and shut down over disappointment or anger towards their parents, resulting in a resentful or bitter state.

Benzolum

Children who have low red and white cell counts (neutropenia), fatigue, and who bruise easily can benefit from this remedy. Consider it when there has been high exposure to benzenes from tobacco or car exhaust. I have given it to children with low immune function who live in highly polluted cities.

Causticum

This is a key remedy for many children with nervous system sensitivity due to a strong sense of injustice and is similar to Phosphorus, Natrum mur, Ignatia, and Carcinosin. These children are particularly sensitive and sympathetic to abuse in the world; and more than that, they feel they must do something about it. They may also be sensitive to the emotional pain and suppression in their family and focus their energy on something highly idealistic—such as becoming vegan or organizing rallies. This sensitivity eventually wears their nervous systems down and they get exhausted, sometimes developing tics, twitches, and hardening of tissues. It's an important remedy for compulsion, slow and gradual paralysis especially on the right side (and Bell's palsy), tremors and numbness, a constant desire to clear the throat, incontinence and bed wetting, asthma or bronchitis that is better from cold drinks, joint pains, and warts.

Formaldehyde

Because formaldehyde is a vaccine additive, this remedy can help detoxify vaccine-damaged children who have a poor memory and mix up or slur their words.

Glonoinum (Nitroglycerin)

For sudden irregularity of circulation, similar to Belladonna, causing explosive sensations, headaches, rage, fainting, or postural orthostatic tachycardia syndrome (POTS). Stress such as exercise or panic causes an adrenaline storm—the heart rate goes up, the child gets heated, and then a fight or flight situation ensues. They may get dizzy and faint and need to lie down. Glonoinum can also heal past trauma from a childhood spent around someone with an explosive temper. A child needing this remedy may have meltdowns on hot days.

Gunpowder

Kids who need Gunpowder are black and white thinkers (due to the Kali component in gunpowder) and have strong, knee-jerk reactions and meltdowns. They are EXPLOSIVE, similar to Sulphur but more intense. I have found it to be useful in PANDAS cases with ritualistic behaviors and sepsis infections. It can also be given at the onset of an acute infection as a preventative.

Kreosotum

Excoriating urination, vaginal discharges that are very itchy and offensive, and itchy eczema can be helped by Kreosotum. This is a popular remedy for people who are woken up by the need to go to the bathroom throughout the night, especially if the urine is offensive in nature.

Lapis Granites Murvey (Granite)

For people who feel like a ROCK—lifeless, weak, extreme exhaustion, closed, shut down, dull, dragging, exhausted, and cold. Detached and indifferent, all thinking is logic based and the body feels hard. A child who needs Lapis may be introverted yet arrogant and feels that other people are trivial. It's a useful remedy when someone in the family has died and the person who is grieving feels as though they are being dragged down into the earth. Compare with Graphites, Sepia, and Ammonium carb.

Petroleum

The body stores oil-based toxins and some infections in fatty layers and Petroleum can reach and detox those layers. It is also useful in drawing out the stuck layers of deep, chronic infections such as herpes and Lyme. Petroleum is a good remedy for dry, cracking, and fissured skin that you might use over-the-counter petroleum-based products to soothe, and the remedy helps people detox from the toxicity of these products. It's also very useful for motion/car/plane sickness with an empty feeling in the stomach that improves with eating.

Polystyrene

People who have been exposed to heated plastic water bottles, baby bottles, and plastic factories can use this remedy to help detox polystyrene from their bodies. High environmental exposures to plastics (including food microwaved in plastic) can lead to spaced out, vacant states or a rush of ideas followed by collapse.

Terebinthina

Similar to Kreosotum, Terebinthina treats severe urinary tract infections with burning, bloody, or dark urine, and also edema.

Conclusion

My hope is that this chapter gives you a broad perspective on the mineral remedies available, beyond classic homeopathic materia medica, that you can use to treat your family. A tip to prescribing these remedies is understanding where a child is stuck in his or her development (often this reflects where a parent is at). Is the issue that they are stuck at the level of incarnation (hydrogen series), that they need help with their sense of self/ego (carbon series), help with their relationships (silica series), help with their schoolwork (ferrum series), or help with their creative contribution (argentum series)? Are they overly autonomous (lanthanide series), do they feel responsible like an adult (aurum series), or are they wise beyond their years (uranium series)? Each element has unique chemical characteristics which are reflected in the physical symptoms of the materia medica, so refine your choice by making sure it matches aspects of their physical symptoms as well.

Chapter 7

Nosodes

Our human microbiome is designed by nature to be a teeming, diverse collection of organisms with a system of checks and balances; viruses, bacteria, yeast, and parasites, living in a state of symbiotic harmony that benefits our larger organism. Modern medicine, with its arsenal of pharmaceuticals, has effectively carpet-bombed this ecosystem, drastically altering its terrain, and we are just beginning to recognize the consequences this is having on childhood development and immunity. However, pharmaceuticals can also save lives when our body is losing out to a foreign invader. So at what point do we draw the line with an overreactive fear of germs and excessive prescribing, causing drug resistance, and how can we safely develop healthy immune responses without the fallout damage from pharmaceuticals? In my view, our society needs to adopt a radically different perspective towards infectious disease, which homeopathy can provide.

There are several different ways that homeopathy can effectively treat infectious disease:

1. Prescribing a constitutional remedy strengthens the core constitution of the person so that when the person encounters a stressful infection, they do so from a place of inner strength. Constitutional remedies can be a plant, animal, mineral, or even a nosode (such as Carcinosin or Tuberculinum). Effective prescribing requires time and individualization.
2. A nosode is a homeopathic preparation made from diseased tissues, such as a breast cancer tumor or isolated pathogens themselves. Prescribing a nosode can heal chronic infections that may have been suppressed by Western medicine, or infections that were never fully recovered from.

3. Prescribing a nosode can heal a disease that was never healed in a previous generation and is passed down to the next generation "miasmatically."
4. Epidemic infectious disease can be prevented through training the body to recognize and understand a specific disease state through the prescription of either a nosode (a remedy made from disease/infectious disease tissue samples) or "genus epidemicus," which is a remedy (can be a plant/animal/mineral) that fits a picture of the disease state. This can be applied on the level of public health by treating large groups of people with single remedies.

Despite homeopathy's documented success in treating massive outbreaks of infectious disease, it's unlikely that mainstream medicine will embrace this form of healing anytime soon. The best way to become unflinchingly fearless in the face of infection is to educate yourself and become your own best homeopath.

Many parents of complex kids already understand the value in a child getting the normal fevers, colds and flus, as well as already have a sense of what is immunologically out of balance in their child. I once got this comment from a parent: "My kid is like a bull in a china closet when she's yeasty and she giggles like a maniac! But then if I treat the yeast with Diflucan, the strep takes over and she just gets super angry with me." A quote such as this demonstrates the personality of the pathogen impacting the personality of the child, as well as the interdependence these pathogens have on each other—you kill one pathogen off and it allows another to thrive. Homeopathy allows us to respond to these pathogens in a softer, more balanced way.

The onset of particular fears and delusions in children can point to the nature of the pathogenic material itself. For example, children who fear insects at an extreme level to the point of not going outside often have contracted a zoonotic infection through an insect vector, such as Lyme disease. Other children, who have a fear of germs and a great desire for hand washing, often have some level of viral or bacterial infection. On the flip side, when that disease state is prevalent in the child, sometimes the child is obsessed with arenas where they can contract or disseminate that pathogen. Often children with bacterial, parasitic, or fungal infections are interested in masturbation, playing with stool, or licking things in public. The pathogen has so taken over the child that it seemingly directs the child's activities to increase its chances of spreading itself.

Not all children require the prescription of a nosode, but they can be helpful, especially in the beginning stages of treatment, to help the body recognize and respond to infections it had been ignoring. This gives a chance for immunity, our core sense of self, to gain a greater foothold.

Some core sensations that indicate the use of a nosode can be:

- Feeling that there is something wrong—may be expressed by the feeling "I am abnormal, I am not myself, something has come onto me"
- Poor sense of self identity, low self-esteem, a suppressed sense of self
- Everything feels out of control
- Unusual fears and delusions, perhaps about death or germs
- Intrusive thoughts
- OCD and stimming behaviors
- Mood swings, tantrums, rage, hitting, violence
- Suppressed emotions (anger, sadness, etc.) in child and often in parent

Physical Symptoms That Indicate Nosodes

For a healthy person in an acute infectious state, physical symptoms are usually easy to spot. For a child with an autoimmune disorder, it is more difficult to differentiate, most likely because many of them are in a constant chronic state of low immunity and infection. Their behaviors are symptomatic of environmental toxicity and chronic viral, bacterial, and fungal infections. In some of these children, this may manifest as hyperactive behavior, while others may be in a "hypoactive fatigued" state. It is important to know if the child has normal fever responses and how many times a year. Some children may get fevers and pick up "every infection out there" and the illness resolves within a few weeks. But most of the children I treat do not get "normal" cold and flu symptoms; their immune system crashed at some point due to a variety of causes such as poor diet, allopathic treatment, vaccines, and genetic susceptibility.

Physical symptoms include:

- Restless sleep
- Lack of normal immune response (fever, runny nose, etc.)
- Frequent urination, strong thirst
- Poor skin: acne, boils, crusty scalp
- Masturbation

- Fatigued, drained of energy, listless
- Uncomfortable and restless in the body
- Joint pains, muscle pains
- Swollen lymph nodes
- Dark circles under eyes
- Sound, light, touch sensitive; aches and pains
- Headaches

Many children with PANDAS/PANS, ASD, and Lyme disease receive diagnostic testing, including stool analysis and viral titers, which can help identify major pathogenic causes. While this can be illuminating and is a useful place to start, these tests aren't always 100% accurate. Knowing the clinical presentations of diseases is important in deciding to give a correct nosode. However, in many of these cases, the clinical presentation is often very different from the norm. Many kids do not have the strength in their immune system to mount a significant reaction and rarely get fevers or have symptoms of the average cold and flu. Rather, it is their unusual behaviors that signify the presence of pathogens. For example, in my clinical experience, flapping and spinning is linked to fungal infections, while lining up of toys and OCD is linked to strep strains.

Gastrointestinal Symptoms That Indicate Nosodes

Many complex children have some level of gastrointestinal imbalance, often present since birth. This may be due to chronic GI imbalance and food allergies in the mother that get passed on to the child, a heavy toxicity load that the child is exposed to in early development, the standard American diet, and/or vaccines. These symptoms are easy to observe via abnormalities of stool or urine, as deviations from a daily, well formed, brown-colored bowel movement. It's important to pay attention to stool frequency, consistency, whether stools are floating/not floating, and smell—they can indicate a lot.

Nosodes can be incredibly helpful for balancing out the GI flora but are tricky to differentiate. A set of bowel nosodes developed by homeopath Dr. Edward Bach over a hundred years ago are certainly still helpful, but our bowel floras have changed considerably since then. Nosodes I often prescribe that are not included in the group of "Bach/Patterson" bowel nosodes include Clostridia, Klebsiella, and Candida albicans. There are provings for some bowel nosodes, but many symptoms are overlapping so it takes some discernment to know which ones to try. Laboratory stool testing can also indicate which specific pathogens are out of balance and can be a place to start. Common constitutional remedies I have given to "gut kids" along with nosodes are listed in Chapter 10.

I often see children who take many supplements, including probiotics, in an effort to bring balance to the GI. Some of the supplements might be helpful, but often when children are taking too many supplements it can be detrimental. Probiotics can bring a lot of relief to a child in some cases; in other cases they keep the child in a state of continued imbalance and are too much for their systems. Some probiotics can also contain strains that a child may negatively react to.

Gastrointestinal symptoms include:

- Bloating, gas
- Unhealthy, foul smelling stools
- Stools with strange consistency
- Fecal incontinence
- Constipation or diarrhea
- Stomach pain
- Strong food cravings
- Nausea, vomiting, poor appetite
- Food allergies

How to Combine Nosodes with Constitutionals

The majority of children with autoimmune disorders are in such a state of imbalance that a single constitutional remedy, particularly if dosed conservatively, would give a minor boost to an otherwise exhaustive uphill climb in the path towards recovery. Even when a remedy fits all aspects of a child, in most cases the constitutional is merely one piece of a complex puzzle.

In most cases that I have encountered, the level of immune impairment and cellular toxicity will often "block" an otherwise well-chosen remedy. An example of this is when a constitutional remedy such as Colocynthis is given—and we know it helps because the child is no longer pressing into their belly out of pain—but then, after some initial improvement, the child starts to endlessly giggle and flap their hands, which I have since learned is a sign of a candida flare. While the remedy was a good choice, the healing that the body needed to move through triggered a release of bacterial/fungal and viral layers that seemed at first to worsen the state of the child. However, this may merely be part of a normal healing process that is misunderstood by the parent and practitioner. A homeopath specializing in immune disorders should have a good understanding of how the body detoxifies and what can emerge as the result of deep levels of detox in a child.

Prescribing nosodes, organotherapeutics, and sarcodes to detox and strengthen systems of the body will help move through blocks in a case. Using these types of remedies concurrently with constitutional remedies became the next logical step in my pursuit to heal children with the complexities that go along with most neuroimmune and ASD cases. Using remedies prepared from vaccines and other isopathic nosodes, has been popularized and developed into a protocol called CEASE by the late Dutch homeopath Tinus Smits. To successfully heal many ASD cases, vaccine clears such as MMR, DPT, Prevnar, Influenza vaccine, Hep B, and Varicella are crucial. Each of these vaccines can have a specific symptom picture as well. For example, the MMR vaccine, based on clinical experience, often creates a symptom of "lateral eye gazing" and "eye stimming" in a child, and the Hep B vaccine can be related to the mouthing of objects.

Strep nosodes, as well as other nosodes of infectious disease origin, have been critical in bringing the immune systems of children diagnosed with PANDAS into balance. Combining good constitutional prescriptions for PANDAS with strep nosodes became an excellent combination to heal the majority of these cases. Children with other diagnoses revolving around immune weakness, including PANS, CVID, and Lyme disease, also respond well to the right nosode. More than just miasmatic prescription clears, these nosodes are extremely helpful for present state pathogenic infections and bolstering immune systems in children that are suppressed by allopathy. The most consistent variable in all of my clients, across the ASD spectrum, as well as PANDAS/PANS and Lyme disease, is a weakened and suppressed immune system compounded by the toxicity of our modern life and genetic susceptibility.

The traditional miasmatic remedies of Tuberculinum, Carcinosin and Medorrhinum play a big role in my practice, and are essential remedies for

ASD, but they can overshadow other nosodes that deserve greater attention. In addition to these three, the most common nosodes that I prescribe include Streptococcus strains, Candida albicans, Clostridium difficile, Mycoplasma pneumoniae, and Influenzinum. I also often utilize the Lyme disease remedies (Borrelia, Bartonella, Babesia), Herpes viruses, Staphylococcus aureus, Coxsackie, and Klebsiella.

Dosing Nosodes

Most nosodes can be effectively and sufficiently prescribed in 30C and 200C potencies as frequently as once a day for a short period of time, or dosed just one time only. Some nosodes are so deeply impressed within someone, possibly ancestrally, or through excessive use of suppressive pharmaceuticals, that higher potencies like 1M, 10M and CM can be of use, and usually these do not need to be dosed more than a handful of times.

What to Expect After Dosing a Nosode

Some people fear dosing nosodes because of the potential of bringing about an immune or detox response. It's important to remember that, while powerful, nosodes (in 12C potencies or higher) do not contain the physical substance itself. If they trigger an immune response, this is not a forced response, it is naturally coming from the vital force of the body establishing balance. If an immune response is triggered such as a fever, rash, or sleepiness, this response usually lasts 1-2 days and is easily managed with a hands-off approach or low intervention natural medicine. If a strong fever response is triggered this likely can be managed with 1-2 doses of Belladonna 30C.

SUPPRESSED EMOTIONS

Our emotional health and immune health are intimately intertwined. When we recognize our own emotions and express them in the moment, we are likely to have a strong immune system. People with weakened immunity often have a difficult time recognizing their own emotions, or those of others, deeply suppressing their emotions and allowing too much information/toxins/infections from the outside to come into them. From a holistic perspective, strong immunity means a strong sense of self, strong self-expression, strong boundaries, and an ability to face life's stresses with unflappable ease. It is crucial that parents recognize that working on your own emotional health will improve the immunity of the whole family.

༄༅ Bacterial Nosodes ༄༅

Bacteria are relatively complex, single-celled creatures, many with a rigid wall and a thin, rubbery membrane surrounding the fluid inside the cell. They can reproduce on their own. Most bacteria are harmless, and some actually help by digesting food, destroying disease-causing microbes, fighting cancer cells, and providing essential nutrients. Fewer than 1% of bacteria cause diseases in people.[1]

Symptoms of bacteria out of balance can vary, but in general you may find:

- smelly discharges
- yellow/green/grey discharges
- intermittent fevers
- gastrointestinal symptoms, especially sharp pain, diarrhea, and foul stools

The most common bacterial nosodes I use with ASD are:

- Streptococcinum and its variant nosodes (Strep faecalis, Strep pneumoniae, etc.)
- Staphylococcinum/Staph aureus and MRSA
- Mycoplasma pneumoniae (walking pneumonia)
- Clostridia difficile
- Lyme nosodes: Bartonella henselae, Borrelia burgdorferi, and Babesia microti

Many of the classic homeopathic miasmatic nosodes are from bacteria as well, such as Medorrhinum, Tuberculinum, and Syphilinum.

Bacterial Nosodes	
Remedy Name	*Classification*
Anthracinum	Anthrax (rabbit)
Babesia microti	Spirochetaceae
Bacillus faecalis	Burkholderiales
Bacillus gaertner	Salmonella enteritidis
Bacillus No 10	Enterobacteriales

Bacterial Nosodes	
Remedy Name	*Classification*
Bacillus No 7	Citrobacter, enterobacter
Bartonella henselae	Parasite
Bifidobacterium adolescentis	Probiotic
Borrelia burgdorferi	Spirochetaceae
Botulinum	Clostridia class
Brucellosis	Coccobacilli
Chlamydia	Chlamydiales
Cholera toxin	Cholera
Clostridium difficile	Clostridia class
Clostridium perfringins	Clostridia class
Colibacillinum	Enterobacteriales
Corynebacterium pyogenes	Acne bacteria
Diptherinum	Cornybacterium diptheriae
Dysentery co	Shigella dysenteriae
Escherichia coli	Escherichia coli
Enterococcinum	Bacilli class
Flavus bacillus	Neisseria subflavus, meningitis
Gardnerella vaginalis	Bacterial vaginosis
Haemophilus ducreyi (AA)	Bacteria, STD
Haemophilus influenzae	Pfeiffer's bacillus
Helicobacter hepaticus	Helicobacteraceae
Helicobacter pylori	Helicobacteraceae
Johneinum	Crohn's disease nosode
Klebsiella pneumoniae	Enterobacteriales
Legionella	Legionella pneumophila
Leprominium	Mycobacterium leprae
Listeriosis	Listeria
Lyme disease	Lyme + coinfections
Medorrhinum	Gonorrhea
Medorrhinum americanum	Gonnorhea American
Meningitis	Neisseriales
Meningococcus nosode	Meningitis spinal fluid

Bacterial Nosodes	
Remedy Name	*Classification*
Morgan gaertner	Morganella morganii
Morgan pure	Morganella morganii
MRSA	Antibiotic resistant staph aureus
Mucotoxinum/Mucobacter	Klebsiella pneumonia
Mutabile/Mutabilis	Enterobacteriales
Mycoplasma pneumoniae (AA)	Walking pneumonia
Paratyphoid A/B	Mumps nosode
Paratyphoidum B	Salmonella paratyphi
Parotidinum	Mumps, paramyxoviridae
Pertussinum	Whooping cough
Pneumococcinum	Streptococcus pneumonia
Poly bowel nosode	Combination nosode
Proteus	Enterobacteriales
Pseudomonas aeruginosa	Pseudomonadales
Pyrogenium	Rotten meat
Rickettsia (AA)	Parasite
Saxitoxinum	Cyanobacteria class
Shigella dysenteriae	Dysentery
Spirulina	Cyanobacteria class
Staphylococcus aureus (Staphylo-coccinum)	Bacilli class
Strep combo	Combination nosode
Strep AB hemolytic (AA)	Combination strep
Streptococcus faecalis	Strep from stool
Streptococcinum	Bacilli class
Streptococcus agalactiae	Group B strep
Streptococcus dysgalactiae	Groub C strep
Streptococcus pyogenes (Strepto-coccinum)	Group A strep
Streptococcus uberis	Strep from cows
Sycotic co	Neisseria mucosa
Syphilinum	Spirochetaceae

Bacterial Nosodes	
Remedy Name	Classification
Tetanus	Clostridia class
Tuberculinum avis	Mycobacterium avium
Tuberculinum bovis	Mycobacterium bovis
Tuberculinum koch	Mycobacterium tuberculosis
Typhoidinum	Rickettsia
Yersinia	Black death/plague

Strep Nosodes

Streptococcus is a genus of spherical (coccus) bacteria containing over 50 distinct species (e.g. Streptococcus pyogenes). Streptococcus is so named because they form chains or pairs—the Greek streptos means "easily bent or twisted," like a chain. Interestingly, ASD children with strep infections seemingly act out this formation of chains through the desire to line things up in an orderly way.

Various streptococcal species are responsible for a broad range of illnesses, including pharyngitis (strep throat), pink eye, meningitis, bacterial pneumonia, and endocarditis, and are implicated in more complex autoimmune conditions like PANDAS. Of course, many streptococcal species form part of the healthy human microbiome in the intestines, upper respiratory tract, mouth, and skin.

Streptococcus is not classically taught in standard homeopathic education as a miasm, but in my experience it is possibly the most common miasm in children today. This is likely due to the current generation of parents having had strep infections systematically suppressed through overuse of antibiotics.

PANDAS is currently thought to be caused by human antibodies generated when GAS (group A strep) infection strikes certain genetically susceptible individuals. The autoimmune aspect is thought to be a harmful cross-reaction of these antibodies with specific, but currently unknown, neuronal cells in the central nervous system, resulting in widespread cellular/neurological dysfunction.

The clinical picture most classically associated with PANDAS is OCD and/or tic disorder, though one distinguishable from Tourette syndrome or chronic tic disorders. In addition, other diagnostic criteria include a temporal association (less than 6 weeks) between known GAS infection and symptom onset, episodic waxing and waning of symptoms in relation to GAS infection, and acute onset between ages 3 – 12 (or puberty).

Because of problems with the GAS-related diagnostic conditions (such as the large prevalence of GAS infections in children and the possibility of other infections causing similar acute-onset neurological and psychological symptoms), a National Institute of Health working group in 2010 developed the related diagnosis of PANS—Pediatric Acute Onset Neuropsychiatric Syndrome. PANS is clinically defined by:

- Sudden onset of OCD or severely restricted food intake
- Two or more additional acute onset neuropsychiatric symptoms from the following categories:
  o Anxiety
  o Emotional instability and/or depression
  o Irritability, aggression, and/or severely oppositional behaviors
  o Behavioral (developmental) regression
  o Deterioration in school performance (related to ADHD-like symptoms, memory deficits, or cognitive changes)
  o Sensory or motor abnormalities
  o Somatic signs and symptoms, including sleep disturbances, enuresis, or urinary frequency
- Symptoms that aren't better explained by another known neurologic disorder (schizophrenia, bipolar disorder, etc.)

The point of introducing these diagnoses is simply to point out that there is a much greater range of clinical symptoms associated with the effects of streptococcus infection (and other infections) than is normally associated with the common conditions of streptococcal pharyngitis (strep throat) or streptococcal pneumoniae, etc. Clearly, dysfunctional immune relations with streptococcal and other infections is resulting in new manifestations of severe clinical symptoms on the behavioral/emotional, mental, and physical levels.

Parents have shared the following about when their child became symptomatic with PANDAS/PANS:

- "He was suddenly emotional and defiant. Before that he was perfect, just SWEET. This was literally overnight."
- "We had to remove strings on clothes, tags on clothing and stuffed animals."

- "'I'm having bad thoughts, I'm thinking about someone killing me, I'm thinking I don't want to kill myself.' These were recurring themes that progressed, [but] he had never even seen a violent movie before."

Streptococcal species are sub-categorized into three groups called alpha-hemolytic (which oxidize hemoglobin in blood cells, but do not rupture them), beta-hemolytic (which cause complete rupture of blood cells), and gamma-hemolytic (which cause no hemolysis). Below are the most important streptococcus strains, all of which are found in the alpha- and beta-hemolytic groups.

Alpha-hemolytic (α-hemolytic) Streptococcus
Streptococcus pneumoniae is also known in homeopathy as Pneumococcinum (a name relating to its old categorization apart from streptococcus). It is a leading cause of bacterial pneumonia, and occasionally implicated in cases of sinusitis, meningitis, peritonitis, and otitis media. These infections tend to focus on inflammation as the major cause of resulting illness.

Streptococcus viridans is a group of commensal (part of the normal flora) streptococcal bacteria found most abundantly in the mouth. Two species, streptococcus mutans and, less commonly, streptococcus sanguinis, are implicated as a cause of dental caries (cavities). Others may also be involved in various mouth infections, and occasionally heart inflammation when introduced to the blood stream. Generally, their pathogenicity is considered low. Homeopathically, Streptococcus viridans is available as a single remedy, but really it is one that consists of multiple similar strains of streptococcus.

Beta-hemolytic (B-hemolytic) Streptococcus
Beta-hemolytic streptococcal species are further classified by alphabetically lettered groupings (A to V, with no I or J), relating to identifying molecules found on the cell walls. You will see these subgroups of beta-hemolytic streptococcus designated by the abbreviations GAS (group A strep), GBS (group B strep), etc. Here, we focus on those groups most commonly used in homeopathy.

Group A streptococcus (GAS)—streptococcus pyogenes is implicated in a large range of both invasive and non-invasive infections. Pharyngitis (strep throat), impetigo, and scarlet fever (the source of scarlatinum) are notable non-invasive infections, while streptococcal toxic shock syndrome, necrotizing fasciitis, pneumonia, and bacteremia are some of the severe invasive infections related to streptococcus pyogenes.

Other diseases that relate to GAS arise as complications of GAS infection, including acute rheumatic fever (caused by cross-reaction of the antibodies used by the body to respond to GAS) and glomerulonephritis (kidney inflammation/infection). Globally, GAS is one of the world's leading infectious causes of death.

In homeopathy, streptococcus pyogenes is synonymous with the remedy Streptococcinum. It is also found in the form of Scarlatinum, although this remedy is created from infected tissue from a patient suffering from scarlet fever, while Streptococcinum is created from lab-isolated streptococcus pyogenes.

Group B streptococcus (GBS)—streptococcus agalactiae is known to cause pneumonia and meningitis (in infants and the elderly), systemic bacteremia, and is implicated in some complications of pregnancy (rupture of membranes and transfer of infection). Women who test for GBS in the 35-37th week of pregnancy are given prophylactic antibiotics to prevent transmission during labor. In homeopathy, Streptococcus agalactiae is available as an individual remedy. It is possible that giving this remedy to pregnant women can help avoid the use of prophylactic antibiotics.

Group C streptococcus (GCS)—streptococcus dysgalactiae (and others) is comprised of multiple strains. The main human-disease causing species is streptococcus dysgalactiae, which is implicated in some pharyngitis and other infections with fever similar to GAS/streptococcus pyogenes. In homeopathy, Streptococcus dysgalactiae is available as an individual remedy.

Technically, many of what were once called group D streptococcus (GDS)—streptococcus faecalis and streptoccocus bovis—have been reclassified to the genus enterococcus. Streptococcus faecalis, useful in homeopathy, is now known as Enterococcus faecalis, or more commonly seen as Enterococcinum. Enterococcus faecalis is a commensal bacterium found in healthy intestinal tracts in humans, but can cause life-threatening infections including endocarditis, bacteremia, urinary tract infections, and meningitis. Enterococcus faecalis has high levels of naturally occurring antibiotic-resistance and is particularly problematic in hospital environments.

Streptococcus bovis is a true group D streptococcus that is commonly found in the alimentary tract of ruminants—cows, sheep, etc. In humans, it is associated with endocarditis and colorectal cancer.

Strep Remedies		
Alpha-Hemolytic Strep	Streptococcus pneumoniae	
	Streptococcus viridans (group of species)	
Beta-Hemolytic Strep	GAS/Streptococcus pyogenes (also called Streptococcinum)	
	GBS/Streptococcus agalactiae	
	GCS/Streptococcus dysgalactiae	
	GDS/Streptococcus faecalis (also called Enterococcinum or Enterococcus faecalis)	
Other/Combos	Streptococcus combo (includes pyogenes, uberis, bovis, and agalactiae species)	
	Streptococcus AB hemolytic (combo of GAS and GBS strains)	
	Streptococcus uberis (a strep strain found in the environment)	

Streptococcus Materia Medica

Our culture's obsessive fear of strep infections manifesting in the ubiquitous throat swab and subsequent and swift prescription of antibiotics is captured by the materia medica of Streptococcinum with its perfectionistic, OCD nature.

Suppressed strep on the mental/emotional level creates a feeling of, "I am negative about myself and attack my sense of self. I suppress my natural feelings because of expectations of how I am supposed to be. I need to be perfect but am not good enough, I am a failure." Many children who were happy-go-lucky, after experiencing chronic strep infections, will start to become much more self-critical. For example, a child who typically has fun playing soccer will start to say, "I am terrible at soccer" and fault themselves over every mistake after chronic strep is treated with antibiotics. Sadly, for many kids, cognitive decline follows chronic strep infection, further exacerbating their OCD nature.

The following materia medica applies generally to the streptococcus remedies, although the majority of it is built upon cases in which Streptococcinum (Streptococcus pyogenes) was the main strep remedy used.

Mental State
- Obsessive Compulsive Disorder (OCD)—lining up things/toys, closing of doors
- OCD throat clearing, OCD handwashing
- Meltdowns, defiance, angry if they don't get it right or their way
- Ritualistic; bedtime rituals to calm fears at night
- Major separation anxiety, meltdown when separated from parent
- Poor handwriting and difficulty with math skills
- Germaphobia
- Perfectionism
- Self-talk, "baby voice" talk and verbal stims
- Age regression
- Tantrums if rituals are disturbed
- Gets angry at the sound of people chewing, breathing, blowing their nose, babies crying, etc.
- General oversensitivity to noise, other stimuli, and touch
- Poor self-esteem, turning away from positive attention
- Putting oneself down with negative self-criticism, self-hate
- Suppressed grief in the family/mother

Physical State
- Tics/twitching and Tourette syndrome; pacing, vocal stims
- Poor fine motor/handwriting
- Excessive thirst, drinking at night and increased urination
- Swollen tonsils and glands, halitosis/bad breath
- Frequent sore throat, sinus infections, upper respiratory infections
- Eye fatigue and photophobia
- Keratosis pilaris/chicken skin
- Thick mucus in the back of throat
- Fever
- Stomach ache with or without vomiting
- Headache
- Throat pain

Health History/Etiology
- History of repeated strep infections in mother or child
- History of autoimmune disease in the family, or rheumatic fever
- History of repeated rounds of antibiotics and steroids, worse after vaccines

- Repeated infections such as ear/sinus infections, dental caries or UTI's
- History of acne treated with antibiotics/strong medications
- History of repeated use of antibiotics
- Underlying Lyme infections, or chronic immune deficiency

Streptococcus Pyogenes (Streptococcinum)
- Tics stem from the face, mouth, or throat
- Stomach pains can be prominent (in Strep faecalis also)
- When there is a history of throat/glandular swelling and sinus infections
- Children having a "teen attitude" towards parents
- Irritability from emotional pressure; will snap and yell when feeling pressured

Streptococcus Pneumoniae (Pneumococcinum)
- Coughing tics, tics involving the chest/breathing
- History of bad coughs/upper respiratory strep infections, breathlessness
- Sinus infections

Streptococcus Faecalis (Enterococcinum)
- When primary issues center around GI system; nausea, anorexia, anal rashes
- Anorexia, loss of appetite
- Red ring on anus, gluteal rashes
- Anger
- Stomach pains can be prominent (Strep pyogenes also)
- Chronic sinus issues, scar tissue in sinuses
- Tics less prominent, but oppositional behavior and confrontational behavior more pronounced

Streptococcus Viridans
- A secondary strep remedy sometimes needed after treatment with one of the major strep remedies (pyogenes, pneumoniae, faecalis)
- When parasites are a concomitant issue

Streptococcus Dysgalactiae (Group C Strep/GCS)
- Group C streptococcus is comprised of multiple strains (Streptococcus dysgalactiae is available as an individual remedy). The main human-disease causing species is Streptococcus dysgalactiae, which is implicated in some pharyngitis and other infections with fever similar to

GAS/strep pyogenes
- Also indicated when skin and eye issues or acne are prominent

Streptococcus Agalactiae (Group B Strep/GBS)
- When there has been infant infection or neonatal transmission of strep or possibly to clear antibiotic suppression of GBS during pregnancy

Scarlatinum
- This nosode is prepared from swabs from the pharynx or squamae (epidermic scales) of scarlet fever patients
- When there is a strong family history of autoimmunity
- Cardiac and circulatory disorders, angina
- Chronic arthritis, joint pains
- Dry skin diseases with red outlines, psoriasis

> DIFFERENTIATING STREPTOCOCCUS REMEDIES
>
> The particular strep remedy can of course be determined based on positive lab test results for a specific strain. If labs are not available, you can also use a form of applied kinesiology (muscle testing) to choose one strain over another. Close attention should be paid to the results of using any one remedy—if the streptococcus picture is a good fit but one strain does not seem to have a strong effect, it may be worth trying other specific strains or one of the combination strep remedies.

Remedies Commonly Given Concurrently with Streptococcus Nosodes

- When grief/sadness is prominent: Nat Mur, Ignatia, Carcinosin, Aurum
- When self-suppression and self-hate are prominent: Thuja, Lac maternum, Carcinosin, Anacardium, Staphysagria, Lac caninum (and other Lac remedies)
- When GI issues and/or gut pains are prominent: Cina, Dioscorea, Euphorbium, Colocynthis
- When rage/tantrums are prominent: Belladonna, Hyoscyamus, Stramonium, Cina, Snake and Spider remedies
- When tics and twitches are prominent: Ignatia, Zincum, Causticum, Tarentula
- When fears and/or panic are prominent: Aconite, Arsenicum, Calcarea carb, Gelsemium
- When behavioral inflexibility/rigidity is prominent: Ferrum met, Cuprum met, Calcarea carb, Kali carb, Calcarea mur, Kali mur
- When poor detoxification ability is prominent: Sulphur, Sulfamilamide

Staphylococcinum/Staph Aureus and MRSA (Bacteria)

The mental/emotional state of Staphylococcinum presents very similar to Streptococcinum, and the primary differentiation are the physical symptoms. The mental state is an overall negative, self-attacking energy and can trigger neurological symptoms such as tics and twitches as well. For Staphylococcinum, the majority of cases are ones where there are boils/pustules/acne, often on the face, thighs, or buttocks areas.

It can also help with suppurating skin wounds that don't heal easily such as crusts around nostrils. This nosode can also help decrease hormonal acne and may coincide with sexual suppression and puberty. It helps with new feelings of shame or disgust around being sexual similar to Staphysagria. There is a separate MRSA (antibiotic resistant staph aureus) nosode available.

Mental/Emotional State
- Self-hate, self-negativity
- Overemotionality
- Shame around sexuality

Physical State
- Fever and chills
- Skin abscess, vesicles, pustules, folliculitis, furuncles
- Impetigo

Klebsiella/Mucotoxinum

Klebsiella is also known as bacterium pneumonia and has also been produced into a nosode called Mucotoxinum. It can be a urinary tract pathogen and also cause pneumonia with sticky, brown or red sputum. Klebsiella also seems to have an impact on GI flora, and has proved useful in kids with very disordered digestion who have a tubercular taint. Klebsiella can cause intense rage and kids can get caught in these cyclical patterns of infections, as described by this mother: "He started Eric on once or twice weekly azithromycin which helped PANDAS a lot but also caused a klebsiella infection of the gut. Klebsiella caused severe rages/aggression beyond anything we had ever seen with PANDAS. I freaked out and stopped all antibiotics cold-turkey and increased probiotics. Over the next 6 weeks klebsiella cleared up, but he got strep during that time of being unprotected. This lead to starting antibiotics again, and several interventions to reduce brain inflammation: steroids, IVIG, spironolactone, LDN (low-dose naltrexone). These did bring down the PANDAS symptoms effectively but left us battling more gut infections (klebsiella, clostridia, yeast)."

Mental/Emotional State
• Rage, aggression, self-abuse

Physical State
• Sinusitis
• Pancreatitis
• Bronchiectasis
• Chronic bronchitis
• Pleuritis
• Disturbed flora from many pharmaceuticals

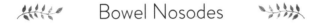 Bowel Nosodes

Bowel nosodes are isolated pathogens that are made into remedies. Some of these remedies were developed over 100 years ago by Edward Bach (the homeopath who created the Bach flower essences). There are thousands of bacteria in our gastrointestinal tract, only a small percentage are considered pathogenic.

Below is a table of general keynotes for common nosodes (bacterial, protozoal, and fungal) that can help heal GI flora:

Nosodes for GI Flora	
Bacillus No 10.	Bach nosode. Anxious, active, irritable, depressed. Cannot digest eggs and fat, warts, lipomas. Headache above left eye.
Bacillus No 7/ Citrobacter	Bach nosode. Mental and physical fatigue, rheumatism, low blood pressure. Brain abscess. Like Kali carb, Iodum.
Candida albicans	Giddy, sillly behaviors. Sugar cravings. Spacey and clumsy. Bloating and gassy. Thirst and frequent urination/eneuresis.

Nosodes for GI Flora	
Candida parapalosis	Like Candida alb (above) but more irritable and tantrums if opposed. Mixing up words. Thrush.
Clostridium difficile	Green, foul-smelling stools. Self abuse. Strong history of antibiotics.
Colibacillinum / E coli	Travellers or infantile diarrhea, hemorrhagic colitis. Strong history of antibiotics. Irresolution. Loss of memory.
Dysentary co/ Shigella	Bach nosode. Anticipatory nervous tension, hypersensitive to criticism, shyness. Like Arsenicum album.
Entamoeba histolytica	Loose stools, stomach pain, stomach cramping.
Enterococcinum (Strep faecalis)	Diarrhea, loss of appetite, stomach pains, allergic, hypotension, weary. Similar to Streptococcinum but gut related.
Faecalis	Bach nosode. Irritable and impatient, retreat from loved ones, like Sepia.
Gaertner	Bach nosode. Overactive brain, undernourished body, chews nails, malnutrition, poor fat digestion. History of antibiotics. Like Silica.
Giardia	Cramping, foul smelling stools, gas, fatigue, dehydration, heartburn, indigestion.
H pylori	Stomach aches, stomach acidity, heartburn, ulcers.
Hep B vacc / Hepatitis	Jaundice, anorexia, nausea, bloating, poor fat digestion, floating stools, postural hypotension
Morgan bach	Bach nosode. Congestion of lungs, skin, head, constipation, gall stones, etc. Introspective, depressive.
Morgan gaertner	Bach nosode. Irritable, tense, fears crowds. Acute inflammation of kidney or gallbladder. Like Lycopodium.

Nosodes for GI Flora	
Morgan pure	Bach nosode. Marked skin eruption, disturbance of liver, gall stones. Like Sulphur.
Mutabile	Bach nosode. Strong changeability of symptoms. Food allergies. Like Pulsatilla.
Parasite nosodes	(See section on parasites.)
Poly bowel nosode	All the Bach nosodes in combination.
Poly bowel plus	All the Bach nosodes plus enzymes and candida nosode. Created by Ton Jansen.
Proteus Bach nosode	Suddenness of all complaints, outbursts of temper, lies on floor and kicks, screams. Brain storm. Like Chlorum.
Pyrogenium	Nosode from rotting meat. Putrefaction in GI. Sharp pains in GI that radiate to the head causing headaches.
Salmonella	Not part of normal human flora. Gastroenteritis/food poisoning. Nausea.
Sycotic co	Bach nosode. Nervous irritability, irritation of whole digestive tract, joints, lungs. Desires limelight, like Thuja, Hyoscyamus or Veratrum.
Torula Bakers yeast	Allergies, Crohn's disease. Worse bread. Irritable, nervous, workaholic, worn out. Gassy.

Most bowel nosodes have a mental/emotional state described as: irritable, tense, anxious and depressed, and prone to outbursts, which can make it hard to differentiate among them, although there are some particular keynotes for each. Intuitive testing and lab testing can also aid with a decision to prescribe a homeopathic bowel nosode.

Bowel nosodes can be particularly helpful when there is a miasm of strong antibiotic use in the family. Clearing antibiotics with a homeopathic remedy such as Poly antibiotic, developed by European pharmacies such as Helios or Hahnemann Apotheck, can be helpful as well (see Chapter 9).

Clostridia Difficile

Clostridia difficile (C. diff) commonly affects people after the use of antibiotics. Each year in the United States, about a half million people get sick from C. diff, and in recent years, these infections have become more frequent, severe, and difficult to treat. Recurrent C. diff infections are also on the rise.[2] Many complex children will have clostridia flagged on lab tests, but clinical symptoms and a worsening after antibiotics can also lead to a prescription of the clostridia nosode.

Mental State
- Significant anger and aggression that is particularly self-injurious
- Wanting to wear hooded sweatshirts, wrap up head, cover the ears
- Hitting themselves in the head or face to the point of bruising
- Pinching themselves to the point of bruising
- Going off on their own—wanting isolation, crouching up in isolation
- Grey complexion
- Threatening violence, no remorse
- Demanding that parents should be doing things for them and if not there is internal resentment
- Instigating fights; purposely making other people upset and finding humor or satisfaction in it; wanting that negative reaction and then laughing about it
- Self hate

Physical State
- Worsened bowel movements and behavioral issues after antibiotic or antifungal use
- History of long-term diarrhea; diarrhea with blood and mucous
- Extremely bad smelling stools and gas—makes you vacate the building
- Discolored/green stools, mushy or frothy stools
- Sensory seeking like jumping intensely on a trampoline
- History of prolonged hospital stays in child or someone in the family

Other Remedies That Coincide with Clostridia
- All other gut nosodes, particularly strep
- Plant remedies for gut issues/pain/parasites like Cina, Disocorea, Euphrobium, etc.
- Remedies for suppressed or self-hating states like Carcinosin, Ignatia, Anacardium, Thuja

Mycoplasma

Mycoplasma pneumoniae is a type of "atypical" bacteria that commonly causes mild infections of the respiratory system. Pneumonia caused by mycopasma pneumoniae is sometimes referred to as "walking pneumonia" since symptoms tend to be milder than pneumonia caused by other germs. It is a common coinfection found in many PANDAS/Lyme cases and has a subtle picture of depression, weepiness, and desire to isolate.

Mental State
• Puts up walls
• Going within themselves; a quieter and withdrawn sense of self
• Becomes distant from the other, communication goes down
• May state they are suicidal, but it doesn't seem serious

Physical State
• Fever
• Dry cough
• Headache
• Chills
• Heavy sweating
• Scratchy sore throat
• Sore trachea (the large airway between the mouth and the lungs)
• Sore chest

Other Remedies that Coincide with Mycoplasma
• Natrum mur
• Carcinosin
• Pulsatilla

Lung-Associated Nosodes	
Pertussinum (whooping cough)	Dry spasmodic cough. Asthma. Restlessness. Anorexia. Cough causing vomiting. Histamine sensitivity.
Tuberculinum avis (source chicken)	Similar to Tuberculinum bov. Great for acute bronchitis in children, acts on lung apices.

Lung-Associated Nosodes	
Tuberculinum bovinum (source cow)	Classic tuberculinum preparation. Defiance, wanderlust, restlessness, hyperactivity, changeability, weak immunity, allergies, worse wet weather.
Mycoplasma pneumoniae	Walking pneumonia. Fatigued, depressive, isolating, weak lungs.
Strep pneumonia	Anger, OCD, oppositional (strep symptoms) with breathlessness, history of upper respiratory infections.
Mucotoxinum/ Klebsiella	Rage, tantrums. Sinusitis. Indigestion after sour food. Pancreatitis. Bronchitis.
Medorrhinum/ Gonorrhea	Precocious, fearless, angry and sensitive children, prone to chronic infection, asthma, green discharges.
Bacillinum (Tubercular lung tissue)	Essentially the same as Tuberculinum bov. Mentally precocious, weak physically. Ringworm. Teeth grinding.

Viruses

Children often have many unresolved chronic viral infections due to weakened immune systems and suppressive medical treatments, leading to symptoms such as fatigue, tics, stimming, anxiety, depression, and decreased cognitive abilities. Viral nosodes are particularly helpful in clearing up and unsuppressing these infections.

Homeopathy has a proven history of success in the treatment of epidemic viral infection in both humans and animals:

- Around the First World War, Spanish flu was rampant and 30% of those who fell ill succumbed despite regular treatment. During this epidemic, 26,795 sick people were treated homeopathically instead of conventionally, and in this group only 1.05% died.[3]
- During the epidemic of cattle plague in 1866-1867, the Dutch government used the services of a Belgian homeopath. Before homeopathic

help, 75-85% of the cattle died; with the aid of homeopathy the number dropped to 10%.[4]

Acute Versus Chronic Viral Infections

Many neuro-immune kids no longer mount acute reactions to viral infections, meaning they don't develop a fever, runny nose, sore throat, cough, or malaise. Instead of the body working through and expelling the virus as it was designed to do the virus does not resolve and becomes chronic, resulting in long-term ill effects. When encountered with a viral infection, these children have more neurological symptoms such as increased irritability, sensory sensitivity, tics, and stimming. In homeopathic terminology this etiological state is often referred to as "never been well since x." Unresolved infectious states can even be passed through the generations from parent (mother or father) to child. When a child with immune dysfunction starts experiencing more physical symptoms of colds and flus it is considered a positive sign of the immune system functioning normally.

Acute Viral Infection Treatment

Nosodes can be used at the very onset of an infection to get the body to respond to the infectious state more effectively. The use of the remedy Oscillococcinum for the flu is well known for helping people stave off the infection when taken at the first sign of illness. However, as the infectious state peaks, the homeopathic remedy to bring about a cure can also be a plant or mineral remedy. Well known remedies for treating the following infections in their acute stages include:

- Chickenpox/Varicella Zoster: Antimonium crud, Mercurius, Rhus tox, Stramonium
- Meningitis: Aconite, Apis, Belladonna, Bryonia
- Pneumonia: Apis, Bryonia, Ferrum met, Phosphorus
- Rotavirus/stomach flu: Arsenicum, Phosphorus, Podophyllum, Veratrum album

A healthy constitution has the capacity to fight off the majority of viral infections. Therefore, providing the best constitutional homeopathic treatment is often all that is needed for acute infections.

Chronic Viral Infection Treatment

Immuno-deficient people who have many low-level viral infections often do well with constitutional treatment using remedies that are well known for treating the flu, such as Arsenicum album, Bryonia, Eupatorium perf, Gelsemium, Nux vomica, China off, Natrum mur, Rhus tox, and Sulphur. The two most common remedies I give in conjunction with clearing viral infections are Carcinosin and Thuja, which help strengthen the immune response to fully clear the virus and can be extremely useful for chronic fatigue associated with viral infections. There are also remedies for boosting a weak and slow-responding immune system in a child who has constantly recurring viral infections with low-level symptoms like coughs that never seem to clear, such as Kali carb, Hepar sulph, or Calcarea carb.

In addition to constitutional treatment, the use of nosodes for chronic treatment can be useful in the following situations:

- A child tests positive for a certain virus and it matches with the clinical presentation of the child
- The inheritance of a viral infection from the parents via neonatal transmission
- History of suppressing the infection with pharmaceutical treatment
- The sequelae of vaccines which often seem to create a picture of suppressed viral infection deep in the nervous system
- History of a weak and depleted immune system, or genetically weak immunity such as a diagnosis of CVID
- When constitutional treatment does not work well
- To antidote the lingering effects of acute infections such as fatigue and depression
- When the whole of the patient is worse ever since a certain infection

Treating chronic viral infections with nosodes can lead to improvement in energy levels, clarity, provide a greater sense of calm, and lead to cognitive gains. For example, parents have told me that their child gets new words when they do the Varicella clear, or that their child is more calm and focused when they do the Influenza clear.

The Energy of Viruses

The excessive "doing" energy of our mainstream culture tips us out of balance into viral overload. The excessive media influence in our lives in particular seems to have a toxifying viral effect on us—I often see people with many chronic viral infections who are addicted to media and can't put down their cell phones or turn off the news. When the body finally succumbs to a viral infection, our bodies ask us to crawl into bed, shut down, and rest. Shifting between being active and doing nothing is part of the cyclical nature of life, and the attempt to vaccinate viruses so we can keep working, keep making money, keep our kids in school, and keep the economy going is slowly breaking down the immunity of our bodies.

Perhaps there is societal fear of viral infections because for centuries a simple common cold could kill someone and bring about infant mortality. However, improvements in nutrition, hygiene, and our standard of living, as well as knowledge of natural medicine, will sufficiently support our bodies to fight off the vast majority of viral infections. Our fear of illness and the subsequent suppression of viruses via vaccination is creating a whole other subset of chronic issues that modern medicine does not have answers for. Natural treatment for viral infections include hot baths to bring on an induced fever/sweat, taking more antioxidants (Vitamin A, C, Zinc, etc.), increasing electrolytes, bedrest, and reduced sugar and dairy consumption.

People with chronic viral infections often have the following patterns of behaviors:

- Overdoing to meet the expectations of others
- Going…going…going…burn out
- Taking in too much information—information overload—body is wound up and wired
- Information is scattered and disorganized in the head
- Don't know what information to keep and what to throw out
- Then like a computer, we crash; need to be shut down and be cleaned out
- Not taking care of yourself to meet other people's expectations
- Taking on a thought/behavior that is not authentically yours
- Kids enrolled in too many sports and activities to "stay busy" or impress others, and getting rundown as a result

These behavioral patterns are prominent themes in Carcinosin, which also happens to be a great remedy for viral infection. The desire to fit in and meet other people's expectations is similar to Thuja ("what will people think of me"), or Calcarea carb ("I am anxious to do everything right so I will fit in").

Mental Symptoms of Viruses
- Boisterous and talkative, sassy, precocious, in your face
- Wound up, can be easily brought to tears
- Repetitive thoughts (monomania), OCD, desire for perfection
- ADHD—unable to stick to one activity for long
- Hyperlexic, dyslexic
- Can take in a lot of information, memorize a lot of facts
- Neurotically anxious and sense of overwhelm
- Intrusive thoughts, such as to lick things
- Masturbation, sexual thoughts
- Vocal stimming, iPad stimming, scripting, watching movies over and over, obsessive interests —stuck on certain toys, movies, and behaviors; ritualistic
- Increased rigidity

  Alternating with:
  - Foggy thinking and spaced out, heavy head
  - Wiped out, exhausted, laid out, "leave me alone"
  - Depressed, don't want to leave the house
  - Flat, apathetic

Physical Symptoms of Viruses
- Mouth ulcers/cold sores/canker sores, sometimes cyclical
- Wound up, hard to relax, hard to fall asleep
- Sneezing with no cold or cough
- Photophobia
- Easily fatigued
- Frequent urination—viruses seem to detox through urine
- Bed wetting
- Insomnia—brain constantly going, can't turn it off
- Vaginal discharges
- Tingling sensations
- Physically hyperactive, restless
- Restless legs
- Achy muscles in the back and legs
- Bone ache
- Limping
- Tics
- Unable to sit in one place to eat

- Visual stimming
- Transient rashes
- Intermittent fevers
- Enlarged lymph nodes
- Low white blood cell counts
- Increased noise sensitivity; tinnitus

Viral Nosodes	
Remedy Name	*Source/Type*
AIDS	Retrovirus
Coxsackie virus	Picornaviridae
Cytomegalovirus	CMV
Dengue fever	Flaviviridae
Hepatitis A	Picornaviridae
Hepatitis A + B nosode comb.	
Hepatitis B	Hepadnaviridae
Hepatitis C	Flaviviridae
Herpes progenitalis	Genital herpes
Herpes simplex	Mouth herpes
Herpes zoster nosode	Herpes zoster
HHV 1 and 2 nosode	Herpesviridae
HHV 4	Epstein-Barr/Mono
HHV 5	CMV
HHV 6	Roseolovirus
Influenzinum	Orthomyxoviridae
Lyssinum/Hydrophobinum	Rabies, dog saliva
Malandrium	Grease of horse
Measles/Morbillinum	Paramyxoviridae
Molluscum contagiosum	Water warts
Mononucleosis	Epstein-Barr
Oscillococcinum	Infected duck liver
Parvovirus	Parvoviridae
Poliovirus	Picornaviridae
Psorinum	Scabies itch
Rotovirus	GI virus

Viral Nosodes	
Rubella nosode	German measles
Vaccinium	Poxviridae
Varicella nosode	Chicken pox
Variolinum	Small pox
Virionum	Retroviridae

Key Viral Remedies

Influenzinum

The most commonly used and useful viral remedy is Influenzinum, which can be used for prophylaxis of the flu as well as to help heal from any lingering effects of it such as fatigue. This remedy should be in everyone's medicine chest. A similar remedy, Oscillococcinum (Anas barbariae), is a proprietary remedy manufactured by Boiron that is well known and well distributed. It is a 200C potentized preparation of duck liver and heart that carries infectious agents known to carry the flu. When taken at first onset it is known to either stave off or reduce the period and severity of the flu. It sells $15 million per year in the US and also sells widely in Europe. I tend to use these two remedies interchangeably.

There are several different flu prevention dosing protocols. I generally use Influenzinum 30C and find it very effective.

- Dissolve 1 or 2 pellets in your or your child's mouth once a week for 4 weeks, and then repeat 3 weeks later.
- Dissolve pellets in 1-2 oz. of water and take one teaspoon once per week for 4 weeks, and then repeat 3 weeks later.
- If you feel the onset of the flu: put 1 pellet in one tablespoon of water and take 1 drop under the tongue every 20 minutes for 2 -2 ½ hours. Then continue to take 2 drops twice a day for a week.

Influenzinum is also a key remedy for treating chronic viral infections. Instead of developing average cold symptoms when exposed, these kids can get irritable, develop tics, or act on edge when their body is struggling with a virus. This remedy can really take the edge off their irritability and malaise, and can even reduce stimming. It can be a good remedy to try when a child is generally seeming "viral" or an active virus is being passed around the family.

Coxsackie

Coxsackie is an enterovirus that lives in the GI tract and is responsible for hand foot and mouth disease with symptoms of painful blisters on the throat, mouth, hands, and soles. This infection seems to be growing in prevalence in both children and adults.[6] While self-limited, it can result in complications such as meningitis or viral heart disease. This viral infection shows that while we can rid society of one group of viral infections, other infections like coxsackie will come in to take their place, perhaps because we need viral infections to play a role in developing our immune systems.

In neuroimmune cases, coxsackie frequently shows up positive in viral titers. I have not seen an obvious and strong response to this nosode when prescribed to children with high viral titers for coxsackie, although it seems to help a bit in reduction of tics. Constitutional prescribing when coxsackie is present seems to suffice in clearing this virus. Several acute coxsackie infections I have seen resulted in extreme skin sensitivity and responded well to China off. Other remedies to treat acute coxsackie infections are ones well known for the flu, including Rhus tox, Arnica, and Bryonia.

Herpes Strains

Remedies from the herpes strains include Cytomegalovirus (CMV), Epstein-Barr Virus (EBV), Herpes simplex, and Herpes zoster or Varicella. A unique characteristic of herpes viruses is their ability to become latent in their hosts and they can become activated at any time, such as herpes simplex cold sores coming out at the same time as an influenza infection. In Western medicine these infections are treated via antiviral medications such as Valtrex; varicella vaccines are also given.

Most people encounter these viruses at some point in life and are subsequently lifetime carriers of them. For immunocompromised individuals, herpes infections can seriously contribute to chronic fatigue. Dosing nosodes such as CMV or EBV seem to help with improvements in energy levels. Nosode remedies exist for the following:

- HSV-1: primarily causes oral herpes, and is generally responsible for cold sores and fever blisters around the mouth and on the face, especially when immunocompromised.
- HSV-2: primarily causes genital herpes, and is generally responsible for genital herpes outbreaks. Requires intimate contact for transmission.
- Varicella causes chicken pox (in children) and shingles (usually in adults). It is highly contagious and causes a vesicular rash and nerve

sensitivity. It is now regularly vaccinated against, although the vaccine's effectiveness lasts for 10-20 years and booster shots are required. I have seen a handful of pediatric cases who received the varicella vaccine get cognitive and speech gains following a clear of either the Varicella nosode or the varicella vaccine nosode. This suggests that there is the possibility of an unrecognized effect of this vaccine or virus on the speech centers of the brain.

- CMV causes enlarged spleen, rash, fever, malaise, sore throat and central nervous system complications. Its presentation is very similar to the Epstein-Barr virus, for which it is commonly a concomitant infection. According to Frans Vermeulen, "About 10% of infants with congenital CMV infection are symptomatic at birth; manifestations include intrauterine growth retardation, prematurity, microcephaly, jaundice, petechiae, hepatosplenomegaly, periventricular calcifications, chorioretinitis, and pneumonitis. Symptomatic newborns have a mortality rate of up to 30% and more than 90% of the survivors have neurologic impairments including hearing loss, mental retardation, and visual disturbance."[7]

- EBV causes classic mononucleosis and enlarged lymph glands, and is transmitted via intimate contact (particularly via exchange of saliva). Young adults in college most frequently manifest acute symptoms, whereas in children who are infected it causes little or no illness. Most people become infected with this at some point in their lives and ideally it resolves within 1-2 months; however it will remain dormant in the body and can reactivate. It is one of many diseases listed as contributing to chronic fatigue.

- HHV6 is associated with roseola and commonly comes up positive in titer tests in PANDAS/PANS and ASD children. Acute infection with HHV6 will result in a fever, rash, swollen lymph nodes, and sore throat. I have seen only subtle shifts when clearing this

> CLINICAL STUDY ON INFLUENZINUM
>
> In 1998 the French Society of Homeopathy conducted a survey of 23 homeopathic doctors concerning their use of Influenzinum for the prevention of the flu (Coulamy, 1998). The survey included use of Influenzinum over a 10-year period (1987-1998) in 453 patients. Results of the survey were remarkable. In approximately 90 percent of the cases no instances of the flu occurred when Influenzinum was used preventively for all ages 2 and older. In the survey, no side effects were noted in 97% of the cases, while 3% experienced mild nasal discharge. Influenzinum has been used throughout the world by millions of people for decades.[8]

virus with the HHV6 nosode and its possible that most children who have positive titers for this infection are effectively fighting it off for the most part.

Vaccininum

This is a nosode created from cowpox, a virus used by the founder of vaccines, Edward Jenner, to create the first ever vaccine for smallpox. It is no longer administered because smallpox is no longer epidemic. However, I have found this an invaluable remedy for clearing what seems to be the miasm of deeply rooted viral infections that are undiagnosable. And indeed, perhaps through taking it, we are clearing an imprint of the cowpox vaccine that our ancestors received.

Materia medica lists this remedy as useful for low white blood cell counts, other viral infections like herpes, neuralgias, skin eruptions, general malaise, restlessness, a tired-all-over feeling with a need to stretch (a sensation common to chronic viral infection), scars, and whooping cough.

Lyssinum (Hydrophobinum or Rabies)

The nosode of rabies falls under two homeopathic names, Lyssinum or Hydrophobinum, and I am usually cautious when telling people they are getting this remedy because it elicits fearful thoughts of brain-infected, saliva dripping animals. This is not a remedy I have ever given to someone who actually had rabies. But I have given it to a good handful of ASD children at later stages of treatment and it seemed to help with a certain level of brain disorganization, allowing for more executive thinking and linear patterns of expression.

The materia medica of this remedy can seem extreme, with fear of running water, striking, hitting, and convulsions. I have not seen a case with these specificities, however, I have had two cases of people who needed this remedy grasp the hair on their head and with eyes wide open say "I feel like I am going CRAZY!!" These were both women who were highly anxious, empathic, and even psychic and felt totally disorganized in their thinking—much like Carcinosin. In one case the woman also needed Lac caninum (dog milk), which was an interesting overlap since all dogs are vaccinated for rabies. In another case it helped recover a completely bedbound person with chronic Lyme. The remedy may also help with a sore back, sore abdomen, headaches, diarrhea, and difficulty swallowing.

Hepatitis B

I generally dose the Hepatitis B vaccine clear and rarely dose these nosodes directly unless there was a worsening after an obvious infection with hepatitis, which I have only seen once in a family who contracted it while in India. There are also nosodes of Hepatitis A and C, which are rarely encountered although some children are vaccinated against hepatitis A as well.

That being said, I employ a Hepatitis B clear when there are obvious liver issues following vaccination such as floating stools or jaundice. One woman who cleared the hepatitis B vaccine saw her blood sugar issues, extreme fatigue, and heart palpitations disappear. The feeling of blacking out from postural hypotension or low blood sugar also seems related to the hepatitis B vaccine.

Morbillinum

This is the measles nosode and we might see an increase in its prescribing these days with the return of epidemic measles. A few doses of it in high potency (in 200C and 10M) can be taken as a prophylactic against infection (see section on homeoprophylaxis). It can also be given to clear up after-effects of an infection.

I have given this nosode to some ASD children who got the MMR vaccine and seemed very loaded down with viral infections. Morbillinum has a peculiar keynote, "fear of the sea," which I once saw in an ASD child who refused to go near the ocean and the remedy actually did clear that fear up! The materia medica of this remedy also lists it as useful in cases of weak eyes, and eye symptoms such as conjunctivitis or eye pus (the MMR nosode clear also seems to help with children who have eye stimming symptoms). May also help with poor weight gain, seizures, mental dullness, swollen glands, ear infections, irritated throat, etc.

AIDS

I have given this remedy only two or three times to the children of parents who were extremely promiscuous, to the level of prostitution. In one of the cases it cleared up Tourette syndrome in the child, who had also been sexually abused by a parent. In another case it was for a child who was adopted, extremely psychic, and had a lot of strong emotionality. This fits some of the materia medica of this remedy which is listed as "Desire for extravagance, youth, beauty; shameless behavior; poor boundaries; intense emotionality—easily crying, feels forsaken, discouraged; sympathetic, empathetic, open alternating with hard-hearted and irritable behavior; desires solitude, to live apart from society in a beautiful home."

Molluscum Contagiosum

Molluscum contagiosum is in the pox family of viruses and is an infection of the skin characterized by small, smooth, painless pink nodules with a central depression that can give off a milky fluid when squeezed. It is generally a mild infection treated in the mainstream by topical therapies.

I have only given this nosode once in a PANDAS case who had molluscum warts on his knee, and it helped to clear up some facial tics. Constitutional remedies such as Natrum mur have successfully cleared up other cases of this infection in children.

Variolinum

This is the nosode of smallpox. It can help to clear up deeply embedded viral infections, similar to Vaccininum. The materia medica of Variolinum differs from Vaccininum in that it fits a presentation that is more intensely fearful, with great fear of death causing much excitement. It can also be useful for aching in the legs, excruciating backache, and to help clear up shingles.

HPV

Human Papillomavirus (HPV) is considered a sexually transmitted infection that is generally harmless but can, in some cases, contribute to cancer or genital warts. It is now routinely vaccinated against in teenagers, both male and female, and I am giving this remedy only as the vaccine clear nosode thus far. Adverse symptoms that occur following the HPV vaccine include complex regional pain syndrome (CRPS), postural orthostatic tachycardia syndrome (POTS), and autoimmune disorders.

The handful of HPV vaccine damage cases I have seen have been devastating, with extreme mental effects such as suicidal depression, bipolar disorder, severely debilitating migraine headaches, encephalopathy, and regression of an average teenager into autistic-like behaviors. These cases all needed constitutional treatment and an opening up of detoxification channels as well.

Fungus

Fungal and mold sensitivity is perhaps the second most common "new" miasm, after the strep miasm, that is commonplace in complex kids, possibly because of the onslaught of antibiotics in our culture which has changed our inner terrain. Fungal or yeast overgrowth is responsible for a broad range of reactions including:

- Every day low grade allergies and sneezing
- Anaphylactic allergies (often to foods containing molds)
- Spaciness, out-of-body behaviors, cognitive impairment
- Loss of appetite
- Neurological inflammation causing tics/twitches

An environmental reason for what seems to be a rise in mold sensitivity are post-industrial building techniques using methods and products that make buildings more susceptible to mold deterioration. Like a dark shadow, this deterioration is often hidden beneath tiles and paint and works its way below the surface in human hosts as well. It's not uncommon for families to leave everything behind and move when their house is troubled with mold. This fleeing behavior is reflective of a deep connection between the tubercular miasm and mold. Tubercular people with their poor immune boundaries tend to get mold/fungal/ringworm infections easily and it further exacerbates their inner restlessness and desire to move.

The overall themes for fungal remedies confirms this tubercular overlap: "Desires exploration, expansion, extension, colonization, invasion, lack boundaries, constant activity, nothing ventured, nothing gained." Many of the explorers of the Americas and its west coast were people suffering from tuberculosis as well as poor living conditions in east coast cities where they were likely suffering from mold toxicity.

Fungal Remedies	
Agaricus (amanita mushroom)	Excitable, ecstatic, fearless, too open, delusional, anxious. Twitching/tics, allergies.
Aspergillus (black musty mold)	Skin, lung, ear, and sinus infection. Facial swelling and redness reaction to mold.
Blastomyces	Most cases are in Southeast USA, dogs can be a vector. Dry hacking cough, looks like tuberculosis.

Fungal Remedies	
Boletus (white agaric)	Gloomy, irritated, profuse perspiration at night. Aching liver and cutting pains in abdomen.
Bovista (puffball fungi)	Distended (puffiness). Greatly sensitive, takes offense. Contains aluminum and has crossover symptoms with Alumina.
Candida albicans	Giddy, silly, spacey, bloated, increased thirst, eneuresis, thrush.
Candida auris	Drug-resistant form of candida recently discovered in hospitals.
Candida parapalosis	Like Candida albicans but more irritable and reactive if opposed. Thrush fungus.
Cryptococcus neoformans	CNS/brain/meningitis affinity, inappropriate speech/dress. Bird vector. AIDS coinfection.
Histoplasma	From bird/bat droppings. AIDS coinfection. May be asymptomatic, or lung symptoms that resemble tuberculosis.
Lentinula (Shiitake mushroom)	Sense of responsibility in neck/shoulders. Pulled from all directions at once. Determined. Uncoordinated.
Mixed moulds	Alternaria alternata, Aspergillus niger, Aspergillus fumigatus, Fusarium sap, Merulius lacrymans, Mucor mucedo, Penicillin, Rhizopus nigricans, Sporobolomyces, Tricophyton rubrum, Ustilago, Cladosporium herbarum
Mucor mucedo (black pinmould)	Chronic sinusitis, otitis, growths in nasopharynx, phlegm and growth of tonsils. Asthma, anemia.
Penicillinum (drug derived from mold)	History of antibiotic use. Allergies. Fatigue. Loose stools.
Ringworm / Trichophyton	Tinea infection. Period of hope alternating with periods of giving up. Worse consolation.
Secale cornutum	Burning and heat, hot feet. Bloody noses, gushes of blood, clumsy, awkward.

Fungal Remedies	
Solanum tuberosum aegrotans	Fungi from the rotten potato. Anal/rectal prolapse. Bad temper.
Stachybotrys (toxic black mold)	Allergies. Acute idiopathic pulmonary hemorrhage.
Tree fungus	Unknown specifics, from Helios.
Yeast/Torula	Weary and workaholic. Bloating/gassy. Cradle cap/dandruff.

Candida

Candida albicans, the most common candida species in humans, is one of the most important pathogenic fungi. It can reside for a long time without causing symptoms of disease and is found as a commensal on skin and mucosa in up to 70% of the human population. Its pathogenicity can emerge when alterations in the host environment (such as antibiotic abuse, hormonal imbalance, poor nutrition, immunosuppression, and surgeries) lead to activation of virulence. Candida is characterized by the ability to take on many forms (polymorphism), of which the most important in the intestines are the yeast-like state (non-invasive and sugar-fermenting) and the fungal state (long, root-like structures that penetrate the mucosa). The general term for the pathogenic states arising from candida is candidiasis, which can occur in many distinct locations on and within the body.

A quote from a parent whose female child had chronic yeast problems is as follows: "This is what yeast causes for her: 1) Constant bloating gas and tummy upset. 2) Severe appetite issues—used to have big appetite because of yeast; gave her antifungals, which controlled the issue of laughter, giggling and yeast issues, but aggravated her bad appetite issues; she is a very picky eater—feeding her is a struggle on a daily basis. 3) Tiptoes, skips, doesn't walk properly;

> ### Mixed Mold
>
> The Mixed mold remedy (sold by Helios pharmacy and others) is very useful for clearing mold sensitivities and mold allergies that create a broad range of physical symptoms including asthma, allergies, headaches, sinusitis, tinnitus, joint pain, and fatigue. Mental symptoms can include irritability, spaciness, and mood swings (from giggly/spastic to crying). The remedy contains the following mix: Alternaria alternata, Aspergillus niger, Aspergillus fumigatus, Fusarium sap., Merulius lacrymans, Mucor mucedo, Penicillin, Rhizopus nigricans, Sporobolomyces, Tricophyton rubrum, Ustilago, and Cladosporium herbarum.

cognition is very bad—it's getting slightly better but still very low for an 8-year-old. 4) Sleeping issues, can't sleep without melatonin. 5) Giggles a lot when happy and overly excited, like a drunk person; easily excited, then can't control it, doesn't know how to get herself back, rolling, laughing. The cycle of the giggling is the yeast, and it will go away with the antifungal—grapefruit seed, oregano extract. She will go back to her nongiggling self."

Although candida albicans is the most frequent cause of candidiasis, there are a growing number of cases resulting from non-albicans candida (NAC). Those species of highest clinical importance are: Candida glabrata, Candida tropicalis, Candida parapsilosis, and Candida krusei. Less prominent are: Candida guilliermondii, Candida lusitaniae, Candida kefyr, Candida famata, Candida inconspicua, Candida rugosa, Candida dubliniensis, and Candida norvegensis.

There are more than 20 other species that have also been isolated in clinical settings, but their occurrence is very low. Overall, NAC species implicated in serious systemic infections have risen significantly over the last decades, and may now account for up to 65% of incidents. NAC species do exhibit significant ranges of distribution depending on location. In North America, candida parapsilosis and candida glabrata are the most common.

The most available homeopathic forms of candida are Candida albicans and Candida parapsilosis. Generally, these remedies are the same, while Parapsilosis seems to be the more emotionally explosive and Albicans the spacier of the two. Keep Parapsilosis or other species in mind as remedy choices if Albicans fails to produce the expected effect.

There are also other remedies derived from related fungi that can be considered, such as Torula cerevisiae (brewer's/baker's yeast). Overall, fungi comprise a very large kingdom that is under-represented in the homeopathic materia medica. Learning to use those that are available is particularly important in immune-compromised patient groups.

In clinical presentation, candida infections fall under two major types: candidiasis of the skin and mucosa (cutaneous, chronic mucocutaneous, thrush, vulvovaginitis, peri-anal, etc.), and systemic (invasive) candidiasis (perotinitis, bone and joint, meningitis and other CNS, urinary, biliary, cardiac, pneumonia, hepatosplenic, pancreatic, etc.).

Mental Symptoms and Behavior Indicating Candida Albicans
• Giggling & Silliness
• Drunken or drugged behavior

- Fogginess/brain fog/spaced out/poor concentration
- Masturbation or playing with genitals
- Unhappy, whining, dissatisfied, hard to please
- "Bull in a china cabinet"
- History of long term antibiotic use in the child or the mother
- Strong sugar and carb cravings
- Flapping
- Toe walking
- Spin in circles, looking out sides of the eyes
- Spinning after carb ingestion
- Head butting, head dragging, pushing feet into people's bodies
- Need for weight/deep pressure
- May hit someone and then crack up laughing
- Chewing on things or finger nails

Physical Symptoms Indicating Candida Albicans
- Night waking (sometimes with laughter)
- Bed wetting
- Pimples on bottom
- White coated tongue
- Nasal congestion/cough/ wheezing
- Itchy genitals, discharge genitals
- Puffiness under eyes
- Itchy skin, white spots on skin
- Cradle cap, dandruff
- Teeth grinding
- Chemical sensitivity, spaced out around chemicals
- Ataxia
- Heavy metal toxicity
- Bloating
- White matter/coating on stools or yellowish colored stools
- Fluffy floating stools
- Cramping
- Cold sores
- Constipation
- Bulky stools
- Gurgling
- Hiccups
- Eczema patches that itch; acne and pimples

- Food allergies, worse carbs/sugars
- Light sensitivity
- White tongue
- High-pitched screaming

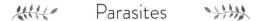 Parasites

Parasites and parasitism may be one of the most under-explored areas of biology. While scientists do not know how many species of parasites exist, they have made the extraordinary estimate that there are four times as many parasite species as there are free-living species. In other words, parasites account for the vast majority of earth's species.

To begin to visualize their extent, consider that more than 1.4 billion people harbor the intestinal roundworm ascaris lumbricoides, 1.3 billion carry intestinal hookworms, and 1 billion have whipworm. Like bacteria and viruses, parasites are a ubiquitous part of the fabric of life on this planet. There is nothing rare about them, though many arguments for unusual and peculiar could be made!

Of course, many bacteria and viruses could themselves fit modern definitions of a parasite. In biology, a broad definition of parasitism is "a non-mutual symbiotic relationship between species, where one species, the parasite, benefits at the expense of the other, the host." Thus parasites can include everything from the helminths (macroparasites such as round-worms and tapeworms) to protozoa, bacteria, viruses, and even plants (such as mistletoe), fungi (such as cordyceps species), and animals (such as lamprey).

Parasites do not typically kill their hosts, but rather reduce their bio-logical fitness through various means such as inhibiting reproductive ability or exploiting host resources necessary for survival (food, water, heat, etc.). Overall, parasites are related to each other via a similar life/survival strat-egy rather than any biological cohesion as species, though large groups of related parasitic species such as intestinal worms certainly exist. This is a conflict poorly addressed in biology, but an interesting one in homeopathy. After all, which pair is more similar, a person who needs Natrum mur and a person who needs Sulphur, or a person and a dog who both need Pulsatilla?

Keep in mind when considering these nosodes that what unites this diverse group of species, and what gives them a somewhat cohesive biologi-cal signature (through homeopathic treatment), is their common survival strategy and associated behavior.

Parasites have a complex and poorly understood interaction with the human immune system, as well as bacterial and viral populations. Important relationships include those between parasites and environmental/food allergies, as well as the ability of certain viruses and bacteria to keep parasites in check. Just as in the complex interactions of the gut biota species, parasites throw an additional complexity into the mix. The topic is too vast to broach here, but from the perspective of natural medicine we should carefully consider the potential effects of antibiotics, antivirals, and antiparasitics (helminth treatment, for example) in affecting this web of interaction. Overall, it is safe to say that parasites provide potential immune benefits (as many challenges to our immune system do), while also potentially placing a heavy toll on the body, whether from parasite-related toxins or various damage to normal growth and development through resource depletion or even physical/mechanical blockages.

In the temperate latitudes (North America, Europe, Russia, etc.) we tend to not consider parasites a large problem, while viruses and bacteria are thought of as the prominent issue. In the tropics it is just the opposite—parasites cause many of the worst and most prolific diseases (consider 2-3 million deaths per year from malaria).

However, the truth is likely less black and white. As populations shift, climates change, and immune function becomes ever more affected by environmental toxicity, poor diet, and other culturally moderated factors, the lines will continue to blur. Consider the Lyme coinfections, which are considered parasitic and which, in some areas, have become endemic. Parasitologists working outside of the tropics are few and far between, but this is an increasingly important area to explore, particularly with immune dysfunction on the rise.

Parasites	
Remedy Name	*Classification*
Babesia microti (AA)	Spirochetaceae
Bartonella henselae	Proteobacterium
Borrelia	Spirochetaceae
Entamoeba histolytica	Amoebiasis
Giardia iamblia	Giardiasis
Hookworm	Worm
Lyme disease	Lyme + coinfections

Parasites	
Pinworm (Oxyuris)	Worm
Fluke	Flukes
Rickettsia (AA)	Bacteria
Ringworm/Trychphyton	Tinea versicolor
Roundworm	Worm
Syphillinum	Spirochetaceae
Toxoplasmosis gondii	Eukaryote

General Parasite Treatment Considerations

The majority of complex children I treat, in the United States as well as abroad, need to clear parasites at some point in their healing process. In children on the spectrum, it is frequently the case that their under-functioning immune systems are unable to keep parasites in check, resulting in overgrowth and increasing interference with normal functioning. I have even seen a correspondence between the severity of ASD and the severity of parasite infestation, demonstrating at the very least that parasites can aggravate and exacerbate autism symptomology. I find parasites, when out of control, to be perhaps the most immunosuppressant of all infections. Despite what I consider strong clinical presentations indicating their presence, laboratory tests often come up negative for parasites, so treatment is based primarily on presenting symptoms.

Of all the infectious "layers" I treat in children, parasites require the most multi-faceted approach, and quite often the strongest treatment. Parasites are unlike treating other layers such as bacterial or viral infections—it is not necessarily effective to use parasite nosodes plus constitutional prescriptions, more help is often needed.

The goal is not to rid children of parasites altogether, an impossible task, but rather to find a point of balance. This requires strengthening the body's natural ability to keep new generations of parasites in check while simultaneously purging/clearing existing parasite overgrowth that is creating problematic roadblocks for healing.

I have found all spectrum of parasite therapeutics useful, from herbal medicines, to homeopathics, castor oil, pharmaceuticals, diet, and more. My first-line approach is most often one or more homeopathic remedies plus a targeted antiparasitic herbal formula. For severe cases, pharmaceuticals are sometimes required. Parasites are one of the few infections for which I consider pharmaceuticals sometimes neccessary. In naturopathy a general rule is to treat with the least force, and increase the force as necessary. Often the forcefulness of a robust parasitic infection is such that great force is needed to put them in check.

Frequent modification of the treatment modality and approach is often necessary. Parasites are highly adaptable and can accommodate themselves to certain therapeutics readily, so staying ahead of them is important. Many parasites (particularly macroparasites like the helminths) not only have high mobility within the body, but also possess the ability to adaptively shift through life cycle stages as needed. In this way they are much more dynamic than many viral and bacterial infections.

Parasites have strong cyclical patterns, particularly around the moon cycle (new moon/full moon), so having cyclical treatment approaches is important. Generally speaking, the full moon is the best time to aggressively attack the parasites, while the new moon is an important time for detoxification support and purging the dead parasites. Note that it is not just the specific day of the new and full moon, but the days leading up to and after these events as well. Parents tend to notice this trend. As one mother told me, "He is worst right before the new moon—can't focus, loses focus or interest fast, gets obsessed with a topic and can't let it go."

Children plagued by parasites often have concurrent high levels of viral, yeast, and strep/bacterial infections as well as high heavy metals. To a varying degree, these infections keep each other in check. When we aggressively treat one layer of infection, it is quite possible that one of the other infectious elements will spring up in response, because of reduced competitive pressure or new territory or the additional resources freed up. The point is that in these situations treatment can be a bumpy ride indeed, and knowing the clinical symptoms of each prominent infection as they rise and fall is critical to dynamic treatment that keeps up with the complex interplay of these infections. It also quickly demonstrates to everyone involved that extreme patience is required, as each small step forward tends to quickly highlight the next of a seemingly endless array of hurdles. Keeping a big picture perspective on progress is a must.

When treating parasites in a child, consider parasite treatment in the whole family, including pets. Other family members, even if not symptomatic, provide potential sources of re-infection and shelter for parasites.

Parasite Energetic Picture/Malarial Miasm

Parasitic infections and the main homeopathic remedies used for treating them fit under the malarial miasm. Sankaran described them as a state exemplified by the following terms: stuck, intermittent attack, persecution, unfortunate, colic, periodicity, disobedient, worms, harassed, hindered, obstructed, and alternation between excitement and acceptance of the state.

The malarial miasm could also be identified as the feeling that someone, or some life situation like a job, person, or institution, is holding you back, persecuting you, and you don't have the power to get out of it—you are stuck in it. Given the familial nature of miasms, this state may be present not just in the parasite-infected child but in the whole family, holding them back from growth and happiness. A father, for example, could be extremely unhappy in his job, feeling harassed by his boss, and takes that energy home and harasses people in the household. Circulating amongst the family, this state may greatly affect an energetically susceptible child on the spectrum, manifesting mentally, emotionally and/or physically. Or, a mother stuck in a constant state of trying to find something wrong with the children or husband, complaining constantly, and persecuting and disempowering the rest of the family with this attitude. This is why it can be important to look at the whole family dynamics when a child is stuck in their healing—where is the family stuck in their growth and evolution? The two often relate.

If there is a prolonged and difficult-to-resolve parasite issue, look for relationships that lead to a state of disempowerment, negative codependency, whining, and blaming. Bolstering physical and immune health often involves establishing better boundaries and being stronger within oneself, with the ability to say no to situations and people whom one feels persecuted by. It is easy to see how this energetic state may relate to parasitic infections in the body—a relationship defined by one species living at the expense of another. It appears as though these inner conflicts often play out on an external, behavioral level in parallel. As you will see below, clinical symptoms found in children with parasite problems demonstrate a clear outward reflection of exactly how the parasites are operating inside the body.

In exploring these energetic patterns, the following are important questions to ask:

- How is a family's empowerment and happiness being taken away, hindered?
  - Is it occupation?
  - Is it where they live?
  - Is it over-criticism within the family of each other?
- Who am I blaming for my situation, how can I stop blaming? How can I take back my power?
- Am I being passive in my power in order to receive something in return?
- Do I have negative codependent relationships that limit my full potential?
- Am I allowing people to take from me, while not standing up for myself—and am I resentful and blaming of someone for that?
- Are my thoughts and desires coming from my higher self, or are they being hijacked by a "lower mind?" Am I in a mental/emotional state of "possession" by something that is not my true and most loving self?

The core of healing is to transform and release negative energetic states that bind us, bringing us into a greater state of self-love, self-empowerment, and the ability to provide and receive love unconditionally. When parasites are discovered in the body we often project disgust and anger onto the parasites themselves, becoming obsessed with disinfecting and purifying our whole system, but this just adds more negativity to the problem. Parasites are a life form wanting to survive just like any other beings, and they have been on the planet even longer than we have. Realizing that parasites are part of the body ecology, and practicing acceptance and non-judgment of its reflection on one's own self-worth, can be an important exercise when dealing with parasites.

The causative pattern is unclear in this instance. Is it the parasites that bring on the malarial miasm? Or is it the creation of a negative and unhealthy energetic state in the body and even the family that creates the conditions under which parasites thrive? In either case, there is a holistic pattern that needs to be reset and unstuck. As with other infections or conditions that correspond to miasmatic states in homeopathy, it is important to recognize and address these patterns on all levels for healing to occur.

This point was beautifully made by the mother of one of my clients. She said, "I am the eternal optimist and thank God I have the positive force to keep driving this forward. I am good at dusting myself off and putting on the armor to get through these spells when the kids flare but it is so hard. I want it to be a chapter from the past. Watching my son slip is so heartbreaking. I will get there. I am not a quitter. I love my children more than life." The message is to stay positive, stay in love, and you will get there.

Parasite Symptoms

I believe the aggression that manifests in a child when parasites are an issue is reflective of the aggression of the parasites themselves within the body, and the body's desire to react in kind. In a physiological sense, it may also relate to toxins released by parasites and/or potential effects on neurochemistry. These species, like bacteria and viruses, do not live inertly inside of us, but rather form complex and deep interactions and chains of effect. Modern research is unveiling some of these complexities. There are also infinitely complex interactions between parasites and other bacteria and viruses—it is truly a vast world within each of us!

The following materia medica is not connected to a specific nosode/remedy, but rather is descriptive of the general symptoms indicative of parasite infections in children, particularly when they are severe enough to shift the child into a distinct energetic state. When these symptoms are at the forefront of a case, it indicates to me that this is the layer requiring prioritized treatment.

Note that while this picture has a lot of overlap with the remedy Cina, which will be discussed afterwards, it covers a more broad manifestation of a diversity of parasite infections. Cina can be considered a sort of miasmatic remedy for parasite infections, and is often useful in some state, but is rarely sufficient on its own. To grasp the overall feel of this state, consider: Hiding, dark undercurrent…lurking in the shadow.

Behavioral Symptoms—Mental/Emotional State
Patterns of violence (very common but not required)
* Randomly hitting people, striking out
* Rage with dilated pupils
* Biting or scratching people, pulling other people's hair
* Worse during full moon and/or new moon—strong periodicity to the behavior, the child can suddenly shift into aggressive behavior
* The child is "not him/herself," more aggressive or violent than usual
* Foot stomping

Whining, irritation, and complaining (second most commonly observed pattern)

- Loud, incessant whining and crying; inconsolable
- Irritable, hard to please, rejects everything, and highly argumentative
- An alternation of the whining/irritated/passive behavior and the aggressive/violent behavior
- Passive aggressive alternating with attacking behavior
- Strong cravings and obsessions
  - Water obsession
  - Craving electronics/internet/iPad/etc.
  - Putting things into piles
  - Strange stimming noises
  - Nose picking
  - Rectal itching/digging
  - Increased nail biting
  - Cravings for sugar and carbs—going to extremes to get them
  - Eating out of the garbage
  - Flashing private parts or masturbation
- Paranoia—the feeling that something is out to get them
- Poor eye contact
- Heightened sensory sensitivities
  - Very touchy, do not want their hair combed, etc.
  - Take clothes off, babies don't want to wear a diaper
- Sensory-seeking behaviors, odd positions and movements
  - Pushing into or lying on abdomen, or sleeping in knee-to-chest position
  - Pushing/digging head into people and objects, trying to wrap around people in an irritating way—acting like a parasite pushing into/against people
  - Wants pressure
  - Hiding behind furniture, squeezing into places, climbing onto things, flip-flopping the body
  - Hitting the head and ears, pushing into the ears
- Restlessness and dissatisfaction
  - Restless squirming of the body
  - Insomnia
  - Walking and talking in their sleep
  - Increased nightmares

These behavioral symptoms are nicely summarized by a quote from one of my clients: "He wraps himself around my thigh and hugs it as hard as he can, or hugs us very hard, like he's jamming his body into ours. Or he needs his own thighs squeezed very hard over and over—he crosses his thighs and bends down like he has to pee, but he doesn't pee he just wants the deep pressure. He jumps so hard on the bed, body slamming himself, or pushing his stomach against the desk extremely hard and gets mad if someone tries to stop him."

Physical Symptoms
- Increased sound sensitivity
- Teeth grinding, gnawing on objects
- Peeling, chapped, or cracked lips
- Bloody nose
- Nose picking—picking the nose and eating it
- Chronic nasal congestion, or periodic nasal congestion
- Discolorations
    - Around the mouth—blue-grey or red ring around the mouth
    - Dark circles under the eyes
- Facial swelling around the eyes
- Loss of vision
    - Periodic loss of vision when parasites wax/wane

Skin
- Open sores, pimples, or cysts in the hair line or scalp
- Strange rashes and pimples on butt, back, scalp, face or trunk
- Hives and increased histamine reactions

Gastrointestinal
- Itchy bottom, picking at butt
- Constipation alternating with diarrhea
    - Explosive diarrhea
- Stomach pain & discomfort
    - Nausea, sharp pains
    - Painful bowel movements
    - Wheezing and coughing followed by vomiting, stomach pain and bloating (with roundworms or threadworms)
    - Full feeling despite not eating all day (with or without bloating)
    - Stomach aches ameliorated by eating sugar/carbs

- Vomiting
  - Around the time of the full moon
- Changes to stool appearance/composition
  - Worms in bowel movement
  - Stringy stools
  - Mucous in stools
  - Strange colored stools
- Round, bloated belly
- Strong food cravings for junk foods
  - They crave what is good for the parasites
- Ravenous appetite but little/no weight gain
- Decreased appetite
  - Perhaps no appetite for breakfast, but appetite may come later in the day by dinner or at night

Urogenital
- Bedwetting
- Excessive touching of genitals
  - Masturbation
- Vulvovaginitis may develop with threadworm infestations
  - Vaginal inflammation, irritation, discharge

Extremities
- Leg pains
  - Most commonly in the shins—thought to be growing pains
- Leg weakness
  - Legs are easily fatigued, often occurs with the full moon

Generalities
- Malnutrition and poor growth, despite proper foods and supplements
- Unexplained weight gain
- Vitamin and mineral deficiencies
  - Magnesium deficiency is most common—when a child's lab work shows vitamin/mineral deficiencies despite supplementation (especially magnesium), consider parasites
- Worse around the full moon or new moon
- Elevated Eosinophils on the complete blood count (CBC) test
- Can be hyperactive, jumping around OR fatigued, poor energy, feeling drained

- Seizures, chorea
- Insomnia, strongly ameliorated by eating sugar or carbs
- Smelling toilet paper or fingers after bowel movements and wiping
  - Licking hands after bowel movements

Clearly the physical symptoms of parasites are extensive as well. As one client put it, "With parasite flares we get anger and aggression, speech problems (mixing words 'chopping shart' instead of 'shopping cart'), teeth grinding, sleeping with bum up, red dots on hands and face, potty accidents with staring (suspected absence seizures), and dilated pupils. His anger and outbursts are like a wild animal. He lashes out at people. He also has headaches, jaw clenching, dark circles under the eyes, and nail biting. It feels like he is being taken over from the inside out."

Cina

Nosodes are available for many major parasites and can be dosed to help the body to recognize and respond to infestations. While they can be extremely important for some parasites such as Lyme and co-infections, I have found them to be less effective for helminth infestations. For round-worms and other GI macroparasites, the use of broad remedies like Cina and accurate constitutional prescribing, as well as the use of herbs and even pharmaceuticals, seems to be the most effective. The problem could also relate to the specificity of the parasite—we rarely have any lab results, let alone accurate and specific ones, to guide isopathic selection. Parasites are notorious for their ability to evade our immune response and this is particularly true for the highly mobile GI macroparasites. The use of constitutional remedies is critical because it is an approach that can strengthen the core vitality and immune response necessary to fight off parasite infestation.

Cina is already well represented in all materia medica, so the following will serve just as a consolidated review of the most important symptoms. Cina also touches on many of the parasite symptoms listed above.

Behavioral Symptoms—Mental/Emotional State
- Hits, strikes out
  - Striking seemingly comes out of nowhere
- Restless
- Whining
- Picking at nose and/or butt

- Tantrums, screaming
- Averse to being touched, but wants to be carried

Physical Symptoms
- May have seizures and spasms
- Teeth grinding
- Insatiable appetite

Additional Important Remedies for Treating Parasites

For acute brain inflammation associated with parasites, rage, fight or flight behavior, dilated pupils, and/or hypersensitivity to lights/sounds triggering nervous system reactions:

- Belladonna—high fevers, need for routine
- Hyoscyamus—strong sexual exhibition urges, need for attention, jealous
- Stramonium—hypersensitive to lights/sounds, strong fears (dark, death)

For a weakened or suppressed immune system associated with parasites:

- Carcinosin—suppressed immunity, no fevers
- Lac maternum—limited breastfeeding, poor coordination
- Silica—body not strong enough to push things out
- Thuja—body feels too fragile, needs to hide their weakness

For severe GI symptoms associated with parasites:

- Chelidonium—bossy, domineering, liver remedy, bile issues
- China—extremely sensitive to touch, periodicity of complaints, bloated, gassy
- Colocynthis—stabbing intestinal pain, suppressed anger in the stomach, don't want to be bothered
- Dioscorea—twisting, pulling sensation of pain and restless in the body
- Euphorbium—wound up sensation of stomach pain and restless in the body
- Sanguinaria—right-sided migraines, terrible nausea, bile issues

For neurological symptoms or seizures associated with parasites:

- Absinthium
- Artemisia vulgaris
- Belladonna
- Hyoscyamus
- Stramonium
- Cicuta
- Cuprum met, Carcinosinum cum cuprum, other Cuprum remedies
- Lyssinum
- Nux vomica
- Zincum met

Remedies with herbal anti-parasitic action that are known to be helpful in homeopathic dosage:

- Artemisia vulgaris (Mugwort)—epilepsy, hydrocephalus
- Chenopodium (Wormseed)—deafness, ear disorders, tinnitus
- Filix mas (Male Fern)—inflammed lymph glands, pale face with blue rings around the eyes, and blindness from atrophy of the optic nerve
- Granatum (Pomegranate)—salivation with nausea and vertigo
- Sabadilla (Cevadilla seed)—hay fever with spasmodic sneezing and strong tickling in the nose
- Teucrium (Cat thyme)—ingrown toenails, desire to stretch
- Spigelia (Pinkroot)—neuralgia, disappointed/heartbroken
- Cucurbita pepo (Pumpkin seed)—intense nausea right after eating
- Ptelea (Hops)—atonic stomach, congested liver, aching behind shoulder blades

For passive aggressive behavior and whining associated with parasites:

- Carcinosin—codependent on parents, suppressed immunity
- Magnesia carb—passive, dislikes arguments/parents fighting, anxious
- Magnesia mur—passive, feels criticized, can whine then go off on their own
- Natrum phos—lonely and wants friends, extremely sensitive
- Natrum sulph—lonely, depressed and wants intense love/connection.
- Natrum mur—sad, emotionally closed off, feels worthless
- Staphysagria—sweet behavior but passive aggressive underneath, sexual suppression

For the detoxification phase after parasites have been killed (with homeopathic, herbal, or pharmaceutical approaches):

- Terebinthina
- Sabadilla
- Sulphur
- Mercurius
- Natrum mur, Ignatia (for emotional catharsis that may come up after parasites have been purged)

Roundworm Nosode (Ascaris)
- Can be used successfully alongside a good constitutional remedy
- Rectal itching is prominent
- Stomach complaints (many and varied) are prominent
- Bedwetting related to parasite infestation
- Strong aggravation at full moon, also possibly at new moon

Hookworm
- Deep parasitic infection causing visual disorders

Fluke
- Lung fluke—Feeling as if you can't breathe well, sense of weakness and oppression around the diaphragm; Tuberculinum is useful for these
- Liver fluke—gall bladder and liver pain, irritability and anger; issues with appetite; Chelidonium is useful for these

Lyme Nosodes: Borrelia, Bartonella, and Babesia

Many chronic autoimmune conditions are exacerbated by underlying Lyme disease, as well as concurrent coinfections such as Babesia, Bartonella, Strep infections, and Mycoplasma. Complex children with underlying Lyme may be more sensitive to sound, have psychotic symptoms, anorexia, achy joints, and rashes. A combination of lab tests, clinical presentation, and energetic testing modalities tend to point to a diagnosis.

Some children who have underlying Lyme disease have the generalized clinical diagnosis of Pediatric Acute-onset Neuropsychiatric Syndrome (PANS) and don't know what specific infection they are fighting. This often happens when Lyme testing has not been done or when the child tests negative for Lyme according to the CDC guidelines. Chronic Lyme is notoriously difficult to test for as it tends to hide deep inside the body. Some doctors will "provoke" an immune response right before the test in order to get a better reading, but even when only one IgG band shows up as positive most Lyme-literate doctors will consider Lyme to be an issue and continue testing or just start treatment.

Autoimmune reactions can develop when the body inadvertently attacks itself looking for Lyme, which is constantly evolving and evading the immune system. Lyme symptoms are often a deep layer that can manifest after addressing streptococcus-related autoimmunity, viral, or mold infections. Lyme symptoms are often indistinguishable from parasite symptoms due to the paroxysmal quality of both. People suffering from both Lyme and parasites are in a state of feeling stuck, as if they can't seem to make progress in life. Lyme symptoms also seem very similar to mold toxicity illness symptoms, which tend to include neurological issues and joint and muscle pains.

There is a parallelism between Lyme and autism with treatment methods based on detoxification, boosting the immune system, improving nutrition, and treating layers of metals, yeast, parasites, and bacterial and viral overload. With some autism cases, it is possible that Lyme disease itself is an underlying layer and shows up as sensory processing issues, waxing and waning symptoms, skin rashes, cherry angiomas, insomnia, night terrors, failure to thrive, leaky gut, thyroid issues, overwhelmed liver/kidney detox, mitochondrial issues, poor exercise tolerance, and headaches. According to Peter Alex, 90% of pediatric Lyme cases present with headaches, especially migraine type headaches worse from light.[10] Lyme disease can also occur in children congenitally/gestationally, meaning it was inherited from the mother in utero. Most often the mother is unaware that she has Lyme disease and issues with the child are not discovered until many years later, but for those who are actively fighting an infection during pregnancy doctors may give the baby antibiotics from birth. In these cases, remedies to release a suppressed immune system will be helpful.

The homeopathic miasm most associated with Lyme is the syphilitic miasm, which refers to its deeply destructive nature, to the point of hopelessness. Syphilitic remedies such as reptile, spider, and acid remedies can turn the tide on this destructiveness, and in some cases the nosode Syphilinum has been used to treat Lyme and coinfections with success. However, it seems that in anyone, regardless of miasm, Lyme can take hold as deep as the dysfunction of the body allows. Lyme is truly an opportunistic organism: if the opportunity is present for that organism to push itself into the body, it will.

There is, however, a predisposing personality of someone prone to developing chronic Lyme. This is described by Marco Riefer, a homeopath in Germany, when he states that people with borreliosis have "a defining characteristic of pathologically overstepping boundaries…they let themselves be used because they feel obligated and are unable to set boundaries, or they cling onto others with the feeling of not being able to exist on their own. Being controlled, used, exploited, sapped and sucked dry is according to my experience a fundamental (and often largely unconscious) feeling in the life of borreliosis patients. Fundamentally there is a massive imbalance of giving and taking, one lives at the expense of the other. In numerous borreliosis cases a clear attitude of victimization can be recognized. In the course of homeopathic healing, the victim identity is dropped as the life force is revitalized."[11]

In addition, the healing of Lyme correlates to our relationship with nature. Lyme patients might be much better in nature or are phobic to aspects of nature. Lyme disease and coinfections are zoonotic, meaning they are contracted from animals; Lyme has been said to represent an imbalance between human society and nature. It flourishes in the suburbs—places where nature has been broken up into smaller, discrete areas which allows small animal vector to predominate and create a weaker ecosystem. Perhaps this breakdown of nature parallels the breaking up and weakening of our own immunity.

Lyme Treatment Considerations

Lyme can require a multifaceted approach including herbs, homeopathy, and pharmacological treatment as well as lifestyle changes. It's important not to get too dogmatic about specific treatment methodologies when treating Lyme. What is important is to strengthen the immune system, as well as empower yourself with a broad base of healing tools and an ability to listen to your intuition.

In the book *The Homeopathic Treatment of Lyme Disease* by Dr. Bill Gray and Peter Alex, it is stated that Aurum ars is the genus epidemicus for Lyme. Dr. Gray's protocol for Lyme prevention dosing after a tick bite is as follows:

- Make sure the tick is removed in its entirety; often the head can be left if improperly removed. The tick can be saved in a plastic bag and sent to a laboratory to be evaluated for Lyme.
- On the day of the bite and for two subsequent days, take 1-2 doses of Ledum 30C (or a lower potency dosed 2-3 times per day)
- On the 6th and 12th days following the bite, take one dose of Aurum ars 200C.

Chronic cases of Lyme should be treated by well-chosen constitutional remedies. However, for the immunosuppressed person, clearing the infection with the nosodes can be useful, especially if the case feels stuck. Babesia, Bartonella, and Borrelia are discussed below, but I have found the nosodes Carcinosin, Lyssinum, Mycoplasma, Psorinum, Ehrlichia, Rickettsia, and Syphilinum to be helpful as well.

Many of the remedies helpful for Lyme are for a state that is worse damp/cold, cyclical in nature, and has shifting symptoms/pains. Treatments that promote warmth and heat—from exercise, to sauna, to breath of fire breathing, to warming foods—all help treat the damp, cold nature of Lyme.

China officinalis and Cina are remedies to help with the cyclical, parasitic quality of Lyme. Also, Vir McCoy, author of *Liberating Yourself From Lyme*, found that spider, snake (particularly Crotalus horridus for babesia) and nosode remedies are useful during the adult/active phase of Lyme; while he intuited that Graphites and Petroleum assist in the dormant phase of Lyme because they help the body clear the Lyme cysts.

Lyme disease can result in a variety of pains that very specific remedies can support. The greater in detail one can dive into the sensation of the pain and visualize what it is, the easier it will be to find a suitable remedy. The remedies below are useful for Lyme pain.

Aconite	Sudden, severe joint pain from exposure to cold/wind, sometimes accompanied by a fever. Joints are hot and sensitive. Fearful and anxious.
Actea spicata	Acute pain of bones in hands and wrists, worse exertion.
Apis	Inflammation with lots of swelling, heat, and itching. Impatient with a desire to be productive.

Apocynum	Acute joint pain with stiffness. Flying pains in different parts. Pains go from top to bottom. Twitching and neuralgia of face.
Arnica	Joint pain with soreness all over. Bed feels too hard, avoids being touched or examined by others. Accident prone.
Belladonna	Sudden, severe inflammation of joints; swelling; better cold.
Bellis perennis	Arnica of the hips and pelvis; achy, stiff feeling in joints, especially the hips. Worse cold, better heat.
Berberis	Pain moves from joint to joint, sudden twinges of pain, worse motion and pressure.
Bryonia	Joint pain with sharpness worse slight motion, better lying on the painful side, irritable upon being questioned. Overworked.
Causticum	Paralysis of parts, Bell's palsy, contracted tendons, loss of muscle strength. Oversensitive emotionally, especially to injustice.
Cimicifuga	Severe neck pain and stiffness, worse motion. Severe drawing pains. Fibromyalgia. Spasms in the back. Loquacious and hysterical, feels trapped.
Dulcamara	Acute joint pain from damp weather, allergies worse change of weather, better motion and warmth.
Eupatorium perfoliatum	Influenza-like pains and aches, fever and chills. Thirsty for cold drinks. Aching of muscles and bones.
Formica rufa	Wandering joint pain with marked swelling, redness, and heat. Pain lasts a day then reappears in another joint. Worse motion.
Kalmia	Sudden, severe, acute arthritis; paralytic pains; cracking joints; worse motion and cold/winter, better hot bath. Pain migrates from joint to joint or moves down the limb. Neuralgia. Confusion of the brain.
Ledum	Acute joint pain with swelling, coldness, and pallor in affected joint. Worse heat, better cold applications. Take directly after any tick bite, up to one month after bite as needed.

Mezereum	Pain in the bones, especially the tibia, worse at night. Inflamed periosteum, eczema, eye tics, cold to the bone.
Ranunculus	Sharp, stitching pains, worse cold air, damp, drafts. Sciatica.
Rhododendron	Highly sensitive and irritable, worse before a storm/cold weather, better heat and motion. Right sided. Affects joints and tendons.
Rhus tox	Worse in the morning on waking, cold and damp, first motion; better after continued motion, hot bathing and showers. Feels restless. Angry and irritable.
Ruta	Extremely stiff joints like they could snap, worse cold/damp and any exertion. Joints are easily strained. Suppressed anger.
Symphytum	Periosteal pain and injury.

Lyme and Coinfections Materia Medica

Below are common symptoms for all varieties of Lyme and coinfections. While these are not specific enough in helping us distinguish which pathogen is problematic, the overall presence of these symptoms can lead us down a deeper path of investigation. Also note that there is a combination Lyme and coinfections nosode that can be used if a specific pathogen cannot be differentiated.

Generals
- Fatigue unrelieved by rest; insomnia; night terrors; night sweats
- Cyclical pattern of symptoms waxing and waning along with the life cycles of the pathogen
- Overwhelmed liver and kidney detox pathways
- Developmental delays, delayed growth, and failure to thrive
- Disruption of pineal gland, hypothalamus, and pituitary—hormonal, emotional, and neurotransmitter imbalance; thyroid imbalance
- Low energy; mitochondrial dysfunction; malaise
- Dizziness; syncope, POTS or neurally mediated hypotension
- Immune deficiencies/dysfunction; increased viral, bacterial, and fungal infections; pneumonia
- Fevers of unknown origin; flushes of heat; chills

Head
- Swollen glands/lymph nodes
- Headaches
- Cataracts and other eye problems
- Increased incidence of ear and throat infections
- Teeth grinding

Gastrointestinal
- Gastroesophageal reflux
- Nausea
- Stomach aches

Musculoskeletal
- Joint pain; wandering pains
- Tense muscles; poor muscle tone; myalgias
- Arthritis; tendinitis

Nervous System
- Sensory sensitivity—incredibly sensitive to lights, sounds, noises, and touch
- Sympathetic over-reactivity
- Sensory Processing Issues—sensory modulation, visual/spacial issues, proprioceptive function, motor planning and function
- PANDAS related symptoms such as tics and OCD
- Seizure disorders
- Decline in cognitive function, speech, and handwriting; difficulty thinking and expressing thoughts; ADHD; impaired concentration; poor short-term memory; difficulty reading and writing; overwhelmed by schoolwork; learning disabilities; confusion
- Mood instability; difficulty making decisions

Skin
- Unusual skin findings like nodules, ulcerations, breaks or holes, blood vessels, cherry angiomas, streaked rashes, persistent rashes, stretch marks
- Hyperpigmentation of skin

Borrelia Materia Medica

Lyme disease is caused by Borrelia burgdorferi, a bacterial species of the spirochete class of the genus Borrelia, and is transmitted by the Ixodes tick. In 2016, Borrelia mayonii was discovered in the midwestern United States as a second bacterium that can cause Lyme disease. The clinical progression of Lyme disease usually (but not always) starts with a skin outbreak such as a rash or bull's eye (stage 1), then moves to arthritis or joint inflammation (stage 2), and finally develops into a nervous system attack (stage 3). Treating someone in stage one or two is much easier than treating someone in stage three. As discussed above, the mental state that primarily needs to be healed in many Lyme patients is a stuck victim mentality that produces inner rigidities and trapped anger, disconnecting them from the flow of life.

One client who needed to clear borrelia painted a clear picture of this state: "I do suffer from migraine headaches, although mostly it's the aura from a migraine that doesn't quite develop. I have severe fatigue, but I can't sleep. I'm taking care of my mother and daughter with Lyme. I do everything for everyone and there is nothing left. Even just the thought of packing for vacation is tiring. I am emotionally numb, just trudging along. It feels like my hopes and dreams are gone and I'm stuck in a rut. I just hold it all in, I am not allowed to be sad. If I let go of an emotion the whole family goes downhill, so I always have to have a smile on."

Mental State
- Explosive irritability and frustration
- Foggy, slowed thinking
- Memory issues, poor concentration, ADHD
- Depression or anxiety
- Irritability and rage
- Irrational fears (of bugs, germs, going outside)
- Paranoia
- Racing/obsessive thoughts
- Lack of motivation, inertia, lost ambition, not present

Physical State
- The presence of a bull's eye rash (although not everyone who develops Lyme disease sees a bull's eye rash after the bite)
- Nerve pain; issues with nerves (Bell's palsy/Meniere's disease/Neuralgias)
- Arthritis, muscle pain, joint pain that migrates, weak extremities, poor coordination
- Rash and flu-like onset

- Temperature disturbances: chills and fevers, flushes of heat, intolerance of hot or cold
- Sound, light, and touch sensitivity; sensory processing issues
- Floaters or double vision
- Headaches (whole head hurts), migraines, and vertigo
- Cardiac symptoms; inflammation of heart, chest pain
- Insomnia and fatigue

Bartonella Materia Medica

Bartonella is a bacteria transmitted by cat scratches and bites as well as insect vectors such as ticks, fleas, sand flies, and mosquitoes. Approximately twelve species of Bartonella can infect humans and animals. The most well-known are Bartonella henselae, which is the organism responsible for cat scratch disease, and Bartonella quintana, also known as trench fever. Bartonella is commonly found with other infections such as Borrelia and is often referred to as a coinfection, although when Bartonella is present, its symptom picture surpasses that of Borrelia and becomes the primary problem. In my experience, Bartonella is the darkest of all nosodes, and one of the most important remedies for treating rage, psychosis, and quite simply what most parents refer to as an "evil presence" in their children. One client shared, "Babesia shows up with her nighttime sweats but I don't think it's a huge player for her. With borrelia she gets stomach aches, the normal body complaints, and some joint pain. But that is also minor. Bartonella makes the biggest mess. Bartonella made her afraid of zombies and other extreme, weird fears that don't make any sense. The fear of zombies started from a game she saw. She had a panic attack in the shower, convinced that I (her mother) was a zombie. It's like she's battling in her head, 'I know you are not a zombie but I really think you are right now.' All her play is violence and death. She wanted to be a deer and me to kill her. I said no, I am not doing that with you."

Bartonella almost seems to take over a child. In the words of a different client, "She got rages twice a week and it got intense, like she's not my kid. She gives me a dead stare as if to say 'don't touch me.' She'll be stomping, throwing, screaming, roaring, and inconsolable. She won't let me go near her when it happens. Then she started adding the phrase 'I am BORED' and then it would start. We had to keep her constantly entertained, and if she wasn't entertained she would go into a rage. She had intrusive thoughts at bedtime with a pink bug with polka dots and snapping claws that disrupted her sleep. She could not make decisions easily. Her beautiful handwriting became poor and she was misspelling words. Her movements were awkward. She was regressing and was okay watching shows like Elmo. Her painting was incredibly abstract, just swirls of color around the paper. She became very sensitive to clothing and could have a rage if she didn't like what she needed to put on."

Yet another client put it this way: "I do think that Bart was attracted to my daughter's underlying sensitivity and then increased her sensitivity greatly. I hate to say it, but there was an exorcist aspect where she was truly possessed at times. Bartonella caused loose thoughts, difficulty differentiating between reality and delusions, auditory hallucinations, and dark paranoia. The handwriting is distinct, it's very similar to schizophrenic handwriting, in fact."

Mental State
- Bartonella seems to be the most intensely psychiatric coinfection of Lyme
- Intense "Bartonella rage" attacks with combative behavior (screaming, flailing, and hitting)
- Mood swings can be cyclical with the full or new moon and can get worse with time
- Delusional fears
- Feels like parasitic control, parasitic possession—something is sucking the energy out of you
- Dark talk about death, devil, zombies, aliens, suicide, killing
- Loss of cognitive function, easily confused, loose thoughts
- A loss of emotional strength; swallowed by victim energy
- No empathy with others, less compassionate, swearing at other people, hostile speech
- Difficulty differentiating between reality and delusion; depersonalization
- Auditory hallucinations
- Schizophrenic states, grandiosity

Physical State
- The induction of vascularized tumors or granulomas—which occur in the region of the skin, the liver, or the spleen—accompanied by a stimulation of blood vessel formation
- Skin rashes (papules, hives, stretch marks, and skin rashes that suddenly appear for no apparent reason and then go away)

- Broken veins, bruises, spider veins
- Flu-like symptoms the same day as the bite
- Prolonged fevers
- Inflammation of the bones (musculoskeletal pains), spine, and brain (neuropathies and paralysis)
- Many GI complaints, enlarged spleen, anorexia, lower abdominal pain, liver disorders
- Many eye disorders such as vision loss, red eyes, photosensitivity, and infections
- Sensation of vibration or trembling; numbness and tingling
- Pelvic or bladder pain; joint or muscle pain

Consider these other remedies in comparison or for concomitant treatment with the Bartonella nosode when there are symptoms of psychosis.

Anacardium	Hallucinations, rigid black and white/right or wrong thinking, hearing voices to do a bad/wrong thing, anxiety of conscience. Attacks of angry rage, deeply depressive with poor self-esteem. Restless in the body.
Belladonna	Acute inflammatory states/fevers/migraines, throbbing vascular symptoms, intense heat. Inflammatory "incredible hulk"-type uncontrollable rage, high energy, hallucinations. CNS inflammation.
Cina	Cyclical rage/aggression with a desire to hit. Whining and irritable behavior. Worse full moon, symptoms of parasites.
Ignatia	Suppressed emotions (deep seated grief) resulting in hysterical rage, edgy sensitivity, resentment and tight sensations in throat and chest. Neurological symptoms.
Stramonium	Same as Belladonna but more fearful. Very sensory sensitive. Tendency to seizures.
Tarentula hispanica	Manipulative aggression, lying, deceit. Likes music and dance—rhythm regulates the nervous system. Hallucinations.
Veratrum album	Delusions of religion and identity, mania, calculated violence, homicide/suicide. Cold and worse from cold, weakness and collapse states, profuse cold sweat, vomiting and diarrhea.

Babesia Materia Medica

Babesia is a genus of protozoa that infect the blood and cause a parasitic, hemolytic disease known as babesiosis. Babesia often seems indistinguishable from Borrelia or Bartonella and often they are coinfections, with Babesia having more respiratory symptoms which may be associated with emotional suppression and depression. Many people who have Babesia experience mild symptoms but for those who are immunosuppressed, its manifestation can be severe cognitive impairment, hallucinations, or extreme feelings of detachment where people and objects seem unreal.

As one of my clients described, "It feels like a protozoan/parasite intelligence takes you over. I got these strange feelings: hot, feverish, lots of anxiety and panic attacks. It gets into your thyroid gland and affects temperature regulation. I had heart palpitations and weird heart stuff. I would wake up at 3am feeling disembodied with generalized anxiety and not knowing where it came from. There was a diffuseness—like your whole head is out in the universe in astral debris. It creates a chemical that results in paranoiac anxiety. I felt unloved, isolated and alone, like I was on the edge of the universe."

Mental State
- Extreme agitation
- Extreme mood swings
- Severe depression
- Anxiety
- Loss of concentration, hard to perform everyday tasks
- Feet and hands issues—staring at hands, obsession with hands
- Unexpressed emotion
- Hallucination, derealization

Physical State
- Onset is gradual and nonspecific
- Drenching night sweats; irregular fevers, chills, headaches, frontal head pressure, general lethargy, pain, and malaise
- Shortness of breath, respiratory failure, gasping for air, ARDS, "air hunger"
- Cardiovascular symptoms such as a sudden loss of blood pressure, chest wall pain, heart attack symptoms, shortness of breath
- Loss of appetite and odd digestive issues; diarrhea, nausea, and vomiting

- Anemia (hemolytic anemia)
- Jaundice; enlarged liver or spleen
- Wasting of body mass; joint pain, muscle pain, stiffness
- Impaired kidney function, dark urine

Homeoprophylaxis

Homeoprohylaxis (HP) is the dosing of nosodes on a systematic schedule to prevent the development of symptoms of specific infectious diseases. HP is a controversial topic in the public health debate as well as within the field of homeopathy. There are classical homeopaths who argue that it is not the purpose of homeopathy to prevent disease in the long term, or that the body should be exposed naturally to infections and to treat holistically as symptoms are expressed. However, there are other contemporary homeopaths who recognize the value of homeopathy in the vaccine debate and the role homeopathy can play in preventing disease without the downsides that vaccines have. It is an interesting fact that vaccination was first used by Dr. Edward Jenner in 1796 and homeoprophylaxis was first used by Dr. Samuel Hahnemann in 1798, and the two methods were developed independently of each other. Vaccination is currently a huge industry raking in billions of dollars and there is a substantial monetary incentive not to allow other disease prevention alternatives to emerge.

Isaac Golden, PhD is a homeopath in Australia who, after his child had a bad reaction to a vaccine, researched the history of HP and developed a HP program (a systematic schedule of dosing nosodes) in Australia, which he implemented over a period of 30 years. His data collection from the program led to him being awarded the first PhD in homeopathic research from a top University. This data is detailed in his book, "The Complete Practitioner's Manual of Homeoprophylaxis." While clearly his study is biased towards the effectiveness of HP, there are studies included in the book on many other examples of HP being implemented around the world that are astounding.

Two American homeopaths, Cilla Whatcott and Kate Birch, picked up on Dr. Golden's program and in 2008 imported its structure with some changes to the nosodes used and schedule of dosing, and implemented an HP program in the United States. They have trained several hundred homeopaths in implementing the HP program that they have developed. (Information can be found at https://freeandhealthychildren.org/about-us/board/).

Dr. Golden makes two points very clear in his book:

1. Nothing can guarantee 100% protection against infectious diseases.
2. HP is NOT homeopathic vaccination. Despite that in concept HP is similar to vaccination, they are totally different methods and pathways of inducing immunity.

Dr. Golden differentiates between short- and long-term HP in his book. Short-term HP can be used in the event of an epidemic, such as a flu epidemic in the winter time, or when travelling to areas where there are epidemic infections (taking the measles nosode in countries where there are outbreaks, for example). His dosing suggestions for taking a nosode in such situations is as follows:

For Short-Term Homeoprophylaxis
- Potencies suggested are generally either 200C or 1M
- Take a single dose (2 pellets) of a remedy every 2 weeks
- If taking multiple nosodes, dose them as far apart as you can
- If there is high exposure, take the remedy more frequently, up to twice a week
- If you are travelling, take the remedy 1 month before travelling and during travel

For example, during flu season, Influenzinum could be taken in 200C or 1M once every 2 weeks, or while travelling to Africa, the Malaria nosode could be taken regularly.

The long-term HP program for infection prevention is seen by some as a relatively new development in homeopathy. Dr. Golden's HP program is a schedule of dosing nosodes of five diseases which he considers the most

---

EPIDEMIC VIRUS INFECTION PREVENTION

The preventative dosing of nosodes, while travelling or during flu season, is a well-accepted practice in homeopathy.

For prevention
- Influenzinum 200C or Oscillococcinum 200C once a day for 1-3 days; repeat every 15-30 days.

At onset
- Arsenicum album 30C three times a day when symptoms include runny nose, restlessness, fear of being infected, dry throat, and burning sensations.
- Bryonia 30C three times a day when symptoms include wanting to be left alone, fatigue, irritability, feeling overworked, needing to veg out.
- Gelsemium 30C three times a day when symptoms include feeling shaky, anxious, weak, and trembling.
- Aconite 30C three times a day if there is panic/fear/racing heart, restlessness and coldness.

threatening (whooping cough, tetanus, Hib, rotavirus, meningococcus, and pneumococcal disease). There is an optional supplementary program for other diseases (polio, hep B, measles, and influenza).

The table below lists examples of large-scale HP programs for the prevention of infectious disease and its effectiveness. The percentage effectiveness refers to the number of people who did not get the infectious disease. It should be noted that the effectiveness of vaccines varies between 40-90%.

Year	Disease/ Researcher	Number of People	Effectiveness*
1963	Influenza/ Gutman	385	86.0%
1974	Meningococcal/ Castro and No-geira	18,640 in Brazil	86.1%
1998	Meningococcal/ Mroninski	65,826 in Brazil	92.4%
1999-2001	Japanese Encephalitis/Dr. Garugu Srinivasulu	20 million children in Andhra Pradesh India	(See below)
2008	Leptospirosis/ Campa and Bracho	2.5 million in Cuba	Infection rate dropped 84%[10]
2012	Isaac Golden's HP Program	2,342 children in Australia	90.4%

* The Meningococcal study in 1998 occurred in Brazil where there was an outbreak of meningococcal meningitis. Many of the doctors in the region were homeopathic doctors and no vaccines were available. The team of doctors homeopathically immunized 65,826 children and obtained a result comparable to pharmaceutical vaccination.

* The Indian intervention was the first large scale administration of homeopathy for the prevention of epidemic viral Japanese Encephalitis (JE), in an area covering 20 million children in the state of Andhra Pradesh, India. This disease had become an unmanageable problem in India, where between 1993-1999 there were 5,308 JE cases and 1,511 children who died in spite of receiving vaccination. Because of the

doubtful efficacy of the vaccine and the cost of vaccinating all children, the local government decided to choose a homeopathic prophylactic program in 1999. The incidence rate of infection from JE drastically dropped, and the death rate dropped to zero.

* The series of remedies given to children for JE prophylaxis was:
  - Days 1, 2, 3: Belladonna 200C
  - Day 10: Calcarea carb 200C
  - Day 25: Tuberculinum 1M

* The Indian government published the statistics and acknowledged the efficacy of homeopathy for preventing epidemic diseases.

It should be noted that not all remedies that are used to prevent disease are nosodes. Other remedies which match a disease state have also been used to prevent infection and these remedies are commonly referred to as the "Genus epidemicus," or "GE," of a disease. This practice goes all the way back to Hahnemann, who systematically and successfully dosed Belladonna for the prevention of scarlet fever. Gelsemium had an extremely high rate of effectiveness in healing the Spanish flu of 1918. Some homeopaths prefer the use of a GE instead of a nosode, however Dr. Golden has a slight preference in using a nosode for more closely matching a disease. At the same time he makes note that the nosode doesn't have to exactly match the disease because similarity still conveys immunity.

Common Genus Epidemicus Remedies		
Disease	*Nosode*	*Genus Epidemicus**
Chicken pox	Varicella	Rhus tox
Influenza	Influenzinum	Eupatorium perf
Measles	Morbillinum	Pulsatilla
Mumps	Parotidinum	Pilocarpus jaborandi
Rubella	Rubeola	Pulsatilla
Rota Virus	Rotavirus nosode	Arsenicum album
Tetanus	Tetanus tox	Ledum
Diphtheria	Diphtherinum	Apis, Mercurius
Haemophilus Influenza	Hib nosode	Belladonna
Hepatitis	Hepatitis nosode	Phosphorus, China
Meningococcal disease	Meningococcinum	Belladonna

Common Genus Epidemicus Remedies		
Pertussis	Pertussin	Drosera, Coccus cacti
Pneumococcal disease	Pneumococcinum	Belladonna

* These are examples, each disease outbreak can have a slightly different GE depending on presentation.

Building Immunity in Today's World

In today's world, we need all the support we can get! Using biomedical support for managing levels of pathogens can complement homeopathy. Most parents learn with time to figure out what works best for their kids, depending on levels of pathogenicity and sensitivity. I also sometimes suggest supplements, examples of this are:

- For bacterial issues – berberine, oil of oregano, garlic, 'Biocidin', fermented foods like coconut yogurt
- For viral issues – antioxidants, andrographis, monolaurin, golden seal, echinacea, lysine, hyperthermic baths
- For fungal issues – caprylic acid, garlic, neem, pau d'arco, binders like bentonite clay, black cumin seed oil.
- For parasites – artemesia, clove, garlic, capsicum, black walnut, neem, pumpkin seed, enemas
- Additional detox support – burdock, dandelion, fiber, milk thistle, zeolite, ocean water, tumeric, broccoli extract, apple cider vinegar, chlorella, glutathione, baking soda, castor oil packs, sauna
- Additional immune support – mushroom extracts, astragalus, camel's milk, colostrum, bone broth
- Additional adrenal support – B vitamins, licorice, vitamin C, beta carotene, rhodiola, ashwaganda, eleutherococcus, glandular extracts

Immunity relies on a bright light of vital force and there are many ways we can boost our vitality and immunity in today's world.

- Know yourself. Boost your inner light and vitality by doing what you love.
- Be in nature and get grounded. EMF is having untold effects on our bodies. Reducing exposure is challenging but you can turn off wifi in your house, connect your devices with ethernet cords, and keep your

cell phones in airplane mode as often as possible. Get grounded by walking barefoot outside. Let the sun shine on your face.

- Be in touch with your body. Listen to its symptoms and be in touch with your intuition to guide you to natural therapies for your body as needed.
- Do hydrotherapy. Take hot baths to elevate body temperature and induce a sweat and "fever" reaction. Do contrast therapy with hot and cold water.
- Forgive your family and love them. The capacity to love your family, especially your parents, is one of the greatest indicators for a happy life.
- Relax. In this go-go-go society we need to let the body recuperate with sufficient sleep and nutritious food.
- Be authentic and express yourself. Suppressed emotions drain the immune system. Express any and all emotions, no emotion is a bad emotion, even anger.
- Don't be afraid to change your life. Quit your job if you don't like it. Switch your kids' schools or homeschool them. Move houses, move states.
- Move your body every day, even if it's just gentle stretching.
- Quiet your mind. Do a media/cell phone/computer fast. Meditate.
- Support your detox and immune systems. Consume nutritive, blood-building food, herbs, and supplements.
- And if all of the above fails, stop everything. Surrender to your higher self and get guidance from above.

Conclusion: The Lessons of Fighting Infection

As you empower yourself with the knowledge to heal your family through homeopathy, an interesting shift begins to happen. Over time you will find that the fear you once had about infectious disease slowly fades away. With this knowledge you will understand how to support the body through the challenging symptoms of an illness. And you will know that each time an infectious disease stresses a system and the body overcomes it, the child detoxifies naturally and develops their immune system. Calm demeanor and steadfast fearlessness in the face of illness, combined with the right remedies and natural medicine, can bring a full return to health.

I have also discovered that each disease has a negative emotional thought pattern that can be overcome, healing then becomes an opportunity for personal growth. Below are the types of lessons that can be learned from diseases.

Lessons from Strep/PANDAS
- Imbalanced thought: I am negative about myself and attack my sense of self. I suppress my natural feelings because of expectations of how I am supposed to be. I need to be perfect but am not good enough, I am a failure.
- Balanced thought: I love myself unconditionally and do not judge myself even when I make mistakes. I am positive about my unique individuality and I allow myself to openly express my feelings in the moment.

Lessons from Mycoplasma/Lung Infections
- Imbalanced thought: I hold on to grief, it's a part of me.
- Balanced thought: I freely express my emotions, I let go of grief.

Lessons from Lyme
- Imbalanced thought: The universe is against me, I am the victim and hold onto anger at the world, I am not in the flow of my natural self, I am not in touch with my inner nature. I am isolated and abandoned.
- Balanced thought: I surrender to the universe and come into the flow of my natural instincts which empowers me, I have the vital force to heal myself, I release anger through radical forgiveness.

Lessons from Parasites
- Imbalanced thought: The world and other people oppress me, take over and control me, and they are to BLAME. I act out my misery and powerlessness by attacking and lashing out at the people and institutions around me.
- Balanced thought: I forgive and send love to the people and forces that oppress me and take full responsibility to address what is holding me back, taking back my power, and making necessary life changes for my own happiness.

Lessons from Viruses/Flu
- Imbalanced thought: I am going, going, going, I have to do, do, do, think, think, think, obsess, obsess, obsess. I have to meet the

expectations of my environment so I ignore the needs of my body. I can't relax. I am in information and sensory overload.

- Balanced thought: I slow down and am in the present moment. I am grounded and relaxed and allow my body to catch up and digest/sort through the information coming in.

Lessons from Candida/Yeast

- Imbalanced thought: I passively let others take over, so I can remain like a dependent child, ungrounded and free of responsibility in a chaotic world. I am OK in a comfort zone, giving into cravings and immediate gratification so I can be spacey and contented.
- Balanced thought: I am in touch with my passion and inner fire which drives me into strong action and self autonomy through will power and clear presence of mind.

There is so much we can learn on our healing journey! The following chapters provide us with more tools to build and support our immunity.

Chapter 8

Sarcodes

Sarcodes are remedies made from specific body tissues and are used to strengthen the holistic function of that particular tissue. They can be helpful when a tissue or organ has an imbalance, whether it is an excess or a deficiency. Giving the remedy alerts the vital force of the body to pay attention to and heal the functioning of that tissue. In addition, these sarcodes, and especially the matridonal remedies explained in this chapter, can be useful when a child has lost or been disconnected from a particular material. For example, the remedy Lac maternum, made from breastmilk, can support a child who never received breastmilk.

The source of sarcode tissues varies depending on the homeopathic pharmacy; most come from human tissue samples, others from animal sources, and some from synthetic hormones. Thyroidinum, for example, is made from the thyroid gland of sheep and helps with thyroid function and thyroid hormone regulation.

Many people with chronic illness or immune dysfunction often have parts of the body that have gone "offline," as if the body has forgotten to pay attention to the needs of that part of the body (like when a printer goes offline despite being connected to the computer). This can happen particularly when there is a strongly suppressed sense of self that doesn't pay attention to certain areas of the body, or when the use of suppressive treatments has damaged and disconnected the body from the full function of certain organs. Chronic stress can also deplete the function of the glandular system, such as adrenals and thyroid, and sarcodes can be prescribed to help bolster the function of these glands. In this function, sarcodes can sometimes take the place of an actual glandular support or thyroid medication. Intuitive assessment will help to assess what level of material substance (such as a thyroid supplement) versus energetic support of a sarcode, is needed in each case.

Prescribing holistically with constitutional remedies, such as giving Silica to strengthen the sense of self, can restore the body to holistic function as well, and most sarcodes are not meant to take the place of constitutional prescribing. Sarcodes are usually dosed in lower potencies (such as 3X, 12X, 6C, 12C and 30C), and given intercurrently with a constitutional remedy to act supportively. A typical dosing of a sarcode may be Adrenal gland in 12C dosed once a day for 1 to 2 weeks, or Adrenalinum 30C twice a week, along with other constitutional prescribing. Different homeopaths will have different dosing guidelines. For example, I often dose sarcodes in 12C or 30C for a balancing effect on the body, while homeopath O.A. Julian developed a formula for prescribing sarcodes for endocrine problems at specific potencies (3C or 5C to encourage functioning of a gland; 7C to modulate/regulate a gland function; and 9C to suppress/inhibit gland functioning[R1]).

A sarcode may be supportive for many weeks or months but is generally not meant to be taken indefinitely like a medication. The purpose of the treatment with a sarcode is to heal the tissue so it can go back to its normal job, not to replace the energy of the tissue, such as with thyroid medication. Sometimes I will give a sarcode in higher potency if it's considerably helpful in a case. I have done this with the sarcode Histaminum (histamine), given in potencies of 1M and 10M, in order to help normalize chronically high levels of histamine. Remember, however, that if the maintaining cause of the high level of histamine is not healed, this sarcode will be palliative at best.

Sarcodes can be used to balance the nervous, immune, and detoxification systems of a child. For the nervous system, sarcodes exist of specific neurotransmitters and areas of the central nervous system such as the corpus collosum. While there isn't well developed materia medica for all of these remedies, there are cases that show promise for their use. A mother of a special needs child who I work with had the intuition to give a homeopathic preparation of the neurotransmitter Acetylcholine 6X to her child, and she found it reduced his overexcitable behaviors. Another child I treated who had years of parasite-associated rage responded very well to the remedy Adrenalinum dosed in 30C to bring chronically high adrenaline down to normal levels. I believe it's safe to assume that modern stressors have dramatically rearranged the norms of neurological systems in children today, and sarcodes offer the possibility of adjusting them.

There are also sarcodes to help bolster the immunity of children. The most well known is Thymus gland, which exists above the ribcage and is most active during childhood, central to the creation and maintenance of a mature immune system. While many sarcode remedies don't have official homeopathic provings, Colin Griffith beautifully describes a Thymus gland proving in his book *New Materia Medica,* where we learn that the word thymos in Greek denotes life force or soul. Griffith states that:

- "The remedy (Thymus) affects the circulation of all the body fluids: blood, lymph and electrodynamic energy. Thus in turn it affects the water balances of the system. It affects the immune system and encourages the development of efficient antibodies. It heals damage to the nervous system from trauma and restores integrity to the five special senses."
- "Thymus Gland is best used to treat vaccine damage when prescribed in conjunction with isopathic remedies, Thuja and Silica."
- "Thymus Gland is one of the most important remedies to consider in cases of brain injury even those of long standing and especially in those who have not responded to other well-chosen remedies."

Griffith prescribes Thymus for "never been well since" childhood illnesses such as chickenpox or measles, in addition to children who:

- "Suffer frequent acute illnesses of the respiratory tract and mucosa, liver and bowels."
- "Are slow learners: slow to walk; have slow dentition, slow physical growth."
- "Suddenly stop developing or who show an obstinate determination to stop learning or to regress."
- "Retreat into themselves after witnessing or experiencing a trauma."
- "Have sudden personality changes especially after acute episodes of illness."
- "Are accident-prone."
- "Are unwilling to meet one's eyes, who sit and look away into the distance with their arms folded; they frown quickly as they think of answers that they may not give."
- "Become obsessive over cleanliness; about little things; about recurrent irritating symptoms."
- "Have sudden weight gain or weight loss or swings in their weight."
- "Are prone to conditions most readily associated with TB and its miasm: infections of the lungs, ears, glands and mucosa; they have weakened bones that break easily."[2]

Lastly, sarcodes derived from organs of detoxification, including the colon, lung, kidney, and liver can also be of great support, especially when there has been particular stress to these organ systems. One child I treated was on multiple pharmaceuticals her whole life starting in infancy, which had a damaging effect upon her kidneys, and giving her the Kidney sarcode in 6C helped to restore function.

For the depleted parents of children who have been suffering years of stress, I often prescribe glandular supportive sarcodes such as Thyroidinum or Adrenal cortex. One mother I was treating had a round, puffy face from chronic stress and weight she could not lose, and the prescription of the remedy Cortisolum (cortisol) helped reduce her puffiness and restore her energy.

Below are two categories of well-known sarcodes, the matridonal remedies and hormones, neurotransmitters, and glands. Other tissues that exist in sarcode form that help to support the physiologic action of that tissue in the body include:

- Artery
- Bladder
- Bone marrow
- Brain
- Calculus biliari (Gall stone)
- Cerebrum
- Cholesterinum (cholesterol)
- Colon
- Corpus callosum
- Frontal cortex
- Gall bladder
- Haemoglobin
- Kidney
- Liver
- Lung
- Microglial cells
- Mitochondria
- Motor neuron
- Stomach
- Thalamus

Matridonal Remedies

The matridonal remedies are a subset of homeopathic sarcodes that are very useful in helping children incarnate and ground into their physical bodies. In other words, these remedies help give the spirit a sense of bodily self, and a sense of physical boundaries that help denote self. In terms of physical health history, these remedies are also useful for birth trauma, preterm delivery, lack of mothering, and lack of breastfeeding.

I learned about these remedies from a sweet and simple book by Melissa Assilem called Matridonal Remedies of the Humanum Family—Gifts of the Mother , in which she includes provings and cases on Lac humanum (human milk), Folliculinum (human estrogen), Placenta humana (human placenta), Vernix caseosa (the substance covering a newborn's skin), Amniota humana (human amniotic fluid), and Umbilicus humanus (human umbilicus). Melissa Assilem prefaces her book with an interesting thought in reference to these remedies. She writes, "I have come to believe that the most profound gift we as humans receive is the sense of self. It is first bestowed in its earthly form in the womb. Could it not therefore be true that when this sense of self is lost, it can be retrieved through the very materials that gave it to us in the first place? These substances are made for the creation of our humanness."[3]

In this book she lists the themes of the matridonal remedies as:

- Lacking in humanity—little empathy, a need to "become more human"
- "I keep floating away" or "I feel in the wrong body"
- Boundary issues "I don't know where I begin and end"
- Poor understanding of self
- Dissatisfied, I am not the person I should be
- I have wasted my life, I want to start over, or I wish I could grow up
- Pregnancy and delivery issues, preterm deliveries
- Female/mothering issues, absence of a mother
- Orphans, adopted children
- Incarnating or grounding into the body

The most commonly used of these remedies is Lac maternum, and a great writeup of the remedy can be found on Tinus Smits's website.[4] Similar to Carcinosin, Lac maternum helps one reconnect to the authentic self and as a result both can have a positive immune effect. Lac maternum is a wonderful remedy for many children who feel overwhelmed and disconnected with a deep desire to "go back into the womb." I once had a case of a raging PANDAS boy who would hide under his bedcovers and refuse to go to school completely turn around with the dosing of Lac maternum. In this case, the mother imagined what it was like to be him and said, "He wants to curl into a dark spot to hide. The world is crazy outside that…its round like in a womb, looks like a brown amniotic sac that is warm and wet and water and cozy…cozy is his word, curled up and safe. You are protected… there is a slight pressure on you that makes you feel safe, curled up and cozy. Someone is taking care of you but you don't have to deal, quiet security…feel only calm and relaxed and that is OK. He is like that when he goes to hide under the bed. I let him fall asleep there, then haul him out. He goes under the bed to try to get there, he is a vortex of chaos in his life and he needs to get there."

Below is a quote from a case of a premature child with a traumatic birth and a diagnosis of ASD that responded incredibly well to the amniotic fluid remedy. His mother used the following to describe him. "He hums. No real words, just sounds. He was premature, sudden thing, his bag broke. The doctor took him out and he had swallowed all the fluid and the doctor had to manually take the water out of him. When I brought him home, he would choke on his milk and it would come up through his mouth and nose. He still needs blended food and struggles to eat, he dislikes drinking but likes water. It feels like he is trapped in something and content in that place. Doesn't think about coming out. It's like he's still in that bag and it never burst. He is struggling to breathe, suffocating in his own water. He is scared of the world around him. He draws shapes that are totally round, it has to be a connected circle, then he scribbles inside that. He likes to pull and stretch on the strings of his toys. Likes to cover himself with a blanket and sleep in the fetal position."

In both of the cases above, these sarcodes did become the constitutional remedy of each child, and helped both cases to drop their respective diagnoses of PANDAS and ASD.

Children who need matridonal remedies may do a lot of pushing their body into mom, as if wanting to crawl back into her. Or on the opposite end of the spectrum, they may be very isolated and emotionally disconnected having missed out on stages of infancy, which can happen with adopted children, preterm babies, or emotionally absent mothers (such as a mother who is in a deep postpartum depression). I have seen many cases of preterm children and children who had significant birth trauma who are "not really here," become more verbal and social in response to the dosing of matridonal remedies. They can be miracle remedies for helping children complete stages of their early development. Also consider the color remedies, Hydrogenium, Helium, Oxytocinum and Hypothalamus gland as remedies helpful for issues of incarnation as well.

Lac Humanum / Lac Maternum

Breastmilk is the first substance that brings us into our body, its core themes are about helping the process of incarnation. Lac humanum is a remedy from one woman that was proven by Melissa Assilem. Lac maternum is made from the milk of nine women (from three days to 10 months after parturition) and colostrum, and was proven by Tinus Smits. This remedy is most comparable to Carcinosin and helps when there is a disconnection to the self, body, and "being here." The child may have poor spatial awareness and is thought of as clumsy, often wanting to hide away or be in a womb-like space. It can soothe challenging mother/child relationship dynamics when there is either over-attachment or lack of connection early in life. As a result, the child might feel forsaken, lost, and have anxiety about where they belong in life. It can also treat stomach symptoms such as body weight issues and eating disorders, addictions, and substance abuse.

Placenta Humana

The placenta is a detoxification organ of sorts and provides a fresh slate for the fetus. It is useful for children who take on too much of their parent's issues or have had so much trauma there is a need for a re-start. Placenta helps people clear out old issues and can unblock a layer for deeper healing. Adults may present with themes of regret, say that they have no future and feel guilty about not achieving enough in life. They have a strong desire to start over again.

Vernix Caseosa

This remedy is made from the substance that coats a newborn baby's skin, a substance whose purpose is to protect. When oversensitive children who feel everything and need an extra boundary take Vernix, they feel less vulnerable and hypersensitive. The child may have poor boundaries, like Phosphorus, and feel overwhelmed perhaps by their environment, allergies, or an environmental illness. In an extreme state the child may feel threatened, paranoid, and even agoraphobic. Children who need Vernix are often disconnected from their own feelings and have no real sense of identity. There can be a lot of mental chaos and the child is easily distracted. Vernix can also treat raw skin and addictive or obsessive behavior.

Umbilicus Humanus

The umbilical cord brings life, and also represents our cord to our original self, our soul. Umbilicus may be useful for children whose birth was complicated by being wrapped in their umbilical cords. Included in the remedy are stem cells, bearing the theme of connecting us back into our primary sense of self and getting back to what is true. Keynotes of this remedy include time distortion, recognition of self, feelings of being included or excluded, angels and wings, and breath issues. It can also help to make children who are in danger feel safe, such as those who are wounded, lost, or abandoned.

Aqua Amniota

The water from which we form, this remedy made from amniotic fluid is also associated with deep emotions and grief. It may be useful for children with pregnancies where there was too much production of amniotic fluid or not enough, or where there were identity issues from the time of formation such as not feeling wanted. Children needing this remedy may have heightened senses or hear pulsations, have a certain innocence about them as though they are lost in time, or are particularly focused on their ancestors or a past life experience.

Oxytocinum

"The hormone of attachment" that is released during labor and breast-feeding, this remedy aids in creating a more flexible bond between mother and child when there is an intense attachment or difficulty weaning. Often the complaints began at birth or around the time of post-partum depression. The child has a feeling of not being allowed to exist and either does not want to talk or talks too much. There may be sleep and developmental issues and slow growth. At their core, the child is searching for love and connection. May also assist in children who cannot progress to toilet training or who fear pooping on a toilet.

Menses

Made of menstrual blood, Menses is similar to Sepia and may be useful when there is bitterness or resentment towards one's family, a familial history of challenging menstrual cycles, and PMS. This teenager or adult has changeable moods, is awkward and sensitive, and has an aversion to superficial conversation. She feels responsible for herself and others and alternates between sleepiness and activity, and between confusion of mind and clarity. It feels as though time moves slowly and she looks inward with a weariness and heaviness in her heart.

Progesterone

Keynotes of Progesterone include themes of journeys, protection of babies and children, family, and past relationships. It encompasses all generations of girls and women and can help to heal feelings of regret and nostalgia. These women want to rescue babies and children, and there are issues surrounding safe pregnancies versus stillbirths, the cycle of life, and death versus resurrection.

Folliculinum

Many women are estrogen dominant and this remedy can help return the body to balance. It is also very useful for girls going through puberty who lose their sense of self confidence. Mothers who need Folliculinum feel as though they have to mother everyone and take care of everyone in addition to being the perfect mother to their own children. They want to rescue orphans and animals and help others but along the way they lose their sense of self and eventually lose their will. There may be a history of mental, physical, or sexual abuse. These women tend to feel out of sorts with their body rhythms and suffer from polycystic ovaries, mood swings, excitability/depression, post-natal depression, and have difficulty bonding with their children. Or the children may have separation anxiety, are unable to be separate from mother, and are over-dependent.

Sarcodes of Hormones, Glands, and Neurotransmitters

These signaling sarcodes have broad-ranging holistic effects and rely upon a delicate balance. Many mainstream medical approaches target imbalance in these hormones and neurotransmitters, resulting in prescriptions that can be lifelong or disrupt the body's natural production. While not all of these sarcodes have provings or established materia medica, what is scientifically known of them can guide our use. Themes that may arise during case taking that could indicate the use of these sarcodes include:

- The functioning of the body and the need for perfect functioning vs. failure of functioning
- Being in the flow; like a river, cycling, or loops and circles
- Blocked or trapped from being in the flow
- Contained vs. released (like the release of a hormone from a gland)

Acetylcholine

This is a neurotransmitter that is released by the nerves to cause muscles to contract, activate pain responses, and regulate endocrine and sleep functions. It may be useful for movement disorders, muscle cramping, paralysis, and twitching. Because its role is both excitatory and inhibitory it may calm down overexcited states or bring about arousal in paralytic states.

Adrenalinum (Epinephrine)

The hormone that causes fight or flight response, this remedy can be helpful for down-regulating adrenaline in children who have frequent dilated pupils, rage, rapid heartbeat, heightened senses, nervousness, and other symptoms of an over-adrenalized system. Adrenalinum can complement the nightshade remedies well (see pages 171-176). Themes of Adrenalinum include emergency states (fear/fight/flight, pounding heart), danger and being drawn to dangerous situations, needing to respond quickly to an emergency, and adrenaline rushes such as extreme sports or panic attacks.

Adrenal Gland

An extract from a whole adrenal gland containing both adrenaline and cortisol, this is one of the most common sarcodes used for adrenal fatigue and can be used in conjunction with or in place of biomedical adrenal support. It is useful in low potency such as 6C or 12C daily for adrenal fatigue, chronic stress, lowered resistance to illness, chronic infection, severe allergies, eczema, psoriasis, and rheumatoid arthritis.

Cortisolum

Released by the adrenal gland and regulated by the pituitary gland, this steroid hormone regulates metabolism, blood sugar, blood pressure, and immune responses as well as produces the fight or flight response (similar to the hormone adrenaline). Chronic stress as well as long-term use of pharmaceutical corticosteroids may disrupt the workings of the pituitary and adrenal glands, decreasing natural cortisol production. This remedy may help with weight gain, rounding of the face, acne, easy bruising, fatigue, and muscular weakness. Especially for special needs moms who are natural trouble-shooters but are exhausted from sorting out and solving everyone's problems, it can calm down that trigger response to panic and react quickly.

Dopamine

A neurotransmitter and a hormone, dopamine is stored and released in the brain and is responsible for transmitting signals in-between the neurons. It is released during pleasurable activities and linked with happiness and "reward." Low levels of dopamine can result in depression, apathy, chronic fatigue, and no desire to move the body. High levels of dopamine are associated with mania, extroversion, pleasure seeking, paranoid suspicion, dread, and emotional eating. Imbalance in dopamine is also associated with ADHD, and many ADHD medications such as Ritalin and Adderal work by increasing dopamine levels. This sarcode is also useful for healing the effects of ADHD medication use, which may disrupt the body's natural production of dopamine.

GABA

Gamma aminobutyric acid (GABA) is considered an inhibitory neurotransmitter because it blocks, or inhibits, certain brain signals and decreases activity in your nervous system. GABA enables the body and mind to relax and fall asleep, and to sleep soundly throughout the night. Low GABA production is associated with seizures, movement disorders such as Parkinsons, ADHD, anxiety, mood disorders, and insomnia. This sarcode may help reduce over-excitation of the nervous system.

Histaminum

Histamine is a capillary vessel dilator, an arteriole vessel constrictor, and a hypertensive. It constricts the bronchi and stimulates digestion. Well-established in homeopathic use, this sarcode helps reduce allergic reactivity such as with hives, itching, rashes, and asthma, as well as stomach ulcers. People who need Histaminum are often oversensitive, impatient, and restless. They often have stomach aches when recalling a painful experience and ailments from bad news; they seek to protect, contain the situation, and limit the damage. Because of these protective functions there will be local swelling, for example when a bee sting cannot circulate through the body. Histamine is highly reactive, it causes a reaction but overdoes it, too much is released, and this reaction is triggered by white blood cells.

Hypothalamus Gland

Hypothalamus gland is made up of the hormones vasopressin and oxytocin, which are released when in pain or when there are changes to blood chemistry or blood pressure. Its materia medica is similar to the remedy Pulsatilla, showing high emotionality, poor decision making, changing ideas, and sudden sexual impulses creating overall nervous instability. There may also be issues with water metabolism such as water retention and bedwetting.

Insulinum

Insulin is a hormone responsible for sugar metabolism in the body. This remedy is useful for diabetes, enlarged liver or hepatitis, and chronic diarrhea in children with enlarged livers. It may also be useful for children with strong sugar cravings, worse from sugar, who have a family history of diabetes.

Themes arising for this remedy include obesity, storing up fat in the body, hoarding and collecting, fear of poverty, saving up, and making sure there is enough for the future.

Pancreatinum

Pancreatin is a preparation of several digestive enzymes produced by the pancreas, and this remedy assists in dyspepsia or abnormal digestion of food from the impaired secretion of these enzymes in the body. It is useful for gout, diabetes, hypoglycemia, and pancreatic disease.

Parathyroidium Gland

This hormone plays an important role in the regulation of phosphorus and calcium in the body. It may be useful for bone disorders and demineralization of the bones.

Pituitaria Glandula

The control center of the body, the pituitary gland produces eight different hormones. Someone needing this remedy may express the desire for the whole body to function perfectly; wants everyone to do their job perfectly, and is a commanding (possibly bossy) organizer of the family.

Serotonin

Serotonin is a neurotransmitter produced in the brain and stored in the gut that helps to regulate mood, body temperature, and appetite and is associated with happiness much like dopamine. Medications for depression known as SSRI's have a direct effect on serotonin levels through increasing the availability of serotonin to the brain. Use of SSRI's may disrupt the body's natural production of serotonin and this remedy may also be of use to people with a history of SSRI use.

As a sarcode, it may assist in disorders including ADHD, bipolar disorder, compulsive disorders, learning disorders, depression, seasonal affective disorder, substance abuse, and schizophrenia.

Testosterone

This remedy can be helpful for boys who are having issues with masculinity and puberty. These boys desire a role of protector, they want to take care of their family, worry about being "masculine" enough or doing a good enough job, and there is a strong desire to be aggressive and fight. There may be themes of reproduction, adventure (journeys, voyages, maps, boats) and water themes such as the sea or stagnant water.

Thymus Gland (Thymuline)

Supportive in chronic infection in children, the thymus gland encourages the development of efficient antibodies. I often use it for vaccine damage and head/brain injuries as it heals damage to the nervous system from trauma and restores integrity to the five senses. These children have poor nutrition and often food intolerance, hypersensitivity in the nervous system or are abnormally free of pain, and can be spaced out and have disoriented feelings. The remedy acts on circulation of all the body fluids: blood, lymph, and electrodynamic energy. It is particularly useful for the tubercular miasm, asthma, delayed sexual development, bones that break easily, and hair loss.

Thyroidinum

The thyroid gland supports the thyroid and balances its regulation. This remedy may assist thyroid disorders, goiter, mania, obesity, malnutrition, hair loss, tachycardia, and psoriasis. It's also useful for "bedwetting in weak children" and undescended testicles in children, plus those who show swings in energy and activity such as frantic and overactive versus slow, sluggish, inactive, exhausted, and tired.

Conclusion

Sarcodes are known to play a supportive role in homeopathy; they are given in conjunction, or intercurrently, with constitutional remedies. However, there is not one way to use these remedies, and some intuitive parents and homeopaths have experimented with the use of sarcodes to beneficial effect. For example, people have tried putting the remedy Vernix into a spray bottle and misting it onto children when they are extra sensitive to their environment to give them a better sense of energetic boundaries. Others have experimented with dosing low potencies of homeopathic Dopamine and Serotonin to improve the attention spans of children. For more information on the homeopathic use of sarcodes, refer to Ton Jansen's *Fighting Fire with Fire*.

The use of sarcodes suggests that the human body has a native understanding of how to balance its own systems and dosing the sarcode is a way of helping our body remember its original template. The matridonal remedies, for instance, are based on the idea that there are universal mother energies that are imparted into children to help their spirits incarnate. We can reconnect with aspects of the divine mother through taking remedies like Lac maternum and Placenta. Trusting that our bodies have the wisdom and vital force to heal is fundamental to the application of sarcodes, as well as all holistic systems of medicine.

Chapter 9

Tautopathy

Tautopathy is a subtype of isopathy in which a homeopathic preparation of a given allopathic medication or toxin is prescribed in order to counteract ill effects caused by that same substance. The most common groups of substances include vaccines, pharmaceutical drugs, heavy metals, and manufactured toxins like pesticides. The most common application of tautopathy is in a situation where the patient was "never well since" exposure to a particular substance, yet there seems to be no homeopathic remedy that matches the totality of the symptoms (the similimum).

Tautopathy is at the core of what is known as CEASE therapy: Complete Elimination of Autistic Spectrum Expression and Similar Modern Diseases, developed by the late Dutch Homeopath Tinus Smits. CEASE evolved from the basis of the first 50 pages of Tinus Smits's *Inspiring Homeopathy* and is essentially based on the systematic clearing of pharmaceutical medications and vaccines along with some constitutional prescribing. The term "clearing" is not the removal of the intended effects of a medication or substance; if you have positive titer/immunity from a vaccine, that titer will not go away after a homeopathic clearing. Rather, a clearing is a way to help the body fully resolve or detox any unhealthy residues or toxic effects from that substance. For example, if someone chose to clear birth control pills, they would take a remedy of that specific drug and the body would focus energy on detoxing the residues of birth control and help recalibrate homeostasis to where the body was prior to taking this medication. During the course of this clear the person might feel lighter, happier, more stable, see a shift in hormones, and begin to have more regular and pain-free periods.

To clear damage, toxins, and traumas, the following isopathic remedies are available:

- Medications—especially antibiotics and steroids. Vaccines, either in combination (Poly combination vaccine) or individually, or individual nosodes of the pathogens within vaccines (Measles virus, Tetanus virus, Pertussinum, etc.)
- Ingredients from toxins within vaccines (Aluminum, Mercury, Formaldehyde)
- Metals, either in combination (Poly combination metals) or individually
- Nosodes (see Chapter 7)
- Ultrasound
- Car exhaust, Poly environmental toxins
- Glyphosate/Roundup
- MSG
- Corn syrup and sugar (Saccharum officinale)
- Alcohol (Alcoholus/Ethylicum)
- Polystyrene/plastic, Plastic softeners and Petroleum (from baby bottles/food containers)

Combination clear remedies created by homeopathic pharmacies include:

- Poly antibiotics
- Poly anesthetics
- Poly antacids
- Poly antifungals
- Poly auto toxins (Toluene, Xylene, Ketones, Glycol ethers, Chlorinated hydrocarbons, Benzene, Titanium dioxide, Petroleum solvents, Asbestos)
- Poly benzodiazepines
- Poly birth control
- Poly environmental toxins (Glycol ethers, Acetone, Benzene, Methylene chloride, Tetrachloroethene, Perchloroethene, Formaldehyde, Toluene)
- Poly hormones
- Poly in vitro fertilization meds (IVF)
- Poly intestinal parasites
- Poly labor meds
- Poly narcotics
- Poly NSAIDs

- Poly plastic softeners
- Poly radiation
- Poly SSRI
- Poly steroids
- Poly tricyclic antidepressant

Indications for Prescription of Tautopathic Remedies in Complex Kids

Tautopathy can be a fundamental aspect of homeopathic treatment in kids who have autoimmune or behavioral issues. Most special needs cases usually do well with vaccine and antibiotic clearings at some point in their treatment. However, I do not prescribe tautopathic remedies simply because a child has been exposed to a given vaccine, toxin, or pharmaceutical; rather, I look for a notably negative reaction, whether acute or chronic. The characteristic situations in which I will prescribe tautopathic remedies include when there were strong negative side effects from a medication or toxin; when there was significant developmental regression following a medication or toxin; when there was an excessive amount of a medication given (based on my experience of normal use); and when a medication given during pregnancy or used during delivery had a strong impact on the mother and produced lasting side effects or symptoms.

Sometimes a parent will intuitively feel that a medication or procedure was problematic for their child. For example, one family that I treated wanted to clear ultrasounds in their autistic daughter because they felt they could have been problematic for her and she had a good response to the remedy. "We dosed ultrasound 30C one week apart. After the first few doses her behavior and mood improved and it lasted for five days at a stretch, then there was a dip. Before this, she was getting scores of 3-4/10 for behavior. After the ultrasound remedy she's getting 7-9/10 for behavior. When we redose it goes up to 9 again. During these days her teachers were able to sit down with her and do things. We are seeing small cognitive improvements and she's doing better socially," her parents shared.

Vaccine clears, pharmaceutical drug clears, and heavy metal clears are described in this chapter. Even though clearing heavy metals isn't technically tautopathy, some metals that kids are exposed to through vaccines or other products can leave a toxic impact that can be treated homeopathically in the same manner. I have included a section on remedies for radiation toxicity, and remedies made from energy sources such as 5G can also be dosed as clears.

Our world is filled with environmental toxins from plastics to pesticides. If you live in farm country and pesticides are sprayed regularly in your area, consider clearing them. If you live in a polluted area, consider clearing carbon dioxide. For one autistic child whose family lived near a highway overpass in Los Angeles, we suspected that all the car exhaust had likely affected her negatively. After dosing the remedy Car exhaust in 30C she developed a fever response, which was a rare (and positive) occurrence for her.

The Use of Homeopathic Vaccine Clears

The debate around the safety and efficacy of new and existing vaccines is gathering considerable attention, with opposing viewpoints developing a steadily widening gap accompanied by considerable hostility and plenty of bad information.

Much could be debated on the theory and clinical outcomes of vaccination. In homeopathy, any chronic condition which can be traced to vaccination is called vaccinosis. In the book *Vaccinosis* by J. Compton Burnett, there are detailed cases which demonstrate the profoundly disturbing effects vaccines can have on susceptible people. Greek homeopath George Vithoulkas writes in his book, *The Science of Homeopathy,* "Vaccination is cited as an example of the Law of Similars—because vaccines are small amounts of material which are capable of producing disease in normal people. This is incorrect. Vaccines are administered to entire populations without any consideration of individuality. Each individual will have a unique degree of susceptibility to any vaccine, yet it is administered without regard to the uniqueness of the individual. Therefore, the concept of vaccination is almost the precise opposite of the principles of homeopathy; it is indiscriminate administration of a foreign substance to everyone, regardless of state of health."[1]

Healing cases of vaccinosis have been recorded in homeopathic literature since the origination of vaccination itself. At the end of this chapter there is a table of remedies recorded in homeopathic literature known for helping heal the negative sequalae of vaccination.

My intention in writing this section of the book is to focus simply on what I see in practice and what I do to help children who are the guinea pigs in this chaotic experiment with the human immune system. On the theoretical side, I will only restate what I believe is the most important, over-arching point: childhood infections have definitive roles in priming and maturing the immune system, helping to develop long-term immunity to other diseases and conditions, and even help to promote aspects of developmental progress. When the natural or full expression of these diseases are avoided or modified via vaccination, the consequences are predictably complex.

Homeopathic vaccine clears are but one tool I apply in practice; I do not give them ubiquitously or prescriptively, but rather when there are clear indications to do so. Strongly consider clearing a specific vaccine homeopathically if after the vaccination there was:

• Shrieking, wailing, seizures, or signs of encephalopathy or CNS disturbance
• A strong and obvious regression in cognitive and emotional development
• A prolonged and problematic immune reaction such as persistent asthma or cough
• Digestive changes, such as loose, stinky stools
• A strong reaction at the site of the injection—like an open wound, or large hard swelling
• A series of shots, especially flu shots, given annually and the child stopped getting sick with colds and flus altogether and developed more behavioral problems in turn

The vast majority of children I see have had a full schedule of vaccinations. Some have had clear setbacks or the onset of significant side-effects after vaccination; many have not had obvious consequences. In my experience, the general issues vaccines seem to contribute to include poor immunity, poor detoxification ability, and imbalance and dysbiosis in the GI system. Even when they are a contributing factor, however, they are often only one layer of many.

Timing and Dosing of Vaccine Clears

In my experience, stronger reactions from vaccine clears are more likely to occur when given close to the time of vaccination. In general, older kids do not seem to have the same level of reaction to the vaccine clear even when they had definitive signs of worsening after the vaccination. On the other hand, vaccines that adolescents or teenagers receive, such as flu vaccines, HPV, or various boosters, can yield negative reactions that respond well to homeopathic vaccine clears.

General Dosing of Vaccine Remedies

Some of the methodologies that are centered on clearing vaccines and using tautopathy utilize a relatively prescriptive approach to dosing vaccine remedies. Here is the general dosing guideline utilized by CEASE therapists:

- Dose starting with the most recent vaccine going backwards
- 30C twice a week for 1-2 weeks followed by
- 200C twice a week for 1-2 weeks followed by
- 1M twice a week for 1-2 weeks, followed by
- 10M twice a week for 1-2 weeks
- Along with supportive supplements such as Vitamin C and zinc, and a weekly dose of a supportive constitutional remedy, if known

Using this dosing guideline and systematically dosing remedies for all the vaccines that a child has had can be a useful approach when it is not feasible or practical to implement a more personalized approach. However, strong reactions can occur if a child receives too many doses for them, or the potencies are too high. It can also take a lot of time to move through the list systematically in reverse chronological order. If there are strong indications that a specific vaccine caused particularly bad reactions, it often makes more sense to start there. Specific indications or symptoms may suggest one vaccine clear over another, and these are important to consider for the most individualized treatment.

Vaccine Side Effects and Possible Indications for Isopathic Detox		
Vaccine	*Bacteria/Virus*	*Possible Indications*
Vaccines in general		• The development of that illness in full blown form (where measles symptoms, chicken pox symptoms or flu symptoms develop after the vaccine) • In children with compromised immune systems: • Loss of fever/immune response going forward • Loss in eye contact and social connection • Reduction in speech

Vaccine Side Effects and Possible Indications for Isopathic Detox		
Vaccine	*Bacteria/Virus*	*Possible Indications*
DTaP	diptheria/ pertussis/ tetanus	• Continuous crying after the vaccine, particularly shrieking, indicating possible CNS inflammation • Convulsions or shock after vaccine • Persistent cough or asthma (Pertussis component) • Poor motor development • TMJ/issues with the jaw/tight jaw (Tetanus component) • Hyperactivity, jumping • Bed wetting • SIDS • Blood sugar issues
HIB	haemophilus influenza type B	• Frequent strep throat • Blood sugar issues • Anaphylactic allergies
Hep B (and Hep A)	hepatitis B virus (and hepatitis A)	• Liver/fatty food issues, bloating • Jaundice • Lethargy • Multiple sclerosis symptoms, especially optical • Mouthing, sucking, and chewing on things
Influenza	influenza virus	• Hyperactivity/ADHD • Repetitive thoughts • Insomnia • Symptoms of heavy metal toxicity
IPV Polio	polio	• Muscle weakness, particularly in limbs • Fatigue
MMR	measles, mumps, rubella	• Febrile seizures or encephalitis after vaccine • Skin rash after vaccine • Joint pain or painful arthritis

Vaccine Side Effects and Possible Indications for Isopathic Detox		
Vaccine	Bacteria/Virus	Possible Indications
MMR (cont.)		• Unusual eye movements/stimming (side gazing, rolling eyes) • Photophobia • Swollen glands
PCV	pneumococcal conjugate	• Chronic upper respiratory complaints • Constipation
Rotavirus	rotavirus	• Profuse diarrhea after vaccine, GI not normalizing
TB/PPD test	tuberculosis test (uses tuberculinum toch)	• Chronic upper respiratory complaints • Discontented and restlessness
Varicella	herpes zoster	• Febrile seizures or encephalitis • Loss of muscle coordination • Flu-like symptoms • Joint pain or arthritis • Rash • Hyperactivity/ADHD • OCD
HPV	human papillomavirus	• Progressive paralysis • Sudden chronic fatigue • Seizures • Menstrual irregularity • Genital warts • Infertility • Mental instability, depression, bipolar
MCV	meningococcal conjugate	• Loss of concentration • Listless

Possible Reaction Scenarios for Vaccine Clears

It is important to realize that every child is unique and will react differently to a vaccine clear. In general, it can range from no reaction to some level of immune reaction. The most extreme reaction will likely be a fever, which can be managed homeopathically.

A parent of one particular ASD case who did many vaccine clears for their child summarized reactions to each vaccine clear as follows:

- Hib 30C, 200C—increase in speech clarity
- Hep A 30C, 200C—daily bowel movement for a week (an improvement)
- Tetanus 30C, 200C, 1M—OCD relating to urination/bathroom use, using it every 5-10 minutes, twisting of tongue, mild fever after first dose, stopped needing to put pressure on her jaw (she was in a habit of doing so previously especially when upset)
- Pertussinum 30C—throat congestion and cold, running nose
- Pneumococcal 30C—noticed increased perspiration after first dose
- Diptherium 30C—upset the next day
- Hep B 1M, 200C, 30C—loose bowel movement, hyper, and increased stimming
- Polio 30C—increased use of speech and interaction

In my practice, the most common type of reaction to a well-chosen vaccine clear is an immune reaction characterized by fever, skin rash, mild cold-like symptoms, nasal discharge, swelling, and sometimes a skin reaction at the site of the vaccination. Generally, these immune reactions are followed by overall gains.

There can also be an overall improvement with no obvious immune reaction. Overarching improvements tend to include increased speech and eye contact, better cognitive function, and improved fine and gross motor ability. The extent of these improvements is highly variable. A more subtle form of improvement after a vaccine clear, as in other isopathic remedy prescriptions, is better response to well-chosen constitutional remedies.

In other cases, a vaccine clear is given and nothing happens. Most likely this means that the particular vaccination was not problematic, or the current symptoms do not relate to that remedy. Lastly, there can be an overall worsening of symptoms.

How to Manage Fever Reactions

In general, fevers are a positive sign of immune stimulation in children with chronic immune deficiency. The ideal response is to wait the fever out because children often get great developmental gains after fevers. Homeopathic treatment, such as Belladonna for a very high fever, is helpful and will not interfere with the vaccine clear. Supplemental natural treatments are also helpful, such as cool compresses, "wet sock" treatment, and good hydration with electrolytes. I tell parents that if a fever gets above 103.5° F (40° C), they can have an anti-febrile medication on hand to give them peace of mind, but this rarely occurs in my practice.

The most likely time for this to occur is when vaccine clears are given too aggressively, in too high a potency, or when there is no support from a good constitutional remedy that is helping to balance/improve the overall immune function. Worsening of symptoms can include temporary increases in pre-existing behaviors, such as stimming. Generally, these aggravations will go away on their own over a relatively short period of time.

It is important to note that the overall reactivity of a child to these vaccine clears tends to fall in line with their reactivity in general—an attribute strongly correlated to specific constitutional types. Whereas a constitutional Sulphur child may have strong detoxification reactions, for example, a constitutional Silica child may have more subtle and mild reactions.

Homeopathic Protocol Before Vaccinations

If a child is going to get vaccinated, the most important advice is to spread out the vaccination schedule and make a strong attempt to maximize the child's health before each vaccination. Although I give more individualized advice based on knowing a given child well, such as making sure they have taken their constitutional remedy recently before the vaccination, these are my general suggestions:

- Take immunosupportive supplements such as Vitamin C (1000 mg per day) the week of the vaccine.
- Take 2-3 pills of activated charcoal the day of, and the three days following the vaccine (pills can be opened and stirred into water or applesauce if the child does not swallow pills as charcoal is tasteless).
- Take one dose of Thuja 30C the day of the vaccination and one dose per day for the next three days.
- If there is a negative reaction to the vaccine, consider giving the homeopathic preparation in order to "clear" it.

Remedies for Vaccinosis

Below are remedies that can be useful for vaccinosis. The most well-known are Thuja, Silica, Malandrinum, Sulphur, and Calcarea carb. Many of these remedies are well known for the treatment of injections or bites (like Ledum and Echinacea) or wounds (like Arnica). Of course, all vaccine nosodes should be included in this differential as well.

Remedies for Vaccinosis	
Ammonium carb	Eczema suppressed after vaccination. Weak and exhausted. Mentally sluggish. Oppressed in chest. Congestion in lungs.
Antimonium tart	For bad effects of vaccination when Thuja fails and Silica is not indicated. Boils that discharge pus after vaccination. Irritable and peevish. Pulmonary conditions like rattling wet coughs.
Apis	Redness, abscesses, swollen and sensitive to touch after vaccination. Stinging pain with great swelling. Active, busy, easily angered. Anaphylactic allergies after vaccination.
Arnica	Reduction of pain and swelling at site of vaccination.
Belladonna	High fevers and seizures following vaccination. Hallucinations, coma, throbbing migraines. Great sensory sensitivity. Right sided otitis media or tonsillitis. Craves sour.
Calcarea carb	Should be considered for children who develop seizures after vaccinations.
Calcarea ovi testae	Skin eruptions after vaccination, especially warts and long-lasting blemishes at the site of injection. Poor sense of balance.
Carcinosin	A history of severe reaction to vaccination. Asthma in children after vaccination; heat, long-lasting after vaccination. Worse after antibiotics.
Crotalus horridus	Pustulous eruptions after vaccination. Haemorragic purpora after vaccination. Skin inflamed and thickened on the 9th day after vaccination.
Echinacea	Symptoms of sepsis; weak and tired, aching, confused and depressed following vaccination.
Gelsemium	Worse since flu vaccinations. Fainting, shakiness, weak, anxious, low stamina.
Graphites	Eruptions on forehead after vaccination.

Remedies for Vaccinosis	
Gunpowder	Preventative for various kinds of inoculations. Bites, blood poisoning, wounds, worms. Sepsis. Intense sudden outbursts.
Hypericum	Spinal taps, vaccinations, trauma from a pinched nerve with needle-like pains that shoot from the area.
Kali mur	Eruption/eczema after vaccination.
Ledum	Heals puncture wounds with much swelling and inflammation. Persistent skin discoloration after injuries, injections, vaccinations. Better cold application. Chronic joint pain.
Malandrinum	Dry, rough, unhealthy skin remaining for years after vaccination.
Mercurius	Sore throat/uvula from vaccination. Increased salivation, night sweats after vaccination. Increased violent behavior after vaccination. Chronic otitis media or pharyngitis with offensive breath.
Mezereum	Post-vaccination injuries and itchy eruptions, depriving the child of sleep.
Psorinum	Burning, itching skin or pustules after vaccination.
Rhus tox	Skin eruptions and itchy eczema after vaccination.
Sarsaparilla	Lithic diathesis, itching eruptions following hot weather and vaccinations. Rheumatism. Clears the complexion.
Silica	Recommended in high dilutions after bad effects of vaccinations. Pain, discharge, nausea, diarrhea, abscess, backache, swellings, and convulsions.
Skookum chuck aqua	Dry eczema after vaccination. Hay fever-like sneezing with profuse coryza.

Remedies for Vaccinosis	
Sulphur	Crops of crusts upon the scalp, arms, legs, since vaccination. Helps to detox the body/move toxins out, particularly if the child has poor methylation.
Thuja	Swelling, emaciation, cough, asthmatic respiration, diarrhea, stomach pain, restlessness, neuralgia, trembling, sleeplessness after vaccination. A good choice if there is a history of adverse reactions from vaccines.
Tuberculinum	Prolonged local reaction after BCG vaccination. Insidious infection due to diffusion of BCG in the body after vaccination.
Vaccininum	Scars break open every year at the same time the child was vaccinated. Restless sleep. Severe pains in left upper arm at the vaccination mark; arm cannot be raised the next morning. Keratitis after vaccination.
Variolinum	Post-vaccination encephalitis affection. Chronic eczema following vaccination. Vaccination prophylactic.
Zincum	General aggravation from vaccination. Suppressed discharges, worse music, worse pressure, worse being touched, better rubbing.

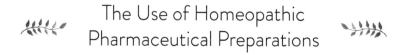

The Use of Homeopathic Pharmaceutical Preparations

The homeopathic philosophy on drug suppression recognizes that pharmaceutical drugs have a suppressive effect on the body's natural vital force, which always seeks a healthy equilibrium.

According to George Vithoulkas, in The Science of Homeopathy, "Since allopathic drugs are never selected according to the law of similars, they inevitably superimpose upon the organism a new drug disease which then has to be counteracted by the organism. Furthermore, if the drug has been successful in removing symptoms on a peripheral level, the defense mechanism is then forced to reestablish a new state of equilibrium at a deeper level. In this way, the vibration rate of the organism is disturbed and weakened by two mechanisms: 1) the influence of the drug itself, and 2) by interference with the best possible response of the defense mechanism. Consequently, if the drug is powerful enough, or if the drug therapy is continued long enough, the organism may jump to a deeper level in its susceptibility to disease."

An example of this is a child with eczema who is treated with a steroid cream. The eczema is the child's best attempt at pushing inflammation to the exterior, but the steroid cream suppresses the defense mechanism's skin-level response. The inflammation then moves to a deeper place in the body, which is often the lungs, and the child then develops asthma. The child is given a steroid inhaler which is used for a long period of time and then develops behavioral issues including ADHD and ODD, which are recognized side effects of steroid drugs. This child is now a candidate for psychiatric medications, which are also suppressive in effect. Scenarios such as this of a mild peripheral symptom being suppressed into a more complicated syndrome is seen far too commonly, and because modern medicine divides itself into specialties, the causative relationship between the development of these syndromes is not well recognized.

Are there ever times when allopathic medicine is the optimal tool? Of course, there definitely are, such as in emergency medicine situations or when bodily systems are overacting to such a degree as to limit the whole person (such as the rejection of a kidney donation, or dangerously high blood pressure). For common, everyday illnesses such as rashes, sore throats, and influenza, supporting the strength of the defense mechanism with natural medicine should be the primary goal of every healer. When healing chronically disturbed and complex patients, pharmacy should be cautiously approached knowing that it can ultimately weaken an already faltering defense mechanism. When people choose to treat with homeopathy, faith is given to the restorative power of our vital force.

Drug Remedy Clears

In the United States, it is estimated that 27% of children have a chronic disease,[2] and most have been on many medications. Does this mean that we should use homeopathy to clear all medications? In my experience this is not necessary because supporting someone constitutionally will often help with subtle impressions left by drugs. Also, not all medications leave a negative taint on the body.

Drug clears can be helpful, however, when there are persistent side effects or a drastic shift in the constitutional profile of the person following the prescription of a drug. Actively suppressive drugs such as psychiatric medications, steroids, hormonal contraceptives, seizure medications, and tranquilizers are good candidates for clears. Also consider clearing medications taken over a long period of time, such as contraceptives, or in many successive rounds, such as antibiotics in children with recurrent infections.

The most common reaction when clearing antibiotics or steroids is a fever. I once had a mother tell me that when she cleared Prozac she felt a deep, nervous system need to stretch, like a full body yawn. Women who clear contraceptives will often feel a fuller range of their emotional expression. If a child has taken ten different types of antibiotics, we do not have to clear all of them individually because homeopathic pharmacies carry combination remedies of major categories of drugs, such as Poly steroid clear, Poly antibiotic clear, Poly contraceptive clear, and so on. Homeopathic pharmacies can also make a remedy from a medication if it's not currently available.

The following drug clear remedies may be indicated when the side effects of those drugs (listed on the right-hand column) are lingering.

Drug Clear Remedy Name	Side Effects of Drug to be Healed
Tylenol/Acetaminophen clear	Loss of fever response. Liver symptoms like jaundice, clay colored stools, and dark urine.
Poly anesthesia	Loss of memory and temporary confusion. Shivering and feeling cold. Nausea and vomiting. Loss of pain sensation.
Poly antibiotics	Allergic reaction to antibiotics (rash). Digestive symptoms like nausea, upset stomach, or diarrhea. Hearing damage. Kidney damage. Liver toxicity. Tooth discoloration. Photosensitivity.
Poly antihistamine	Spaciness, drowsiness, confusion, dizziness. Blurred vision. Trouble urinating or not being able to urinate. Restless and moody. Dry mouth.

Drug Clear Remedy Name	Side Effects of Drug to be Healed
Poly contraceptives	Mood changes. Flattened mood. Decreased libido. Weight gain. Breast tenderness. Irregular cycle.
Poly NSAIDS	Stomach ulcers and heartburn. Easy bleeding. Ringing in the ears. Allergic reactions like rashes or wheezing. Liver or kidney issues. Blood pressure issues.
Poly SSRIs	Flattened affect. Agitation, nervousness, restlessness. Sexual problems. Insomnia.
Poly steroids	Appetite issues, weight gain. Mood swings—anxiety, anger, depression, mania, psychosis, pressured speech. Agitation. Fluid retention. Blood pressure issues. Weakness. Nausea and vomiting. Upset stomach. Moon face (rounded face). Acne. Insomnia.

Homeopathic remedies of a drug can also be given to help someone wean off a drug. I have often given a homeopathic preparation of an antipsychotic in 12C or 30C to be taken while weaning off a specific prescription drug. I've seen this work, and also not work, depending on how deeply wired the person's dependency is on the drug.

Isopathic preparations are not the only pathway for drug clearing. The materia medica of many remedies confirm their usefulness for drug overdose situations. Remedies known for clearing the effects of drugs include:

- Camphora: As an antidote to the excess of medicinal action of small doses of a drug. Clearing the effects of being anesthetized and issues with lack of pain response. May be spacey, out of it, total loss of memory after medication.
- Cadmium sulph: Side effects of chemotherapy and radiation treatments.
- Carbo veg: Supports activated charcoal administration as the primary gastrointestinal decontamination procedure after acute drug overdose.
- Cicuta: For drug overdoses with convulsions, paralysis, respiratory failure, twitching, and jerking of the limbs.
- Gelsemium: For drug overdose resulting in a stupor or coma.

- Helleborus: Functional shutdowns of various parts of the brain, particularly since fever, trauma, and drug overdoses. Loss of memory.
- Opium: Coma from drug overdose.

⚜ Homeopathic Heavy Metal Clearing ⚜

Heavy metals are known to disorganize the nervous system, stunt mental development, slow nerve conduction, cause brain fog, increase yeast, and also seem to enable parasite infections. Furthermore, metals will bioaccumulate in the body and this is worsened for people with poor detoxification capacities. Metals also get passed on from mother to fetus possibly causing abnormal development, and via breastmilk, causing issues with nursing and possible developmental delays.

Parents of immune-compromised children often order heavy metal tests (via urine or hair) and have tried some form of chelation supplements to detoxify them. There are also many proven natural treatments for heavy metal detox, from sweating to supplements like cilantro and chlorella. However, the presence of heavy metals on a test is not abnormal and shouldn't always compel a family to pursue intense chelation treatment. If a child's detoxification channels are compromised, even natural chelation treatments can aggravate the child by stirring up and redistributing the metals in an unhealthy way. If this has occurred, work on improving the child's detoxification capacity (possibly with drainage remedies) and at some point consider a low potency homeopathic dilution of a metal remedy that fits the profile of the child.

Well-selected homeopathic remedies are often gentler than chelation agents. Simply the use of strong constitutional prescribing over time will help detoxify metals. I also give homeopathic remedies of metals in low potency (usually 12C) a few times a week to help remove the toxic influence of that metal. If the child has a substantial gain from the remedy and matches the materia medica of that metal, consider giving it in higher potencies as well. But not all metals that show up high on tests need to be given in homeopathic form. It helps to correlate a high heavy metal to the materia medica of that remedy to gauge if a child is overly influenced or toxified by that metal. Intuitive testing can also play an important role here.

I had one case in Malaysia where a 3-year-old girl with an ASD diagnosis had an off-the-chart level of mercury toxicity. I prescribed Mercurius 12C daily and she developed strong eczema, but her autism symptoms of fogginess and regressed speech reversed and she lost her diagnosis. The mother re-tested the mercury level and it had dropped from a 47 to a 4 over a period of several months solely due to this homeopathic treatment.

Another client shared the following: "Our DAN doctor once told us that Trevor had one of the highest levels of mercury in his practice (at the time he had seen over 3,000 metal tests from ASD kids). It was heart breaking. We never did chelation because my gut stopped me. We just had new test results come back and he is now on the very low end for typical mercury range in a kid's body. I am blown away! It's been 6 years of homeopathy, energy work, diets, zero supplements, and goodbye mercury! They tested him for everything under the sun, food allergies, Lyme, all sorts of viruses, candida plus his vitals. I have 10 pages of lab results and he is only low in magnesium and B12, and not super low. Also, he does not show a reaction to gluten or casein, which he did as a kid (not that I plan to bring those back). It was working with homeopathy that got us here. I am so grateful for having found this path. We still have a way to go, but at least his body seems to be stronger and healthier."

For most children, a low potency metal remedy can be given intercurrently with a constitutional. I often prescribe Alumina 12C in this way, which helps reduce spaciness and fogginess and increases response time. One mother stated after she gave her daughter Alumina, "She has grown more, been more coordinated walking, and has better stamina. I've also seen an increase in emotional/cognitive maturity; she's doing less baby stuff." Alumina even seems to support the detoxification of lead, which I have seen in cases where both aluminum and lead were high, but only Alumina seemed to support the child.

> ### ALUMINUM
>
> Aluminum is very present in our environment and we are often exposed to aluminum through what we consume. Aluminum seems to promote oxidative stress that leads to neuronal death, and high levels of aluminum are implicated as the cause of Alzheimer's disease.
>
> Aluminum-based adjuvants have been used clinically throughout the world since 1926 and their safety is typically not questioned. However, severe neurological effects have been seen in patients receiving dialysis fluids containing aluminum, as well as in animals and industrial workers exposed to aluminum. Vaccines with aluminum toxins are found linked to prolonged synthesis of specific IgE and it is hypothesized that regular application of aluminum containing vaccines is one of the factors leading to the increase of allergic diseases. Also, according to Hugh Fudenberg, MD, a leading immunogeneticist, individuals who had five consecutive flu shots between 1970 and 1980 (the years studied] are ten times more likely to get Alzheimer's disease.[3]

Heavy Metal Remedies	
Aluminum/Alumina	Mentally dull, weak memory, slow in answering questions. Cannot be hurried. Disoriented. Dryness of mucous membranes. Constipation. Heaviness of limbs progressing to paralysis. Slow reflexes.
Antimony/Antimonium met	Irritable, grumpy, moody, kicking, hitting, pulling hair, worse looked at or touched. Anger leads to coughing, vomiting, or breath holding. Voice problems, lung complaints. Problems of testes or ovaries.
Arsenic/Arsenicum album	Anxious, hypochondriacal, fear of germs. Panic attacks. Fastidious, compulsive, and perfectionistic. Restless. Gastritis or ulcers with burning. Diarrhea. Insomnia. Coldness of extremities. Thirsty for small sips of water. Anorexia.
Beryllium	Closely resembles Aluminum. Insecure, vague fears of the unknown, fears people, crowds, strangers. Mentally slow, orientation problems, forgetful, dementia. Low energy, dryness of mucous membranes. Swollen glands.
Bismuth/Bismuthum	Violent abdominal pains with great fear and desire for company, similar to Phosphorus. Vomiting as soon as water hits the stomach. Thirst for cold water.
Cadmium	Unstable emotions, socially anxious. Similar to Argentum nit. Forgetful. Voice problems. Lung complaints like asthma. Cancer miasm.
Lead/Plumbum	Contractures of tendons. Emaciation and weakness of limbs. Tremor and twitching of muscles. Drawing sensation in abdomen. Poor memory, slow perception. Distant. Heaviness. Very similar to Alumina.
Mercury/Mercurius viv	Hurried, irritable, impulse to scream. Violent. Destructive impulses. Introverted, closed, and suspicious. Compulsive disorders. Suicidal. Chronic otitis media and pharyngitis with offensive breath. Excessive saliva. Gingivitis. Tongue imprinted by teeth. See comments below on Thimerosal.

Heavy Metal Remedies	
Nickel/Niccolum Carb	Poor at conversation, controls conversation. Unemotional. Quarrelsome. Worse contradiction. Severe periodic headaches. Sleeplessness. Violent sneezing. Intense hiccough.
Platinum/Platina	Highly dramatic, self-absorbed, loves attention. Numbness and tingling sensations about cheek bones and lips. High sex drive. Similar to Ignatia. Band sensations.
Tin/Stannum	Weak respiration, feels empty and hollow in the chest. So weak cannot speak. Feels "unheard." Weakness worse exertion, worse talking, better lying.
Thallium	Hair loss. Trembling. Paralysis of lower limbs. Locomotor ataxia. Similar to Plumbum.
Thimerosal	Thimerosal is ethylmercury sodium salt which was used as a preservative in vaccines since the 1930's, which coincides with the original description of autism. It has been suggested that the emergence of autism is due to mercury poisoning. The materia medica of Mercurius has many symptoms shared with autism, including extreme shyness, socially withdrawn, introversion, mood swings, no facial expression, avoidance of conversation, gaze avoidance, staring spells, speech comprehension deficits, sensitivity to sound, photophobia, aversion to touch, intention tremor, involuntary jerking, tremor, clumsiness, difficulty chewing and swallowing, mental delay, and excessive sweating. In June 2000 the FDA admitted that children were being exposed to unsafe levels of mercury in vaccines, and it has been reported that it was removed from vaccines by 2001. However, Thimerosal is currently listed as an ingredient in some vaccines, particularly flu vaccines. Ask your doctor for the specific brands of vaccines your child was given and research each one to determine whether Thimerosal might need to be cleared.[4]

Heavy Metal Remedies	
Tungsten	Eye complaints, visual disturbances. Headache. Quick to anger and takes offense. Sharp mind. Cheerful, enthusiastic.
Radioactive metals: Uranium, Thorium	Overwhelming sensitivity, living in chaos. Cancer miasm. Many systems of the body challenged, out of order. Otherworldly.

(There is also a combination heavy metals remedy called Poly metals.)

Electromagnetic Field Sensitivity

More and more people are sensing the effects of electromagnetic frequencies (EMF) and radiation on our bodies. Sources of radiation can include cell phones and cell towers, X-rays, Wi-Fi, microwaves, smart meters, power stations, electronic devices, and airplane travel. Let's not forget the sun is a major source of radioactive exposure as well. There are many studies that show our bodies are impacted by radiation, resulting in a greater likelihood of cancer, birth defects, and infertility. In general, the greater the exposure, the more toxic the effect. Increasing numbers of people describe themselves as scattered, easily distracted, and suffering from poor memory, all of which can be attributed to the electronics that people have become addicted to. Many children I treat spend most of their day glued to a device, and if you take that device away from them, the child will rage due to some combination of radiation induced inflammation as well as the dopamine effects of nonstop streaming content.

A proving of the remedy Mobile phone included in Colin Griffith's *New Materia Medica, Volume II* describes the effect of mobile phone energy on the body, which is comparable to most EMF effects. "The central nervous system is affected; there are pins and needles, numbness, tingling and dyspraxic tendencies. Paralysis can set in. Spatial awareness is impaired. Inertia. All the electrical impulses of the body are affected adversely. Mental degeneration. Sensations of pressure and heaviness are experienced. The whole body or just the head can feel heavy. There is an exaggerated awareness of the difference between the two sides of the body: left and right; also of a dislocation between the top and bottom half, above and below the pelvic area. Sensation as if the body is dying. Sensations of both heat and cold; heat is mostly internal and cold is external. Waves of icy coldness creeping up the back. The endocrine glands are impaired; the thyroid and the thymus take up the radiation and become infiltrated and damaged. Kidney energy becomes exhausted quickly, which means the filtration system of the water in the body is affected. The calcium/magnesium balance is disrupted. Spleen energy is affected making it harder to maintain the integrity of the immune system; there is a greater tendency to succumb to infection, especially viral (patients can feel as if they are 'coming down with something' all the time)."[5]

We can also question the effects of radiation on the fetus in utero, and it's possible that children with deformities of body structure, poor growth, or sensory issues may be due to excessive EMF exposure, ultrasounds, or even baby monitors during pregnancy and infancy. Parts of the body most affected by radiation are the thyroid, thymus gland, lymphatic system, central nervous system, skin, bone, blood, liver, kidneys, and sex organs.

Just as homeopathic remedies can be made from forms of light, remedies can also be made of energies such as microwave frequencies. These remedies, which are sometimes referred to as "imponderables," can be given to counter their effects on our bodies, and include X-ray, Sol (sun), Microwave radiation, 5G, Wi-Fi, Broadband emission, Mobile phone, EHF (extremely high frequencies), Electricitas, MRI, and Ultrasound.

While some imponderables like X-ray are established in classical homeopathy, some have been newly proven. Colin Griffith's *New Materia Medica Volume II* contains an appendix on remedies for clearing the effects of radiation, in which he notes, "New remedies that may positively affect radiation toxicity in the body: Ayahuasca, Clay, Emerald, Goldfish, Green, Japanese white oleander, Moldavite, Moonstone, Plutonium, Purple, Rainbow, Rose quartz, Ruby, Sea holly, Winchelsea sea salt, Sequoia, and Yellow. New remedies that may help to lift the radiation miasm: Emerald, Jet, Moldavite, Plutonium, Rainbow, Ruby, Yellow."

Some of the more helpful remedies for radiation toxicity are in the table below. These remedies may fit a person as a constitutional and the gemstone remedies especially can support the clearing of radioactive toxicity by helping the body stay energetically and structurally aligned. Other remedies from radioactive toxic sources, like X-ray, Ultrasound, and 5G can also be prescribed as tautopathic clears.

Emerald	Blocks negative energies and cleanses the body of excessive radiation. Improves circulation, cleanses lymph, and rekindles imagination and intuition. Helps us to express from our heart and our emotions more fully.
Plutonium	Feelings of being slowed down or sped up. Extremely fearful; terrified; fear as if from an indefinite source, from the distant past. A feeling of being externally forced to keep on going and do all kinds of things; cannot live as she likes; a feeling of too much obligation. Urge to put things in order. Feeling of decay, disintegration into different identities. Fear of ecological catastrophes. Learning difficulties associated with neurological developmental problems, poor coordination and lack of balance. Electromagnetic and heavy metal toxicity. Useful for the correcting of geopathic stress disorders. Desire to lie down from feeling of extreme heaviness. Periodical or paralyzing fatigue. Chilliness and shivering.
Clear quartz	Strengthens the sense of self, expanding our consciousness, connecting us to our higher self, and grounding us into the earth. Restores vitality to the digestive system.
Mobile phone/5G	This remedy provides relief from bone tiredness, lassitude, and exhaustion in the limbs and in the mind. A return of suppressed emotional and physical feelings. Cell phone addiction.

One client who took 5G in 30C shared that "My experience was a game changer! I woke up feeling more rested than I've felt in years. I experienced a deeper sense of peace and calm to the core of my being. It was as if there was a part of my physical body that was subtly but powerfully in overdrive finally unplugged and could rest. I felt more connected to the rhythms of the Earth and more of a sense of my true vibration in its purest form. I felt one with nature."

Contemporary homeopath Jeremy Sherr speaks of a new category of disease (or miasm) in today's culture that he abbreviates as "FARC," for the combination pathogenic influence of Fungus, Aids, Radioactivity and Cancer. My experience is that there are many special needs children who fit this category, particularly if we replace the AIDS category with immunodeficiency, viral overload, and vaccine injury.

There is also evidence that the increase in radioactivity in our environment lowers our immunity and potentiates overgrowth of mold and fungi. Therefore some complementary remedies for those suffering from EMF sensitivity include:

- Mold/fungi remedies include Mixed molds and Agaricus.
- Remedies to treat oversensitivity incluce Carcinosin and Tuberculinum.
- Neurologic remedies to treat toxified or burned out nerves include spider remedies like Tarentula; metals like Zincum, Platina, and Argentum nit; and acids like Phosphoric acid and Picric acid.
- Plant remedies for joint pain caused by EMFs include Rhus tox and Dulcamara.
- Remedies to assist with electronic device addiction include Opium, Codeine, Nux vomica, Coffea, and the sarcode Dopamine.
- Gemstone remedies to clear and protect the energy field include Emerald, Clear quartz, Ruby, Jet, and Moldavite.
- Animal remedies for high sensitivity include fish, insect, and spider families, as well as Lac delphinum and Calypte anna.

While radiation is ubiquitous these days, some simple measures can be taken to reduce exposure to radiation including keeping your cell phone on airplane mode, using a headset when talking on the phone, maintaining a landline in your home, using ethernet cords instead of Wi-Fi, and reducing air travel. Spending plenty of time outside, barefoot, and taking extra magnesium supplementation also grounds and protects the body from excessive EMF.

Conclusion

The use of homeopathic remedies prepared from pharmaceuticals is a practice that deserves more exploration, particularly in complex cases which often have a family history of substantial pharmaceutical use. If it seems that a long, chronic history of pharmaceuticals has disrupted organ systems or function, the additional use of sarcode remedies, or homotoxicology, can also help clear up the functioning of the body.

One possibility that has only begun to be explored is tautopathic remedies given not just for detoxification, but to bring about the intended effect of that particular medication. For example, could a low potency of an asthma medication assist in opening the bronchioles of an asthmatic child just as effectively as a material dose? This is a hypothetical realm to be investigated and has the potential to revolutionize medicine.

Interestingly, many bodies of water, especially those near large populations such as the River Thames in southern England, are filled with sewage runoff containing pharmaceuticals that did not breakdown after passing through our bodies, from birth control to antidepressants. Humanity's vast reliance on pharmaceuticals is impacting the ecology of the planet in ways we barely understand. Shifting to a homeopathic model of health and healing is not only gentle for us, but gentle for our planet.

Chapter 10

Remedies by Categories of Complex Kids

Over many years of treating immune-compromised and challenging children I have come up with the following "clinical groups" representing meaningful categories that are useful in finding the right remedy. The groups fall under two large categories: those defined primarily by the chief complaint or etiology of the child, and those that correspond to the main personality trait, even if it's not the main medical complaint. There is some overlap between the groups, and they do not encompass every possible case, but they are helpful in understanding a majority of complex children.

Studying these clinical groups will also help you gain a better understanding of the main complaints, issues, and personalities of the different families or groups of remedies. The remedies listed under each group are not exhaustive; rather they represent the most important and common remedies that I have found to correspond with that group of children. The groups of remedies in this chapter include the following behavioral and physical complaints.

Behavioral Issues
- Children with acute rage and panic
- Highly anxious children
- Angry children
- Insecure, weak children
- Negative, antisocial children
- Sad, serious children
- Precocious, advanced children

- Suppressed, oversensitive children
- Angelic children

Physical Issues
- Physically depleted children due to chronic viral infections
- Miserable gut/sensory children
- Tics, twitches, and seizures in children
- Hyperactive children
- Children with birth/head trauma
- Cognitively slow children

Children with Acute Rage and Panic

These children may fall into what Sankaran calls the "acute miasm," described as sudden, panic, danger, escape, helpless, fright, terror, alarm, instinctive reaction, and reflex reaction. This situation arises often in ASD cases where there is a deep neurological disorder, as the disease pathology either reaches the level of the central nervous system/brain or where there is a mechanical disruption of the central nervous system such as from a traumatic head injury.

The child's rage may present as adrenaline reactions such as dilated pupils, screaming at the top of their lungs, kicking, and fight or flight behaviors; they are often stronger than you would expect. They may look like they are feeling absolute terror with heart palpitations, or they may look frozen in fear. The child may fear death in the moment of their rage or panic attack, can make very violent statements, and swear a lot. There may be tics and twitches. These children often have a strong need for routine so that they have a predictable environment to calm their persistent fears. The parents of children who rage are exhausted, similar to PTSD survivors, just trying to keep their head above water, walking on eggshells around their child because of how easily their rages are set off. The mother is often scared that their child might overpower them when in a rage. There may be a history of an acute emergency situation either during pregnancy or delivery where she felt the baby or she could die, such as a hemorrhage, an accident, or fear of death during delivery.

Diseases tend to be highly inflammatory, including prolonged high fevers, delirium, and convulsions. Often this child has landed in the ER multiple times or needed to be hospitalized and may have been eventually medicated with sedatives or anxiolytics. For many children, the root of the rage or convulsions is deep parasitic infection which causes a high level of inflammation in the system, often impairing vision or causing other neurological deficits. It can be challenging to treat children who are on anti-seizure medications since the drugs are by nature suppressive in their effect, and their convulsions may not respond to homeopathy as a result. It is also not wise for children to be withdrawn from those medications since their systems become dependent on them. However, for children who are not on anti-convulsant medications and who have obvious nervous system-level inflammation that causes the above symptoms, homeopathic remedies can be extremely effective and give their parents a big sigh of relief. I believe that parents should be taught how to dose remedies as needed and counseled on how to go up in potency if necessary, dosing as often as needed. These children also tend to do well with anti-inflammatory supplements such as fish oil, and many have deep-seated parasite infections that need to be addressed as well.

Remedies for Children with Acute Rage and Panic	
Aconite	Pure panic state arising as an adrenaline fight/flight reaction with heart palpitations and need for company. Not necessarily violent. Fear of death, flying, claustrophobia. Shock. PTSD.
Adrenalinum	For children who have been in continuous fight or flight modes. Pupils are often or easily dilated. Helps normalize adrenaline levels.
Atropinum	Tantrums, rage, brain inflammation, especially due to allergies/lung inflammation. This is the alkaloid found in Belladonna, used medically for pupil dilation.
Belladonna	High energy, active children who have brain inflammation, rages, tantrums with dilated pupils, and superhuman strength. Strong fears with a need for routine. Can be used for acute fevers.
Cina	Hitting, striking, biting other people, throwing things. Parasite infections. Outwardly aggressive because inwardly GI system is being attacked. Tantrums, rage. Goes into Belladonna/Hyoscyamus/Stramonium states.

Remedies for Children with Acute Rage and Panic	
Histaminum	For children who are continually in a histamine flare/reactive mode. Helps normalize histamine levels.
Hyoscyamus	Brain inflammation leading to rage. Controlling of mother, very jealous of siblings. Acts with no shame, like showing genitals/butt, masturbating, or swearing (exhibition). Stool/urine accidents.
Red (color)	For imbalance towards inflammation/anger/reactivity/heat. Helps subdue and bring balance to the "red" in the energy system.
Stramonium	Rage. Dark fears, wide-eyed look of terror, fearful of death/dying, strong fear of the dark. Need for company. Tendency to inflammation, tics, Tourette's. PTSD. Seizures. Very sensory sensitive. Childish.

(Also important are all nosodes, snake, and spider remedies.)

Highly Anxious Children

These children are dominated by fears, which can include separation anxiety, fear of leaving the house, fear of flying, fear of heights, fear of being in the car, fear of certain people, and fear of the dark. They are highly reliant on their parent or an adult when they have panic attacks, often contacting them during school and going to the school nurse. Many are hypochondriacal and hysterical about small complaints. They have intrusive thoughts that are fearful. Their nervous systems seem to be on edge from so much anxiety so it is hard to sleep, hard to calm down, and little things can set them off. These children may also be sensitive to EMF and electronics and efforts should be made to reduce their exposure.

Remedies for Highly Anxious Children	
Aconite	Pure panic state arising as an adrenaline fight/flight reaction with heart palpitations and need for company. Not necessarily violent. Fear of death, flying, claustrophobia. Shock. PTSD.
Argentum met/nit/phos	Open, impulsive, connecting, and suggestible. Strong sugar and fat cravings, likes ice cream. Arg nit is more impulsive. Arg phos is more focused on friendships.

Remedies for Highly Anxious Children	
Arsenicum alb	Hypochondriac; fear of germs and getting sick. OCD about cleanliness. Burning GI pains, diarrhea, vomiting, food poisoning, gut bugs with anxious restlessness. Perfectionistic, controlling. Strong reliance on doctor.
Asarum	For hypersensitivity of the nerves or nerves on edge causing hysteria, faintness, nausea, vomiting, and vanishing of thoughts. Great joyfulness alternating with gloominess. Painful menses from oversensitive nerves.
Calcarea carb	Stubborn and anxious. Dislikes changes/new things, fear of heights, cautious on the playground. Doesn't like people observing them. Gets overwhelmed with what is expected of them. Desires to be in their comfort zone.
Carcinosin	Codependent on parent or medication. Needs to exert control over everything because they are so overwhelmed. Can't sleep at night because they can't turn off thoughts. Passionate, loves nature. Family may be overscheduled.
Gelsemium	Weak and trembling in the legs with anxiety, feels like they could faint/collapse, sinking stomach feeling, and vertigo. Anticipatory anxiety. Sad. For chronic viral states, flu, fatigue, CVID, etc.
Moschus	Spoiled children who make up illnesses for the sake of attention. Hysterical and anxious they will die. More common in girls than boys. Hysterical asthma.
Mus musculus	The remedy from a mouse, this child freezes and wants to hide upon strangers approaching. Easily scared. Craving for sugar, especially at night.
Natrum mur	Doesn't make eye contact easily with strangers, and even family. Very anxious about social situations. Has a hard time opening up, introverted.
Phosphorus	Empath. Poor boundaries so emotions of people can easily affect them. Dislikes being alone, always needs someone with them. Open and bubbly or shy; wants friends. Environmentally sensitive. Tubercular, dry coughs. Related to insect, bird, fish, cat remedies.

Remedies for Highly Anxious Children	
Stramonium	Dark fears, deer-in-the-headlights look of terror, fearful of death/dying, strong fear of the dark. Tendency to brain inflammation, tics, Tourette's, nightmares.

Angry Children

The main issues for these children are anger, tantrums, and rage. They often have liver issues or poor ability to detox; many of them may eventually need Sulphur as a remedy to deal with these underlying issues. In other cases, the rage and anger can be a release of suppressed emotions manifested in the nervous system. These children may not have a good ability to freely and easily express their emotions as they come. This group should be differentiated from the acute neurological rage remedies (like Belladonna, etc.); in those remedies there is more active brain/CNS inflammation. Some anger and rage can be manipulative, while in other kids it is reactionary—both are in this group.

Remedies for Angry Children	
Anacardium	Internal split where one voice tells them to do the right thing, another voice says they are bad. Restless, needing to move. Low self-esteem resulting in mean behavior to others. Hallucinations, cursing.
Apis (and other insects such as Culex and Cantharis)	Tendency to be very inflamed; redness, swelling, allergies, asthma, eczema. Histamine reactions. Industrious, organized. Sensory sensitive. Anger from getting too worked up.
Ferrum met	Bossy, emotional, domineering. Acts forceful but hates being told what to do or being pressured. Red lips and flushed cheeks with tendency to anemia. Difficulty breathing. Pushing through hard work.
Gloninum	Made from nitroglycerin, this remedy is very explosive! Known for heatstroke, helps to heal vascular issues leading to rage attacks. The child may suffer from POTS, Raynauds, heart issues, or other issues where regulation of the vascular system is compromised. May have pulsating, bursting headaches similar to Belladonna.

Remedies for Angry Children	
Hydrogenium	Explosive anger. Child is very creative. Out of body feeling. Mother didn't want the baby, considers abortion. Adopted children. Numbness, skin formication, deep headaches.
Hyoscyamus	Brain inflammation leading to rage. Controlling of mother, very jealous of siblings. Acts with no shame, like showing genitals/butt, masturbating, or swearing (exhibition). Stool/urine accidents.
Ignatia	Heartbroken, disappointed, suppressed grief, lump in throat. Idealistic, wanting things a certain way and if that doesn't happen will have a meltdown, act hysterical. Contradictory. Tics, twitches. History of grief in family.
Lac lupinum	Explosive anger like a wild animal. Sees red. Highly energized.
Lachesis (and other snakes)	Passionate, talkative, social, jealous, competitive, moody children. Can have sepsis, parasitic infection, blood stagnation. Can be violent, manipulative, lashing out. Tend to be warm and intolerant of tight clothing.
Lycopodium	Napoleonic complex, feeling small on the inside and acting big, bossy, egotistical, criticizing, intellectual on the outside. Or socially shy. Correlates with liver stagnation, constipation, gassiness, big appetite.
Medorrhinum	Precocious, artistic, passionate children who are advanced early on but have frequent infections, asthma, bacterial dysbiosis, sinusitis. Behavior alternates between extreme states such as shy to social, or empathetic to cruel and destructive.
Mercurius	Advanced, precocious children who are either adult like or introverted. Suspicious someone is out to get them and prone to impulsive but directed violence. Can help with excessive salivation, pharyngitis.
Nosodes	Strep (all), Lyssinum, Staph aureus

Remedies for Angry Children	
Nux vomica	Workaholic, driven, competitive children who get their nervous system worked up and then become sensory sensitive such as to drafts. Irritable, snappy, and spastic. GI symptoms worse from overeating.
Rhus tox	Achy body, back, and joints which feel better with movement. Body feels restless, uncomfortable in their skin. Eczema. Worse dampness. Suppressed anger, particularly at family members. Ritualistic.
Staphysagria	Emotionally vulnerable, easily hurt, bullied, embarrassed, ashamed, especially if people don't like them. Changeable symptoms depending on emotional state. Suppressed anger. Sexual suppression or abuse. UTIs.
Sulphur	Warm, generous, lazy, messy, funny children who like people. They want someone to take care of them so they can have fun exploring their hobbies, collections, or video games. Poor detoxers prone to many infections. Anger in outbursts.
Tarentula (and other spiders)	Speedy, neurological, sensory sensitive children who love rhythmic music, which helps to regulate them. Can be violent, manipulative, lashing out, with hallucinations. Social and competitive or isolated and withdrawn.
Tuberculinum	Sarcastic, cynical, self-centered, dissatisfied, defiant, mean, and destructive. Lung weakness, tendency to fungal infections. Time conscious that life/things will be over fast, so they have to fit it all in; hurried.
Veratrum album	Cold, cruel behavior, very intellectual with no heart. A desire to be the leader of the group with fear of being excluded or looked down upon. Migraines, diarrhea, prostration.

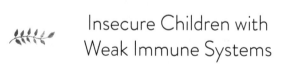

Insecure Children with Weak Immune Systems

This group falls under the psoric miasm, where there is an underlying lack of self-confidence, self-worth, social skills, security, nutrients, strength, and energy. But if they are hopeful and keep making an effort, then they feel they can do it. In general, this is the underlying deficiency state that most kids move towards as pathogenic layers are peeled away. Everyone has this core psoric weakness that needs healing.

Children in this category present as insecure, nervous, or uncertain about new situations and timid when making connections with other children. They may be stubborn out of fear of change and a desire to stay inside their comfort zone. They think that they need a lot of support from others, and often have multiple overlapping infections due to weakness of the immune system, nutrient absorption, detoxification, and metabolism. They don't like to be observed and are fearful of critiques of their performance, taking tests in school, or doing mentally challenging homework. They may also be quite rule bound, simplistically black and white in how they see things, and don't comprehend nuance or the bigger picture. They often have slow comprehension and are slower learners. These children like standard toys such as blocks, Legos, trucks, trains, dollhouses, and puzzles and they're usually happiest while at home. They may be stubborn about sticking with the toys and foods they know and love best and may need extra time to catch up with their peers. Their tastes can also be childish, wanting to play with younger children or toys too immature for their age. Parents of this type of child are usually direct, logical, and family oriented. They are often reticent or sweet. There may have been infertility issues.

Common physical presentations in this group:

- Functional pathologies such as chronic ear infections, coughs, pneumonia.
- Frequent colds/flus, skin rashes, constipation, pathology at mucous membrane level.
- Slow metabolism (either not putting on weight, not growing taller, or excessive weight gain), thyroid issues, cold temperature in the body, energy may be low.
- Poor and weak immune reactivity where infections last a long time; they don't mount high fevers that kick an infection.
- Things invade their mucous membrane boundaries and they don't have the inner strength to kick them out.

Homeopathic glandulars and cell salts can help build the systems of these children up as well. For example, many of these children may have underactive thyroids, for which Thyroidinum 30C dosed daily for a few weeks will help, or malabsorption of minerals causing poor tooth enamel, for which cell salt Calcarea fluor 12X daily will help. Gemmotherapy tinctures can also be quite helpful in restoring function to tissues/organs and boosting immunity.

These children tend to do well with herbal medicines, diets, and other therapies that build up their deficiency states. For example, bone broths, immune strengthening herbs like astragalus and andrographis, adrenal tonics, and hot baths.

Remedies for Insecure Children with Weak Immune Systems	
Calcarea carb	Stubborn and anxious. Dislike of changes, new things, fear of heights, cautious on the playground. Don't like people observing them. Get overwhelmed with what is expected of them. Desires to be in their comfort zone. Major remedy.
Calcarea mur	Cautious and observing, homebody. Similar to Calcarea carb, timid and fearful of doing things wrong but less stubborn. Tends to feel sad and isolated when stressed.
Carcinosin	Codependent on parent or medication. Needs to exert control over everything because they are so overwhelmed. Can't sleep at night because they can't turn off thoughts. Passionate, love nature. Family may be overscheduled.
Graphites	Bad skin rashes with cracking, weeping, honey-like fluid; itchy eczema. Very stubborn children who can be active and energized at night. Like Calcarea carb but less insecure.
Hepar sulph	Very chilly, worse cold, intolerant to drafts. Swelling and induration of glands. Great sensitivity to pain. Anxious and irritable. Pharyngitis with splinter-like pain in throat.
Kali carb	Conformist, rigid, doesn't like to break rules. Wants to stay at home due to insecurity and weakness of immune system. Not very emotional. Black-and-white thinking. Coughs, low back pain.

Remedies for Insecure Children with Weak Immune Systems	
Kali mur	Similar to Kali carb but sadder, more closed off, shut down. Wants to go by the rules but shuts others out due to lack of ability to relate. Feels rejected by the mother.
Lac vaccinum	Suppressed sense of self, wanting to fit in. Worse from cow milk (this remedy is from cow milk). Poor/low immune function. Neutropenia (low white blood count). Lots of ear and upper respiratory infections.
Lycopodium	Napoleonic complex, feeling small on the inside and acting big, bossy, egotistical, criticizing, intellectual on the outside. Or socially shy. Correlates with liver stagnation, constipation, gassiness, big appetite.
Natrum carb	Lonely because of a deep feeling of rejection, often from a father who compares his child to other children and doesn't provide unconditional love.
Natrum fluor	Closed off and introverted, not warm and friendly, a bit mean and hard. They may be loners, but actually like being at parties. Like the bad kids at school. Hardened tissues.
Natrum mur	Lonely, closed off children who seem sad but don't express themselves. Feel on some level rejected by people/family/mother. Introverted. Dryness of mucous membranes, headaches, sensitivities, allergies.
Silica	Mild, sweet children who want everyone to be happy and harmonious so they forgo their own needs and wants. Don't stand up for themselves. Shy. Poor nutrition, hair, skin, nails, and growth. Weak back.
Thuja	Wide acting for suppression. The core sensation is feeling weak/fragile on the inside and acting strong or playing the part on the outside. Not a strong sense of who they are, so things come easily into them. Boosts immunity.

Negative, Antisocial Children with Poor Self-Esteem

The naturally contradictory children in this group tend to negate everything, seek negative attention, and do things wrong on purpose in order to get negative attention. There may be a member of the family unit that is the negative one, where one sibling is always in trouble and the other sibling is perfect. They actually balance each other out. There is often a cycle of negativity within the family where the parent's constant view of one child as negative feeds into that child's chronic negativity, creating a strong victim mentality. A parent's attitude can greatly impact the attitude of the child. These children may fall under the category of Jan Scholten's Stage 17, the halogens (such as Flourine, Chlorine, Bromine, and Iodine), which by nature are ionically negative elements.

Despite their attitudes, the children in this group often have a sarcastic and wry/dry sense of humor and crack good jokes. They may be able to achieve a lot and are not afraid to try new things but can still be very down on themselves.

Metabolism issues, either fast metabolism or thyroid issues, are often at play here making it hard for them to gain weight even if they eat a lot. They can be speedy and sharp in their minds and do well with cell salts.

Remedies for Negative, Antisocial Children with Poor Self-Esteem	
Bromium	Guilty feeling of parent or child. Scapegoat. Cheater. Thyroid issues. Hyper, always moving, running away, not social. Glandular swellings, hoarse coughs. Constipation.
Bryonia	Dislike being asked to do anything, not even to move from their position. Want to be left alone. Can totally "tune out" due to illness. There is an overemphasis on work/making money by parents. Tendency to dryness, upper respiratory infections, constipation.
Chamomilla	Inconsolable and whining. Rejects everything you offer them, but this is mostly due to some body pain/discomfort/inflammation, such as a toothache or ear infection.

Remedies for Negative, Antisocial Children with Poor Self-Esteem	
China off	Super skin sensitive, dislikes changing clothes or brushing hair due to intense sensitivity. Tantrums, tics. Infectious disease. This is the main treatment for malaria and parasitic Lyme coinfections. May be very mental/creative with lots of ideas. There are many versions of China: China bol, China ars, China sulph, etc.
Chlorum	Contradicts everyone, especially their mother, and does things for the sake of getting negative attention. Feels not as loved as the other siblings. Victim mentality. Issues with rejection and saying no. Can follow Natrum mur. Has chlorine sensitivity or thyroid issues.
Fluoric acid	Amoral. Acts naughty without fear of consequences, as if nothing has value to them. Self-centered, hardened. Rebels without a care. May have bad teeth.
Kali brom	Highly rigid, black-and-white outlook with a deep-set fear or guilt that they did something wrong, like have a sexual thought, or that they have "sinned" and are "damned." Religious. Tendency to acne. Helpful for girls who get acne around their cycle.
Kali fluor	Highly rigid, tense in the body, yelling and contradicting if people don't do things the right way. Deep lack of confidence. May align themselves with the naughty child of the class, becomes their sidekick.
Kali iod	Highly rigid, tense in the body, rejects all of society/people and things need to be done a certain way. Can be angry, cruel, and yells at family, bossing them. High metabolism—eats a lot but skinny.

Remedies for Negative, Antisocial Children with Poor Self-Esteem	
Natrum mur	Lonely, closed off, quiet children who seem sad but don't express themselves. Prefers reading or isolated activities versus social ones. Feels on some level rejected by people/family/mother. Introverted. Dryness of mucous membranes, headaches, sensitivities, allergies.
Nitric acid	Peevish. Makes nasty comments, screws their face at you, rolls their eyes, blames others. Selfish. Tendency to ulcers (genital or mouth).
Oxygenium	Consumes all the energy/attention of the household but they feel neglected, unworthy, and that they deserve more. Selfish and overemotional. Will tantrum if they don't get their way. May have lacked oxygen or "support" during delivery.
Selenium	Lazy. It's too much effort to even think, or try, especially with school. No drive, drained, doesn't want to put forth any more energy if they fail. Messy and dislikes responsibility.
Tuberculinum	Sarcastic, cynical, self-centered, dissatisfied, defiant, mean, and destructive. Lung weakness, tendency to fungal infections. Time conscious that life/things will be over fast, so they have to fit it all in; hurried.

Sad, Serious Children

Children in this category are often described as loners who have difficulty forming or keeping friends and can even feel shut out from the rest of their own family. They have an aura of seriousness with a heavy presence that is unlike their peers. Flower essences may help these children on a spiritual level. Also consider clearing lung pathogenicity with Mycoplasma or Streptococcus pneumonia nosodes as grief and lungs are associated. Sometimes there is a lack of love in the family in general or a parent who doesn't know how to love that contributes to the sad and serious state of the child. In these cases, it is important for the entire family to heal in order for the child to heal.

Remedies for Sad/Serious Children	
Adamas	The remedy of diamond, this remedy is similar to Ignatia with feelings of great disappointment and desire for perfection. They may shut people out with resentment, anger, and feelings of worthlessness. Hurried and impatient, there is also a hardness; they can become emotionally cut off.
Aurum met	Serious children with gravitas, connects better with adults than other children and has adult tastes like classical music. Can be deeply sad and feel emotions very intensely. A heart chakra remedy. Can be a leader. May have experienced the loss or death of a father figure.
Calcarea muriaticum	Unsure of how to act, feels observed, and as a result shuts down and goes into bedroom/isolation. Feels lonely due to insecurity and would rather isolate.
Causticum	Sensitive to injustice, empathetic, feels other's sadness/pain/emotions. Becomes angry when something unjust is done to themselves or someone else. Weak lungs.
Cocculus	Exhausted and sick over caring/nursing for a loved one. Anxious and grieving. Feeling vertigo or stupefied. Slowed nerve conduction. Motion sickness. Headaches, migraines. Overly sympathetic people.
Cygnus (swan)	Actively experiences grief even though it happened a long time ago. History of sexual aggression. Preference for the color white. Tightness in throat. Similar to Staphysagria.
Ignatia	Heartbroken, disappointed, suppressed grief, lump in throat. Idealistic, wanting things a certain way and if that doesn't happen will have a meltdown, act hysterical. Contradictory. Tics, twitches. History of grief in family.

Remedies for Sad/Serious Children	
Granite	Heavy feeling as if being pulled down, death of family members, extreme exhaustion and weakness.
Green sunlight	A support remedy to bring self love back to the heart chakra, a natural "lift" remedy.
Lac maternum	For issues with breastfeeding, prematurity, lack of bonding with mother. Helps to incarnate the body, boost the immune system, and improve malabsorption. Seeks womb-like environments, wants to escape.
Natrum mur	Lonely, closed off, quiet children who seem sad but don't express themselves. Prefers reading or isolated activities versus social ones. Feel on some level rejected by people/family/mother. Introverted. Dryness of mucous membranes, headaches, sensitivities, allergies.
Nux vomica	Workaholic, driven, competitive children who get their nervous system worked up and then become sensory sensitive such as to drafts. Irritable, snappy, and spastic. Propelled by a sense of "something missing."
Spigelia	Heartbreak that feels like being stabbed in the heart. Similar to Ignatia with its sense of heartbroken disappointment. Parasitic infection.
Staphysagria	History of abuse, possibly sexual abuse. Easily embarrassed and ashamed. History of UTI's/styes/kidney issues. Resentment. Suppressed anger, indignation.
Strychninum	The acute version of Ignatia/Nux vomica, it is the main alkaloid from these plants. Intense sadness and heartbreak. Spasms, cramps, rigidity.
Upas tieute	Heartbreak, but in malarial miasm. May whine and have worms.

(Consider lung disease nosodes as well: Mycoplasma, Pneumococcinum, Pertussinum, Tuberculinum, etc.)

Precocious, Advanced Children/Sycotic and Tubercular Miasms

Sycotic and tubercular children can be very self-assured, outgoing, and self-reliant. They tend to be high energy, sometimes with ADHD, or wanting to focus on only the things they are interested in. They can be very rigid about how they decide things are supposed to be, but not necessarily black and white like Kali carb children.

Many of these remedies are metals. Like highly conductive electronics, these children are neurologically oriented with minds that can be very "speedy" and "wired," with repetitive thoughts, scripting, and ritualistic behaviors, as well as subtle tics and twitches which they may try to conceal. They can be very social, natural leaders who love to be the center of attention. On the flip side they sometimes do not engage much with others and stay in their own world because they don't feel a need for others. Or they may be so incredibly socially aware that they become anxious about being in public. Sometimes they don't understand how to engage in reciprocal back and forth because their interaction with the world is a one-way street. While this child tends to be more fearless than fearful, sometimes they will not try something new unless they know they can be the best at it. If they are not good at something, they will hide that fact. If they did something they know is wrong, they won't tell their parents.

Sycotic and tubercular children can be very ambitious, competitive, and exacting. These children only respond to strong authority figures because they often see themselves as the authority. They may be very verbal with an advanced vocabulary, even hyperlexic, and act older than their age, perhaps even dressing like an adult. They may engage in constant activity even though their body is run down, and for this reason they can never truly kick some chronic infections which may suppurate in the body.

Terms for the sycotic miasm are: hiding their faults, avoiding dealing with fixed weaknesses, acceptance of things for how they are, neuroses, with ritualistic behaviors based around fixed and rigid ideas. Terms for tubercular miasm are: hectic, intense activity, trapped, suffocation, closing in, change, activity, freedom, desire for change. For more on miasms, see Chapter 3.

Remedies for Precocious, Advanced Children/ Sycotic and Tubercular Miasms	
Argentum met or nit	Very socially sensitive children. Empathetic, but nervous about social gatherings because of how intensely they feel things. Neurotic with lots of fears, can be very silly and attention seeking. Tics, speech issues. Electric shock sensations.
Arsenicum met or album	Hypochondriac—fear of germs, getting sick. OCD about cleanliness. Burning GI pains, diarrhea, vomiting, food poisoning, gut bugs with anxious restlessness. Perfectionistic, controlling. Strong reliance on doctor.
Aurum met	Serious children with gravitas, connects better with adults than other children and has adult tastes like classical music. Can be deeply sad and feel emotions very intensely. A heart chakra remedy. Can be a leader.
Cadmium met	Socially anxious, social anticipation. Acts loud, silly, overbearing, and can be very expressive and open. Fearless, likes to fight. Cancer history in family.
Cuprum met	Very controlled, serious, all business, but feels better when in nature.
Ferrum met	Bossy, emotional, domineering. Acts forceful but hates being told what to do or being pressured. Red lips and flushed cheeks with tendency to anemia. Difficulty breathing. Pushing through hard work.
Ignatia	Heartbroken, disappointed, suppressed grief, lump in throat. Idealistic, wanting things a certain way and if that doesn't happen will have a meltdown, act hysterical. Contradictory. Tics, twitches. History of grief in family.
Lycopodium	Children who want to impress with their knowledge, win at games, be the best at things. But on another level are insecure and likely have symptoms of poor digestion such as gassiness. Big readers but can also be dyslexic.

Remedies for Precocious, Advanced Children/ Sycotic and Tubercular Miasms	
Medorrhinum	Precocious, artistic, passionate children who are advanced early on but have frequent infections, asthma, bacterial dysbiosis, sinusitis. Behavior alternates between extreme states such as shy to social, or empathetic to cruel and destructive.
Niccolum met	High achievers, need to control everything with perfection. Suppressed emotions but can also have emotional outbursts like Ignatia. Mayor of the classroom. Headaches and cough.
Palladium met	Children who can be the center of attention, performers, on stage, getting recognition, but unlike Platina do not act haughty. Can have right-sided issues of genital region such as hernias, ovaries, varicoceles.
Phosphorus	Empath. Poor boundaries so emotions of people can easily affect them. Dislikes being alone, always needs someone with them. Open and bubbly or shy; wants friends. Environmentally sensitive. Tubercular, dry coughs. Related to insect, bird, fish, cat remedies.
Platinum met	Children who love attention and performing in front of others. Feels proud and a bit better than everyone else; haughty. Can act hysterical with many neurological complaints.
Pulsatilla	Sweet and sensitive. Give love to get love. Clingy. Changeable, variable symptoms and moods. Thick mucus.
Sol (sun)	Loving, empathic, with poor boundaries. Can be very self-focused (like astrological Leo) with an inability to see one's own faults.
Sulphur	Warm, generous, lazy, messy, funny children who like people. They want someone to take care of them so they can have fun exploring their hobbies, collections, or video games. Poor detoxers prone to many infections.

Remedies for Precocious, Advanced Children/ Sycotic and Tubercular Miasms	
Thuja	Wide acting for suppression. The core sensation is feeling weak/fragile on the inside and acting strong or playing the part on the outside. Not a strong sense of who they are, so things come easily into them. Boosts immunity.
Tuberculinum	Sarcastic, cynical, self-centered, dissatisfied, defiant, mean, and destructive. Lung weakness, tendency to fungal infections. Time conscious that life/things will be over fast, so they have to fit it all in; hurried.
Veratrum album	Cold, cruel behavior, very intellectual with no heart. A desire to be the leader of the group with fear of being excluded or looked down upon. Migraines, diarrhea, prostration.
Zincum metallicum	Wired and fast in the brain, don't know when to stop, doing work/activity over and over again. Useful for tics, stuttering, and sleep disorders. Unsupresses the nervous system.

(Also consider the lanthanide and aurum series remedies; most animal remedies such as the lac, spider, and insect remedies (except for molluscs); Belladonna and Hyoscyamus; other tuberculinic remedies such as Antimonium crud or Antimonium tart, Calcarea phos, and Baccillinum; viral nosodes; and variations on these remedies such as Aurum sulph.)

Suppressed Children

This child generally falls under the cancer miasm, which Sankaran describes as: control, perfection, fastidious, beyond one's capacity, superhuman, great expectation, chaos versus order, stretching beyond one's capacity, self-control versus loss of self-control, and over the top.

Suppressed children are generally precocious and want to meet your expectations, yet they are anxious under the surface and dependent on their mother for a sense of security and doing things for them because the world is just too much. They experience sensory overload easily, such as at big birthday parties with the lights and sounds, it is all TOO MUCH and too chaotic for them. They are too sensitive to process it all. They want to exert control over their environment by things being done a certain way.

These children are often very sensitive and empathetic with other children or animals. Their sensitivity can even extend to supplements, chemicals, and foods. They may be advanced in one area and behind in another area (usually more mentally advanced and physically stunted), and are often very creative.

Interestingly, suppressed children will pick up on the family stress and act out the suppressed emotions of other family members, perhaps by being defiant or going into hysterics when told no. They can hold it together outside of the home (control), then have a meltdown in the home (loss of control). Highly self-critical and perfectionistic, these children do not need to be disciplined, or the slightest of scolding looks sets them straight.

Because their minds are racing about events of the previous day or anticipation of the next day, these children often suffer from insomnia. There may also be trouble breathing, possible tics and twitches of the face, throat clearing, or shoulder shrugging, etc. The child is emotionally suppressed because the family is also emotionally suppressed. This holding back of emotional expression is a metaphor for the immune system, which holds itself back from fighting against infections.

The parent of a suppressed child often presents as overburdened, juggling a million things, running a house, keeping a job, perfectionistic, doing too much for others, all the while keeping a cheerful façade despite suppressed grief or disappointment. Possibly there is an unhappy marriage or personal drama in relationships. They are list makers, type-A doers. Often the mom is ambitious in her career and possibly heads her own company. Mom is often a fast talker in the interview. The heart chakra area is generally shut down and mom can't really take deep breaths. Possibly a knot feeling in the throat. They will email you typed up highly organized notes of their child before the appointment because they don't want to forget anything. Family history may include cancer, autoimmune disease, and psychiatric medications.

Most PANDAS/PANS and chronic Lyme disease cases in general tend to fall under this category, as their immune systems are generally suppressed. As a PANDAS case becomes less suppressed with these remedies, they often move towards the weak/psoric remedies (see pages 354-357) such as Calcarea carb and Natrum mur.

Remedies for Suppressed Children	
Agaricus	Super excitable, outside of themselves, not centered, reeling, fearless. This is a mushroom and has an effect much like Candida alb and other fungus remedies. For tics and twitches, allergies with itchy palate and ears, and intense sneezing.
Anacardium	Internal split where one voice tells them to do the right thing, another voice says they are bad. Restless, needing to move. Low self-esteem resulting in mean behavior to others. Hallucinations, cursing.
Arsenicum album (and all varieties)	Hypochondriac—fear of germs and getting sick. OCD about cleanliness. Burning GI pains, diarrhea, vomiting, food poisoning, gut bugs, with anxious restlessness. Perfectionistic, controlling. Strong reliance on doctor.
Aurum ars	Heavy, depressed, and suicidal. Always in a hurry, impatient, and restless.
Cadmium met	Socially anxious, social anticipation, but acting loud, silly, overbearing, very expressive and open. Fearless, like to fight. Cancer history in family.
Carcinosin	Codependent on parent or medication. Needs to exert control over everything since they are so overwhelmed. Can't sleep at night because they can't turn off thoughts. Passionate, loves nature. Family may be overscheduled.
Conium	Induration of the glands. Emotionally closed and flat. Sexual suppression. Breast cancer.
Cuprum met	Controlled and ritualistic, closed and on guard. Wants to maintain a steady state. Tendency to cramps, projectile vomiting, rigid body. All business, no fun.
Ferrum met	Bossy, emotional, domineering. Acts forceful but hates being told what to do or being pressured. Red lips and flushed cheeks with tendency to anemia. Difficulty breathing. Pushing through hard work.

Remedies for Suppressed Children	
Gallium met	Withdrawn into the dull routine of life, not responding/answering when people ask them something, like they are deaf. You have to yell to get them to listen. Tendency to fungal infection.
Germanium met	Going through the motions of work, like a robot, drained of all life. Fatigue. Suppressed anger with small outbursts and no remorse. Anemic.
Ignatia	Heartbroken, disappointed, suppressed grief, lump in throat. Idealistic, wanting things a certain way and if that doesn't happen will have a meltdown, act hysterical. Contradictory. Tics, twitches. History of grief in family.
Lac remedies	See pages 94-97.
Natrum mur	Lonely, closed off, quiet children who seem sad but don't express themselves. Prefers reading or isolated activities versus social ones. Feel on some level rejected by people/family/mother. Introverted. Dryness of mucous membranes, headaches, sensitivities, allergies.
Staphysagria	Emotionally vulnerable, easily hurt, bullied, embarrassed, ashamed, especially if people don't like them. Changeable symptoms depending on emotional state. Suppressed anger. Sexual suppression or abuse. UTIs.
Thuja	Wide acting for suppression. The core sensation is feeling weak/fragile on the inside and acting strong or playing the part on the outside. Not a strong sense of who they are, so infections and influences come easily into them. Boosts immunity.
Zincum met	Wired and fast in the brain, don't know when to stop, doing work/activity over and over again. Useful for tics, stuttering, and sleep disorders. Unsuppresses the nervous system.

Remedies for Suppressed Children	
Zincum phos	Restless, repetitive movements, anemia, sleeplessness, changeable mood, tingling sensations. Suppressed nervous system. High anticipatory anxiety. Coughing tics.
Zincum sulph	Tremors and convulsions, restlessness, irresistible desire to laugh.

(Also consider all nosodes [Streptococcus, Candida, etc.])

Specific Suppression	Remedies to Consider
Suppressed anger	Anacardium, Rhus tox, Staphysagria, Ruta, Carcinosin
Suppressed grief	Ignatia, Upas tieute, Strychninum, Nat mur, Causticum, Cocculus
Suppressed pain	Opium, Sanguinaria, Bellis perennis, Arnica
Suppressed nervous system	Zincum, Cicuta, Thuja, Carcinosin, Mezereum
Suppressed immune system	Carcinosin, Thuja, Conium, Natrum mur
Controlling out of fear	Arsenicum, Carcinosinum cum cuprum, Ferrum met, Aurum met

Angelic Children

These remedies will help children who seem to be floating, light, and not quite "in their bodies" become more grounded. Parents often describe these children as "in their own little world" or "living in a bubble." They are physically uncoordinated and seem to have trouble getting into the position they want to be in. They tend to sleep a lot and daydream. They are not in the least bit motivated to do what other kids are doing and have no desire to play with other kids. With poor boundaries and little or no ego, they have few tantrums if any. These are often the most empathetic children in their class and tend to attract people without trying. Below, I include larger categories of remedies that can fit these kids, which you can refer to in earlier sections of this book.

Remedies for Angelic Children	
Plant hallucinogen remedies and the mushrooms	Anhalonium, Cannabis indica, Psilocybe cubensis, Agaricus
Elements	Hydrogen, Aluminum, Baryta carb, Beryllium, Boron, Borax, Phosphorus, uranium series
Noble gases	Helium, Neon, Argon, Krypton, Xenon, Radon
Imponderables	Vacuum, Black hole, Sol, color remedies
Color remedies	Red helps with inflammation and first chakra issues; Orange helps to be more creative and vital; Yellow supports healthy digestive function; Green helps with emotional healing and heart chakra; Blue helps release an overmentalized state; Purple helps to move/clear deeply syphilitic energies; Pink helps to create more softness of being; Turquoise helps open up the throat chakra.
Drug remedies	Alcoholus, Opiates (Codeine, Dilaudid, etc.)
Matridonal remedies	Lac maternum, Placenta, Vernix, Umbilicus, Amniotic fluid
Animal remedies	Goldfish, Jellyfish, Butterfly, and birds

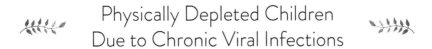

Physically Depleted Children Due to Chronic Viral Infections

Exhausted, burned out children who are lacking in stamina and get tired easily compared to their peers. Perhaps they had years of inflammation, seizures, tantrums; now that has been resolved and they are left depleted. These children have been subjected to chronic viral infections that they cannot kick, such as Epstein-Barr virus/mononucleosis/cytomegalovirus and these infections lead to deep bone aches and even immunodeficiency diagnoses like CVID. Sarcodes, cell salts, and gemmotherapy are other energy therapies that help to rebuild these burned out kids. Therapies that raise the core body temperature such as hot baths, sauna, peat baths and andrographis can help, as well as adrenal support, Chinese herbs to rebuild vital energy, and nourishing foods like bone broth.

Remedies for Physically Depleted Children Due to Chronic Viral Infections	
Ammonium carb	Chronic fatigue, more often in the elderly but can help some debilitated ASD cases. Oppressed sensation in the chest. Resentful, closed, shut down.
Bryonia alba	Dislike being asked to do anything, not even to move from their position. Want to be left alone. Can totally veg out due to illness. There is over-emphasis on work/making money by the parents. Tendency to dryness, upper respiratory infections, constipation.
Carbo veg	Very debilitated states—vacant, weak, and burned out. Food poisoning. Apathetic and depressed. Difficulty breathing with desire for open air, desire for fanning, but feels cold.
Eupatorium perf	Deep bone ache, such as when you have the flu. Viral infections. Periodic headache. Back pain. Thirst for cold drinks. Anxious, despondent, restless.
Gelsemium	Weak and trembling in the legs with anxiety, feels like they could faint/collapse, sinking stomach feeling, and vertigo. Anticipatory anxiety. Sad. For chronic viral states, flu, fatigue, CVID, etc.
Germanium met	Going through the motions of work, like a robot, feel drained of all life. Fatigue. Suppressed anger with small outbursts and no remorse. Anemic.
Kali carbonicum	Rigid, dogmatic, linear thinking. Wants to stay home; gets cold or sick easily. Asthma/pneumonia. Low back pain. Calcarea carb often follows.
Muriatic acid	Weakness and collapse states, issues with hydrochloric acid production in the body.
Natrum muriaticum	Lonely, closed off children who seem sad but don't express themselves. Feel on some level rejected by people/family/mother. Introverted. Dryness of mucous membranes, headaches, sensitivities, allergies.

Remedies for Physically Depleted Children Due to Chronic Viral Infections	
Phosphoric acid	Burned out, flat. This remedy can be needed after too much connecting or the death/loss of a loved one. Collapse, exhaustion, apathetic state—needs to drink juices or sodas to feel refreshed.
Picric acid	Exhausted state with total inability to think. Cannot exert mind. Complete brain fog.
Plumbum met	Heavy, loss of power feeling, especially in the limbs. Feels ignored, in a fog. Arrogance. Slowed reflexes. Similar to Alumina.
Psorinum	Fear of poverty with skin afflictions—especially itchy rashes. Chilly, pessimistic, anxious. History of bed bugs.
Sepia	Emotionally flat, exhausted. Pushes people away, doesn't want to be around family members, feels taken advantage of. Often children need this remedy because their mothers do. Hormone issues, especially stagnation, need to exercise to feel better.
Sulphur	Warm, generous, lazy, messy, funny children who like people. They want someone to take care of them so they can have fun exploring their hobbies, collections, or video games. Poor detoxers prone to many infections. Also consider Sulphuric acid for really burned out Sulphur constitutions. Often there is a deep burning sensation in the GI.
Tuberculinum	Sarcastic, cynical, self-centered, dissatisfied, defiant, mean, and destructive. Lung weakness, tendency to fungal infections. Time conscious that life/things will be over fast, so they have to fit it all in; hurried.

Miserable Gut/Sensory Children

Sensory issues, especially related to digestive distress, typify the main problem for this group. They may be highly sensitive to touch, or twisting, pressing, and pushing into their body to relieve some sense of discomfort. Common symptoms the child may present with include:

- Changeable or abnormal stools
- Systemic infections of candida
- GI dysbiosis
- Parasites
- Bedwetting
- Rashes on the bottom, itchy bottom
- Poor/picky or ravenous appetite
- Frequent nausea
- Stomach pain, pressing on the belly
- Dark circles under the eyes

The child is uncomfortable in their body, restless, and likely moody or whiny. A lot of stereotypical ASD behaviors are the result of a dysbiotic gut, such as running around, vocal stimming, tapping, string shaking, flapping, spinning, pinching, and hitting, which is an outward manifestation of their inner discomfort and possibly the movement and behavior of the pathogens themselves. Aggressive behaviors come and go, often with the full moon or new moon, which are times when GI pathogens replicate. The child may also have a history of rage or convulsions due to parasites.

This child may fall under what is called the malarial miasm described by Sankaran as: stuck and intermittently attacked, persecution, unfortunate, colic, worms, migraine, obstructed, harassed, hindered, miserable, lamenting, and whining.

As a parent you might feel frustrated about your child's progress, like all of your efforts aren't helping and the child is stuck. Children (and parents) who fall into this clinical group can have a strong victim mentality, that the world is set against them, and this can be typical of parasite infections. Often the mother has a history of gastrointestinal symptoms as well.

Various nosodes will be helpful in these cases, as well as vaccination clears. There are many diagnostic tests that the biomedical approach uses to assess GI health, such as OAT tests, Complete Diagnostic Stool Analysis, and so on. These tests are useful as they can identify nosodes that will help these children. But remember that these tests are only a snapshot, and it is still important to try and match up the known materia medica of a nosode to the child's state before giving that remedy.

It is immensely helpful to be able to put yourself in your child's body to feel what they feel in order to determine what remedy will best help them. See pages 28-29 for the guided meditation I use to help my clients get to this place. There are no right or wrong answers to these questions, you are just using imagination and empathy to give words to what the child cannot otherwise describe for themselves. Take some time with this meditation and write down all of the words and thoughts that come up. Then start looking through the remedies below to find one that fits.

Remedies for Miserable Gut/Sensory Children	
Abies nigra	Indigestion, ulcers, acidity. Feels like there's a hard thing, like an egg, lodged in the esophagus, especially after eating. Feeling weak and faint.
Aethusa	Projectile vomiting. Inability to digest milk. Malnutrition and food allergies. Vomiting with sweat, diarrhea, and weakness. Pyloric stenosis. Reserved people with strong emotions who are compassionate towards animals.
Aloe	For diarrhea with rumbling, gurgling, gas, sputtering, involuntary bowel movements. Easily excited and angry. Comparable to Sulphur.
Antimonium crudum	Irritable and gloomy, this remedy is for bloating, white tongue, emotional upset felt in the stomach, and cracked and brittle nails. Similar to Cina, Chamomilla, and Sulphur.
Arsenicum album	Hypochondriac—fear of germs and getting sick. OCD about cleanliness. Burning GI pains, diarrhea, vomiting, food poisoning, gut bugs, with anxious restlessness. Perfectionistic, controlling. Strong reliance on doctor.
Berberis vulgaris	Sudden stitches of intense pain, like there is a blockage in the intestines. Sharp, stitching, colicky pain which radiates downward. Also good for kidney stones. The GI supplement Berberine is the active component of this plant.
Borax veneta	Poor sense of identity and great childish, sweet naiveté. Incredible fear of falling, sensation/fear of being dropped. Discontented, emotional, crying, nervous. A great remedy for infantile/children's complaints, especially cold sores, hernia, indigestion, and nursing pains.

Remedies for Miserable Gut/Sensory Children	
Bryonia alba	Dislike being asked to do anything, not even to move from their position. Want to be left alone. Can totally veg out due to illness. There might be an over-emphasis on work/making money by the parents. Tendency to dryness, skin complaints, UTI's, constipation. Sprains, strains, flus. Top remedy choice for appendicitis.
Capsicum	Intense burning sensations. Bursting headache, inflamed mastoids/pain behind ears. Craves strong tasting, spicy foods. Parasites. At home all the time, spoiled, sluggish, and lazy. Inflammation. Migraines. Compare to Sulphur, Natrum sulph, and Belladonna.
Carbo veg	Made of charcoal, this remedy is useful for a wide variety of complaints. For GI issues, it helps with weak or slow digestion, poor appetite with gassiness, burping, or nausea. Stomach may be greatly distended.
Carcinosin	Codependent on parent or medication. Needs to exert control over everything because they are so overwhelmed. Can't sleep at night because they can't turn off thoughts. Passionate, loves nature. Family may be overscheduled. Sensitive stomach, easily anxious, food allergies, constipation.
Chamomilla	Inconsolable and whining. Rejects everything you offer them, but this is mostly due to some body pain/discomfort/inflammation, such as a tooth ache or ear infection. One cheek red, the other cheek pale. Oversensitive to pain/injury.
Chelidonium	Liver remedy, bossiness and irritability. Scapula pain related to digestive issues. Bossy towards other people because they want what is best for them. Right-sided headaches. Similar to Sanguinaria and Lycopodium.
China off	Super skin sensitive, dislikes changing clothes or brushing hair due to intense sensitivity. Tantrums, tics. Infectious disease. This is the main treatment for malaria and parasitic Lyme coinfections. May be very mental/creative with lots of ideas. There are many versions of China: China bol, China arsenicum, China sulph, etc.

Remedies for Miserable Gut/Sensory Children	
Cina	Hitting, striking, biting other people, throwing things. Parasite infections. Outwardly aggressive because inwardly GI system is being attacked. Tantrums, rage. Main remedy for treating parasites, see page 285. Can be given cyclically in 30C the day before, day of, and day after each full and new moon.
Colchicum	Tremendous trapped gas/bloating. Great sensitivity to smells. Gout with joint inflammation. Uric acid accumulation.
Colocynthis	Sharp/cutting/stabbing feeling in the gut, bending over to alleviate pain. Cannot place demands on or ask anything of the child. Suppressed anger held in the digestive system.
Croton tig	Diarrhea in one sudden, urgent gush, immediately after eating or drinking. Abdominal pain extending downward to rectum. Abdominal pain better from warm milk. Rumbling and gurgling.
Cuprum met	Controlled and ritualistic, closed and on guard. Wants to maintain a steady state. Tendency to cramps, projectile vomiting, rigid body. Attitude of all business, no fun.
Dioscorea	Intestines feel twisted, stretched, and pulled, like the wringing of a rag; stretching backwards, forwards, or side to side to get the pain out. Colicky babies. Housewives who feel confined and limited in the home.
Elaps	A snake remedy that has GI symptoms. Cold sensation in stomach, feels cold drinks moving down after swallowing. Abdominal pains better lying on abdomen. Peptic ulcer. Fear of being alone, fear of rain, fear of snakes.
Euphorbium	The intestines feel all bound up like a ball of rubber bands (these are latex plants). Sensitivity to latex. Feeling restless, wanting to break free. Terrible burning pain like fire in the GI tract. Stomach or GI cancer.

Remedies for Miserable Gut/Sensory Children	
Ferrum met	Feels full and then vomits after eating only small amounts or even during the meal. Worse at night. Feels forced to eat. Oppositional. Anemia.
Gambogia	Severe diarrhea with sudden gushing, diarrhea plus vomiting. Teeth sensitive to cold. Food poisoning, gastroenteritis. Depressed after diarrhea has been suppressed. Yellow, green, or bloody stool. Itchy anus.
Ipecacuanha	For a constant nonstop desire to vomit and a horrible sinking feeling in the stomach. Disgust.
Lac maternum	For issues with breastfeeding, prematurity, lack of bonding with mother. Helps to incarnate the body, boost the immune system, and improve intestinal malabsorption. Seeks womb-like environments (hiding under covers), wants to escape.
Lac vaccinum/ defloratum	Suppressed sense of self, wanting to fit in. Worse from cow milk (this remedy is from cow milk). Poor/low immune function. Bloating. Contractive pain in stomach, better by external pressure.
Lycopodium	Napoleonic complex, feeling small on the inside and acting big, bossy, egotistical, criticizing, intellectual on the outside. Or socially shy. Correlates with liver stagnation, constipation, gassiness, big appetite.
Magnesia carb	Whines about everything, feels like life is unfair to them, anxious about little things, acts babyish. Also dislikes any confrontation, such as parents fighting. Sour sweat, hypotonia, poor digestion.
Magnesia mur	Whining and worried, closed off and seeks isolation, wants to be babied. Passive. Allergies, liver issues, constipation, worse milk. Acts like an orphaned child.
Magnesia phos	Whining and wanting to be taken care of, picked up, babied. Squealing. Baby talk. Cramping that is better with heat and pressure.
Natrum carb	Mild and timid, wanting only one friend at a time, views all other people negatively except for their one best friend. Very sensitive stomach, milk allergies.

Remedies for Miserable Gut/Sensory Children	
Natrum muriaticum	Lonely, closed off children who seem sad but don't express themselves. Feel on some level rejected by people/family/mother. Introverted. Dryness of mucous membranes, headaches, sensitivities, allergies, constipation. Craves salt.
Nosodes	Candida albicans, Torula, Strep faecalis, Strep pyogenes, Staph aureus, Proteus, Morgan gaertner, Morgan pure, Dysentery co., Escherichia coli, Salmonella, Pyrogenium, Giardia, H. Pylorii, MMR vaccine, and Rotavirus vaccine are all helpful for GI conditions.
Nux vomica	Workaholic, driven, competitive children who get their nervous system worked up and then become sensory sensitive such as to drafts or smells. Irritable, snappy, and spastic. GI symptoms worse from overeating. Alternating constipation and diarrhea with gassiness. Colicky babies. Cramping/sharp stomach pains.
Opium	Lacking in pain or temperature sensitivity (gets badly hurt and doesn't complain). A history of opiate use or pain medications in the mother or during delivery. Constipation due to lack of sensation, hypotonia, loss of feeling alternating with rage and hypersensitivities.
Ornithogalum	Gastric ulcer pain. Pain as food passes through the stomach. Food feels as if it's sloshing around like a bag of water. Projectile vomiting. History of stomach cancer.
Phosphorus	Empath. Poor boundaries so emotions of people can easily affect them. Dislikes being alone, always needs someone with them. Open and bubbly or shy; wants friends. Environmentally sensitive. Peptic ulcer. Gastritis with nausea and vomiting. Ravenous appetite. Appetite increased due to headache. Great thirst for cold drinks.
Podophyllum	Cramps followed by watery, profuse, explosive, noisy bowel movements. Gurgling in intestines before stool. Sinking sensation or weakness after stool.

Remedies for Miserable Gut/Sensory Children	
Ptelea	Atonic stomach, worse from lying. Ravenous hunger, empty sensation in esophagus and stomach. Worms. Stomach and liver symptoms causing pain in the limbs. Great remedy for liver congestion.
Pulsatilla	Sweet and sensitive. Gives love to get love. Clingy. Changeable, variable symptoms and moods. Thick mucus. Parasites.
Rheum palmatum	Stools, body odor, and gas are very sour smelling and scalp is moist. Child is gloomy and doesn't want to sleep, eat, or drink.
Robinia	Too much stomach acid and belching. They are sour smelling and very irritable and agitated. Hyperacidity and burning of GI tract.
Saccharum off	Hungry after big meals. Craving sweets. Blood sugar issues, hypoglycemia. Malabsorption. Acting very sweet or lack of being sweet. Issues with showing affection.
Sanguinaria	Gallbladder colic causing nausea and right-sided migraines. Light sensitive. Oversensitivity to pain.
Sanicula aqua	Ravenous and bloated but doesn't gain weight. Irritable, throwing things (like Cina, Chamomilla). Poor absorption of food. Fishy odors.
Staphysagria	Emotionally vulnerable, easily hurt, bullied, embarrassed, ashamed, especially if people don't like them. Changeable symptoms depending on emotional state. Suppressed anger. Sexual suppression or abuse. UTIs.
Sulphuricum acid	Burning, raw feeling in intestines, stool burns. Putting a big personality out there and then getting totally exhausted.
Sulphur	Outgoing, happy, exploring, sometimes irritable, short fuse. Burning butt, lots of infections, high energy (more high energy than Sulphuricum acid).
Yellow color	Supports the digestive function as a whole, boosting the third chakra/solar plexus and helping to develop one's sense of self.

𝒜𝒜𝒜𝒜 Tics, Twitches, and Seizures in Children 𝒜𝒜𝒜𝒜

Tics and twitches are neurological conditions that are the result of either some form of inflammation or a general over-sensitivity in the neurological system. There is a rising prevalence in these conditions likely due to the overall weakening of immunity and the suppression of infection (particularly streptococcus infections) in children.

These children can be quick-thinking and prone to ADHD. I often find that their parents have nervous constitutions. Some children can control their tics while at school and let them all out when they come home, which fits the behavioral tendencies of the cancer miasm. Some examples of tics include throat clearing, eye twitches, mouth grimacing, head jerking, and choreic movements of arms, legs, and shoulders. This group also includes Tourettes-like verbal tics.

Remedies for Tics, Twitches, and Seizures in Children	
Absinthium	Tonic-clonic (grand mal) seizures, with trembling/twitching before convulsions. Facial features distort with seizure/twitch. Paranoia.
Agaricus	Super excitable, outside of themselves, not centered, reeling, fearless. This is a mushroom and has a fungus-like effect. For tics and twitches and allergies with itchy palate and ears, and intense sneezing. Also consider Mixed mold/House mold remedies.
Anacardium	Internal split where one voice tells them to do the right thing and another voice says they are bad. Restless, needing to move. Low self-esteem resulting in mean behavior to others. Hallucinations, cursing. May also be a sweet, sensitive, chronically-depressive, low self-esteem child who deeply fears doing the wrong thing.
Argentum met or nit	Very socially sensitive children. Empathetic, but nervous about social gatherings because of how intensely they feel things. Neurotic with lots of fears, can be very silly and attention seeking. Tics, speech issues. Electric shock sensations.
Artemisia	Seizures. Worms. Worse after fright. Chorea with inability to swallow. Profuse sweat.

Remedies for Tics, Twitches, and Seizures in Children	
Belladonna	High energy, active children with tendency to brain inflammation/rages/tantrums with dilated pupils, and superhuman strength. Strong fears with a need for routine. Can be used for acute fevers or as a general anti-inflammatory remedy for the nervous system in low potency.
Bufo	Mental retardation, slowed mental development, in the "reptile brain," not social, interested in masturbation.
Calcarea carb	Insecure, observing children. Late bloomers/missed milestones. Cramps in feet/legs at night. Seizures after exertion and/or fright, or from dentition. Tonic-clonic (grand mal) convulsions.
Carcinosin	Codependent on parent or medication. Needs to exert control over everything since they are so overwhelmed. Can't sleep at night because they can't turn off thoughts. Passionate, loves nature. Family may be overscheduled.
Causticum	Sensitive to injustice, unfairness, emotionally sensitive, and sensitive to reprimand. Severe headache. Tonic-clonic (grand mal) convulsions. Sensitive nervous system; tendency to tics/twitches. Similar to Carcinosin, Natrum mur, and Phosphorus.
Cicuta	Strange neurological movement tics, chorea. Seizures with horrific contortions and grimacing. History of abuse in the family. Fear of attack. Desire to stab.
Cina	Hitting, striking, biting other people, throwing things. Tics related to parasite/worm infections. Outwardly aggressive because inwardly GI system is being attacked. Tantrums, rage. Goes into Bella/Hyos/Stram states.
Clerodendrum inerme	Wild jasmine as an herbal tincture is known for healing intractable motor tics/twitches in children. As a homeopathic remedy it is also useful for reducing tics.

Remedies for Tics, Twitches, and Seizures in Children	
Cuprum met	Controlled and ritualistic, closed and on guard. Wants to maintain a steady state. Tendency to cramps, projectile vomiting, rigid body. All business, no fun. Clenching tics. Shrieking.
Hippomanes	Averse to being spoken to, wants to be left alone. Involuntary twitching under lip. Weakness in joints of feet, knee, soles, hands, and fingers.
Hyoscyamus	Brain inflammation leading to rage. Controlling of mother, very jealous of siblings. Acts with no shame, like showing genitals/butt, masturbating, or swearing (exhibition). Stool/urine accidents. Tourette's.
Ignatia	Heartbroken, disappointed, suppressed grief, lump in throat. Idealistic, wanting things a certain way and if that doesn't happen will have a meltdown, act hysterical. Contradictory. Tics, twitches. History of grief in family. Throat clearing/neck moving tics.
Lyssinum	Rabies. Violent and hypersensitive to stimulation, biting and growling during convulsions, frothing at the mouth, confused and chaotic in the mind. Feels like "I am going crazy."
Magnesia phos	Wanting to be babied/carried/lots of attention (like Pulsatilla). Tight/clenching/cramping in the belly resulting in screeching.
Mezereum	Eye tics. Eczema. Anxious feeling in the stomach.
Natrum mur	Emotionally sensitive children with poor eye contact and low self-esteem, can act babyish. Very anxious about social situations, introverted. Prone to viral infections, eye tics, sensitive to sun.
Nux vomica	Workaholic, driven, competitive children who get their nervous system worked up and then become sensory sensitive such as to drafts. Irritable, snappy, and spastic. GI symptoms worse from overeating.

Remedies for Tics, Twitches, and Seizures in Children	
Opium	Lacking in pain or temperature sensitivity (gets badly hurt and doesn't complain). A history of opiate use or pain medications in the mother or during delivery. Constipation due to lack of sensation, hypotonia, loss of feeling alternating with rage and hypersensitivities.
Physostigma	Eye tics. Spinal irritation. Chorea. Paralysis.
Stramonium	Rage. Dark fears, wide-eyed look of terror, fearful of death/dying, strong fear of the dark. Need for company. Tendency to inflammation, tics, Tourette's. PTSD. Seizures. Very sensory sensitive. Childish. Strep nosodes, OCD, defiance, negative thoughts, perfectionism, tics, twitches, chorea.
Strychninum	The acute version of Ignatia/Nux vomica, it is the main alkaloid from these plants. Tetanic rigidity. Worse slight touch.
Tanacetum	Abnormal lassitude, a nervous and tired feeling. "Half dead, half alive feeling" all over. It is of use in chorea and reflex spasms due to worms. Ears close up suddenly.
Tarentula hispanica	Speedy, neurological, sensory sensitive children who love rhythmic music, which helps to regulate them. Can be violent, manipulative, lashing out, with hallucinations. Social and competitive or isolated and withdrawn. Also consider other spiders such as Mygale.
Valeriana	Nervous system is worked up causing sleeplessness. Red parts turn white, hysterical spasms, weak stomach/digestion. Feverish and sweaty. Similar to Chamomilla.
Viscum album	Choreic movements like hand scrolling. Fungal infections. Anxious or frightful state.
Zincum met	Wired and fast in the brain, don't know when to stop, doing work/activity over and over again. Useful for tics, stuttering, and sleep disorders. Unsuppresses the nervous system. Twitching limb. Restless legs and feet. Consider also Zincum phos, Zincum sulph.

Hyperactive Children

Hyperactive children are full of energy and on the go. Some are in a high adrenaline state, some are uncomfortable in their body due to pain or discomfort, some have a natural vitality which leads to high energy, and some are hyperactive due to nervous system inflammation.

For those children who are naturally vital and energetic we simply need to adjust to their high levels of energy. But some children who are hyperactive are having an overly strong energy output or release that is detrimental to their growth and cognitive development. Children on ADHD medications can be difficult to treat with homeopathy unless the parents are dedicated to eventually stopping those medications. Our current culture with high media consumption, electronic games, and EMFs can highly exacerbate hyperactivity. The exposure to screens should be controlled and reduced as much as possible. Many of these children also have viral infections that keep them wound up and may crash if they are continually pushed. Effort should be made to slow them down (often the whole pace of the family needs to slow down) so their bodies can catch up. Sarcodes of GABA, dopamine, and serotonin (see Chapter 8) may also be useful for these children.

Remedies for Hyperactive Children	
Adrenalinum	When children have been consistently in fight or flight mode, full of energy, really intense. High adrenaline may show up on labs.
Animal and insect remedies	Children in animal remedy states seem to be reacting more from instincts and are challenged by acting in a more controlled manner (see Chapter 4).
Apis	Intense inflammation, redness, swelling, hives, bad red eczema, asthma, allergies, anaphylaxis. Children who are environmentally sensitive, hyperactive, organized, and may like certain shapes, letters, or patterns.
Argentum met or nit	Very socially sensitive children. Empathetic, but nervous about social gatherings because of how intensely they feel things. Neurotic with lots of fears, can be very silly and attention seeking. Tics, speech issues. Electric shock sensations.

Remedies for Hyperactive Children	
Belladonna	High energy, active children with tendency to brain inflammation/rages/tantrums with dilated pupils, and superhuman strength. Strong fears with a need for routine. Can be used for acute fevers or as a general anti-inflammatory remedy for the nervous system in low potency.
Carcinosin	Codependent on parent or medication. Needs to exert control over everything since they are so over-whelmed. Can't sleep at night because they can't turn off thoughts. Passionate, loves nature. Family may be overscheduled.
Coffea	Hyperactive, insomnia, rush of ideas, neurotic. Sensi-tive to coffee, or overuse of coffee in the family.
Hyoscyamus	Brain inflammation leading to rage. Controlling of mother, very jealous of siblings. Acts with no shame, like showing genitals/butt, masturbating, or swearing (exhibition). Stool/urine accidents.
Iodum	Hurried, always on the move, non-stop kids who are agitated and obsessive. Ritualistic. Child is ravenous, has high metabolism. Thyroid issues in the family. Children of immigrants who lost their culture.
Lachesis	Passionate, talkative, social, jealous, competitive, moody children. Sepsis, parasitic infections, blood stagnation. Can be violent, manipulative, lashing out. Tend to be warm and intolerant of tight clothing.
Medorrhinum	Precocious, artistic, passionate children who are advanced early on but have frequent infections, asthma, bacterial dysbiosis, sinusitis. Behavior alter-nates between extreme states such as shy to social, or empathetic to cruel and destructive.
Stramonium	Rage. Dark fears, wide-eyed look of terror, fearful of death/dying, strong fear of the dark. Need for com-pany. Tendency to inflammation, tics, Tourette's. PTSD. Seizures. Very sensory sensitive. Childish.

Remedies for Hyperactive Children	
Sulphur	Warm, generous, lazy, messy, funny children who like people. They want someone to take care of them so they can have fun exploring their hobbies, collections, or video games. Poor detoxers prone to many infections.
Tarentula hispanica	Speedy, neurological, sensory sensitive children who love rhythmic music, which helps to regulate them. Can be violent, manipulative, lashing out, with hallucinations. Social and competitive or isolated and withdrawn.
Tuberculinum	Sarcastic, cynical, self-centered, dissatisfied, defiant, mean, and destructive. Lung weakness, tendency to fungal infections. Time conscious that life/things will be over fast, so they have to fit it all in; hurried.
Valeriana	Nervous system is worked up causing sleeplessness. Red parts turn white, hysterical spasms, weak stomach/digestion. Feverish and sweaty. Similar to Chamomilla.
Veratrum album	Cold, cruel behavior, very intellectual with no heart. A desire to be the leader of the group with fear of being excluded or looked down upon. Migraines, diarrhea, prostration.
Zincum met	Wired and fast in the brain, don't know when to stop, doing work/activity over and over again. Useful for tics, stuttering, and sleep disorders. Unsuppresses the nervous system.

Children with Birth or Head Trauma

When there has been significant birth trauma, children may be in a more chronic state of head injury presenting as dullness of mind and a stupefied, out-of-it feeling. There is a sensation that something is wrong in the head; they may push on or draw back their jaw or press their forehead into the parent's chin. Some may hit or bang their head violently, signifying horrible headaches. Or sometimes there is just a certain spaciness to the child and knowing that there was a severe birth trauma leads you to consider the following remedies.

Examples of significant trauma may be forceps delivery, preterm delivery, deprivation of oxygen during birth, being stuck for an overly long time in the birth canal, swallowing of meconium, having a large hematoma on the head, having a cord wrapped around the neck, or some sort of head or bodily trauma during infancy that had a lasting effect. Sometimes parents do not realize there may have been long lasting trauma that continues to affect a child many years later, and only via subtle signs can you tell there is trauma. The etiology of these children's issues tends to be more within the structure of the body. They often do well with craniosacral therapy, which allows their bodies to unwind the patterns of trauma held as memories within their fascia.

Children with chronic inflammation, or a history of acute nervous system inflammation such as encephalitis or seizures, can also lead to a state of head trauma. Some of these cases may also be a result of vaccine-induced injury.

Remedies for Children with Birth or Head Trauma	
Abrotanum	Failure to thrive in babies and children. Discharge from umbilicus. Emaciated lower limbs. Fearful of injury/touch.
Aconite	Pure panic state arising as an adrenaline fight/flight reaction, with heart palpitations and need for company. Not necessarily violent. Fear of death, flying, claustrophobia. Shock. PTSD.
Arnica	For body trauma with bruising, contusions, concussion, accidents, sprains, etc. Person can feel out of it after injury. Useful chronically for workaholics who dislike touch or interference with a history of injury.
Bellis perennis	Fear of bodily injury, dislike touch, lameness, soreness, sore breasts, especially useful when there was an injury to the pelvis and/or deeper organs, such as during delivery. Feeling lame after delivery. Also a remedy for cancer/history of cancer.
Bufo	Slowness or dullness from brain trauma. Epilepsy at night. Disposition to masturbation. Desire for solitude. Playing with the tongue.

Remedies for Children with Birth or Head Trauma	
Calendula	Fear of injury, lameness, soreness, especially useful when there was injury to skin or connective tissues, lacerations. History of many bodily injuries.
Camphor	Issues with being anesthetized, lack of pain response. Spacey, out of it, total loss of memory. Freezing cold sensations.
Helleborus	Long-term chronic head injury; for constriction of the cranial bones. There is a pushing of the chin/jaw as if wearing a helmet that they want to get off. Furrowed brow. Great sadness, remorse.
Laurocerasus	Blue baby; cyanosis of a newborn, gasping for breath. Allergies so bad the lungs and head are filled with fluid.
Matridonal remedies	Matridonal remedies help heal trauma from pregnancy and early childhood (see Chapter 8).
Natrum sulph	Headaches with sensitivity to light, wants a relationship only with the mother. Depressed. Head injury. Worms.
Nux moschata	Dreamy, bewildered, confused, spaced out, narcoleptic, dry mucous membranes, distended belly.
Opium or Morphinum	Lacking in pain or temperature sensitivity (gets badly hurt and doesn't complain). A history of opiate use or pain medications in the mother or during delivery. Constipation due to lack of sensation, hypotonia, loss of feeling alternating with rage and hypersensitivities. Seizures.
Oxygenium	Consumes all the energy/attention of the household but they feel neglected, unworthy, and that they deserve more. Selfish and overemotional. Will tantrum if they don't get their way. May have lacked oxygen or "support" during delivery.
Pitocin/ Oxytocin/ Syntocin	Lack of bonding with the mother, can be from the use of Pitocin during labor or if the child did not have the opportunity to bond after delivery.

Remedies for Children with Birth or Head Trauma	
Staphysagria	Indignation that a medical procedure was conducted against your will or choice. Loss of bladder control. Sensitive to what other people think. Easily embarrassed.

(See also Tics/Twitches/Seizures, pages 381-384.)

Mentally Slow Children

Cognitive slowness may exist for many reasons with some cases being amenable to homeopathy and some cases not, depending on the etiology. For some children, cognitive regression is a matter of behavior, where there is an obstinate fear in the child to perform according to expectations—we may see this in Baryta carb or Natrum mur. They simply find life easier if they remain childlike. Giving these remedies helps treat underlying performance anxiety and confidence issues so they can move forward. In other children there is a fog and slowness in perception, such as a slowness in answering questions. This is due to toxicity, such as metal toxicity or drug toxicity, as we see in the remedy state Aluminum. Detoxification protocols will help these children be more present and aware. In more extreme cases, children have suffered some level of brain damage or have a genetic disorder which has functionally impaired their cognitive capacities, and while homeopathy can help ease the life of the child they may not make a lot of cognitive progress.

Children with chronic immune dysfunction may go from being a straight A student to having emotional breakdowns with the simplest of calculations. Clearing suppressed infection with nosodes (such as the strep nosodes) plus providing constitutional care will easily bring their cognitive function back on board. Another childhood complaint, dyslexia, will also resolve with constitutional care. Some well-known polychrests known for helping dyslexia include Lycopodium, Thuja, Natrum mur, Medorrhinum, Calcarea carb, Carcinosin, and Anacardium.

For nonverbal kids, constitutional prescribing may help bring more speech but this is rarely the first thing to improve. For cases of older children who are used to being nonverbal, attempting to learn speech at a later age feels awkward and difficult. For them, learning how to use a letter board can be a beautiful revelation of the depth of communication the child is capable of. I have also seen speech improvements when virus detox, methylation dysfunction, and metal detoxification were addressed. Teaching mothers of nonverbal children to use their intuition to connect with their child can also be a blessing.

Remedies for Mentally Slow Children	
Aethusa	Violent vomiting, convulsions, pains, or delirium. Inability to digest milk. Lacking power to hold body or head up—profound prostration, stupor, and lack of reaction. Restless and crying. Brain fatigue.
Alumina/ Aluminum	Mental dullness and slowness, as if in a fog, dislike being hurried. Easily disoriented and loss of identity, like someone who has Alzheimer's. Constipation. Can be given in 12C potency for aluminum detox.
Aluminum silicata	Slow cognitive development with clay-like stool.
Baryta carb	Mental slowness or regressed mental development with shy, passive behavior, sense of inferiority. Tonsil and gland inflammations. Like a more extreme version of Calcarea carb, but not as common as Calcarea carb. Helps to shift the stubbornness that keeps a child in a backward state so they can have the flexibility to move forward and catch up with their peers.
Baryta mur	Similar to Baryta carb, but more closed off. May help with convulsions.
Baryta phos	Similar to Baryta carb, but more open and connecting.
Baryta sulph	Like Baryta carb, but more hurried and irritable. Wants to remain like a baby, with silly baby talk.
Bufo	Confusion, epileptic seizures. The mind remains childish, only the body grows. Interested in masturbation. Violent colic. Lymphangitis. Lapping or playing with tongue.
Carbon dioxide/ monoxide	Helps with mental dullness, spaced out, not present. Confusion, disoriented, vacant. Also helpful for people living in a lot of smog.
Graphites	Bad skin rashes with cracking, weeping, honey-like fluid; itching eczema. Very stubborn children who can be active and energized at night. Like Calcarea carb.

Remedies for Mentally Slow Children	
Helleborus	Brain disorders, convulsions, head injury, low vitality, muscular weakness, sinking sensation. Pressing on facial bones. Dull, slow perception, slow in answering, apathy, indifference to loved ones. Stupefying headache.
Natrum mur	Child is in his own world, afraid to connect to people. There is a deep sensitivity and sadness inside. Feel on some level rejected by people/family/mother. Introverted. Dryness of mucous membranes, headaches, sensitivities, allergies.
Nux moschata	Entire loss of memory of the past. Thoughts vanishing. Dreamy and bewildered. Intense drowsiness. Dryness of mucous membranes.
Opium	Dreamy, placid, coma state, worse after injury or painkillers, indifferent, drugged out. Constipation due to lack of sensation. Lack of pain response.
Phosphoric acid	Burned out, flat. This remedy can be needed after too much connecting or the death/loss of a loved one. Collapse, exhaustion, apathetic state—needs to drink juices or sodas to feel refreshed.
Picric acid	Exhausted state with total inability to think. Cannot exert mind. Complete brain fog.
Plumbum	Deep loss of power. Progressive paralysis, contracture of tendons. Haughty, poor memory. Empty talk, droning on, hard to pay attention to.
Sepia	Emotionally flat, exhausted. Pushes people away, doesn't want to be around family members, feels taken advantage of. Often children need this remedy because their mothers do. Hormone issues, especially stagnation, need to exercise to feel better.
Silica	Mild, sweet children who want everyone to be happy and harmonious so they forgo their own needs and wants. Don't stand up for themselves. Shy. Poor nutrition, hair, skin, nails, and growth. Weak back.

ᴥᴥᴥ Common Remedies for Parents ᴥᴥᴥ

This chapter is about remedies for children, but to conclude I want to bring things back to the parents. As discussed in Chapter 1, it is of utmost importance for parents to heal themselves along with their children. If parents can identify and resolve whatever physical and emotional problems they've been struggling with, especially anything that has been suppressed, their child's healing will increase. The following remedies are ones that I prescribe to parents frequently, but this is in no way an exhaustive list. Sometimes the remedy that a parent needs is the same remedy that the child needs to heal a layer. Children more likely overlap with a parent's state the younger (and less differentiated) the child is.

Common Remedies for Parents	
Aconite	For clearing PTSD, when parents have had an intense emergency experience with their children that still makes their heart pound with fear and anxiety.
Argentum nit	Neurotic, anxious, extroverted parents with poor boundaries who are oversensitive to others' opinions, have OCD, and present with low impulse control. Impressionable. Can easily have a random thought enter the mind and "take over"—fear of jumping from a height, driving off a bridge, etc.
Arnica	Often an acute remedy, it can become a chronic state when there have been many deep, chronic injuries/car accidents/occupational injuries. I give this remedy to people (often men) who sustain injuries and afterwards say they are "fine" and go back to work. They develop a distance around them that is somewhat protective, but they reinjure themselves easily because they have lost the full integration of their body. Helps people who have had a lot of injuries become more present and aware.

Common Remedies for Parents	
Arsenicum album	Type A perfectionists, OCD tendency about cleanliness. Fear of losing money or work/job. Obsessive about contracting germs and fear of disease, always cleaning, can get OCD. Always researching the newest treatment or doctor, can become very reliant on their practitioners (like Carcinosin). Helps parents calm down and realize that germs and diseases are not the enemy.
Calcarea carb	Feeling unsure, worried, and insecure; sense of being observed and evaluated in what you are doing as a parent; anxious that kids are going to fall and get hurt or sick. Anxious about not following the rules correctly. Conscientious and feel observed doing every-day tasks such as grocery shopping. Feels better when organizing things. Helps parents feel more secure about their kids' safety and their performance at work or in the home.
Carcinosin	For parents who lose their sense of self and become sensitive to everything (other people/their own emotions/toxins), causing them to become very anxious and codependent on others/medications. Overly concerned about meeting the demands of the world. Has an inner sensation of chaos and overwhelm that the body can't handle; becomes hyper controlling in order to manage the anxiety. Feels exhausted but also has insomnia. Helps parents to become realigned with their true authentic self, be more organized mentally, and feel more independent in action and thought.
Causticum	Strongly sympathetic people who acutely sense the feelings of injustice (a mix of anger/indignation/grief), often showing up as some form of societal idealism and action. Intense emotionality about issues such as vaccines or racism. This oversensitivity to others eventually hardens the nervous system and causes issues like paralysis, incontinence, coughing, joint pains, and warts.

Common Remedies for Parents	
Chlorum	Unhappy people who are very negative and always looking for something to complain about. This parent may have lost who they are because they have poured so much energy into their family (martyr complex). They don't know what it means to do something for themselves. I give this often to moms and it helps them remember to put themselves first instead of last and to be less negative.
Cina	Often when children have parasites, parents need to be treated too. This is a common layer that needs to be treated in the healing journey. Often when parents need Cina they whine, blame others (such as their family/job), and feel easily imposed upon. They may present with an itchy butt, nose picking, irregular stools, and bad eating habits. Worse during full or new moon.
Cocculus	Bad effects from nursing a sick loved one. Exhausted, sleepless, grief-stricken, and sick from anxiety. This stress leads someone towards a stupefied state with dizzy spells, a slowed nervous system (paralysis), low back pain, and painful periods (weakened adrenals).
Ignatia	Repressed grief and heartache, lump in the throat from holding back tears. Many parents go into this state from their child's diagnosis, which leads them to shut down emotionally and go into their head and get overly mental. This mentalized state plus repressed emotions lead to insomnia and thoughts spinning in the head. Ignatia helps parents release and process suppressed sadness so they can be more present in their hearts again and express their emotions.
Lachesis	People who need this remedy have an inner duality with a hidden side that is manipulative and competitive. Can be verbally abusive, jealous, controlling, and have bipolar/manic-depressive states. Helps people rise above their lower self and identify with their higher selves.

Common Remedies for Parents	
Lycopodium	Critical parents who are in their heads, who read and research a lot, who are active in their careers and always critical of their spouses (sometimes they have issues with commitment), but they act nice to everyone outside the home. Gassy, liver stagnation, poor digestion, furrowed brow. Helps parents who are overly mental be more in the present moment.
Magnesia remedies (Mag carb, Mag phos, Mag mur, Mag sulph)	Passive people who fear conflict and deeply want peace and harmony. They can get a floating anxiety due to this fear, creating an inner restlessness, and often have an underlying fear of being alone/abandoned/orphaned. This lack of ability to stand up for themselves will come out through whining or a lot of physical complaints such as cramping, headaches, and digestive/liver issues.
Natrum mur	Emotionally closed and distant parents, cool and aloof, not easily connecting. They likely didn't have a close relationship with their own parents or experienced a deep sadness at some point in life. They harbor deep feelings of depression or grief but find it difficult to cry. Helps parents be more emotionally open and connecting, and more naturally joyful.
Pulsatilla	Nice, sweet women (and sometimes men) with soft, emotional eyes who weep easily and need approval. Indecisive, easily pushed around. Better from consolation. They give love to receive love. Lots of hormonal issues—can easily become hormonally stagnant (irregular periods) and do better with exercise or fresh air. Helps people-pleasers not to care as much about what people think, exert their sense of self, and have better will power.

Common Remedies for Parents	
Sepia	Hormonally stagnant people (mostly women, sometimes men) who are resentful towards their families to the point of being mean and/or wanting to escape. Post-partum depression. Emotionally flat, heavy, and exhausted. Feels better with movement, being industrious/busy, exercising, and checking things off their to-do lists. Helps women come back into an emotionally/hormonally free-flowing place where there is joy in connecting with family.
Silica	Mild-mannered people who are averse to conflict and want everyone in the family to be happy. They work hard at keeping the home balanced/harmonious and care a lot about how the family is perceived. Will be kind to everyone but are occasionally stubborn/rigid about their opinions. May be petite with a small appetite and may have unhealthy skin or nails.
Staphysagria	Repressed anger, resentment towards spouse. History of sexual abuse. Indignation. Angry, easily embarrassed. Nervous about what others think of them. Urinary tract infections and styes, worse from any procedures done to them. Helps women stand up for themselves and not be oversensitive to what other people say or do to them.
Sulphur	Warm, open, gregarious people with a sense of humor and decent self esteem. Can be lazy, messy, not care what others think of them, intellectual, philosophizing, and really into their hobbies and collections. Tendency to excess heat symptoms like rashes, gassiness, etc. This is an important remedy for poor detoxers and toxins may surface after dosing.
Thuja	For people who act strong and confident on the outside but are hiding a deep insecurity and weakness on the inside. They may have had a challenging upbringing where they had to learn to act a certain way to get by. Great remedy for viral infection/warts/skin.

Conclusion

Treating complex children is a worthy challenge that leads us down a path of tremendous discovery. Parents who have great success with homeopathy are open-minded and ready to shift how they view health and disease. They are excited to discover holistic systems of health that, though non-conventional, are already well established. Homeopathy is a long-standing system of medicine with a history of well-documented use, a great breadth of supporting literature, and many excellent and highly experienced teachers. These parents learn that homeopathy is a unique and comprehensive way of viewing our journey in health and self-evolution, not a quick fix, a magic pill, or just another pit stop in an attempt to try every possible healing tool. Some of those who dive deep into this form of medicine become inspired to practice themselves, either just for family and friends or by branching out and helping others. There are many ways to continue your homeopathic journey, but here are some next steps worth considering:

- Enroll in homeopathic classes or schools. I offer online classes and other educational resources at www.intuitivehomeopathy.com and www.homeopathyforcomplexchildren.com.
- Invest in some of the important fundamental books and materia medica listed in the Appendix beginning on page 402.
- Get a homeopathic remedy kit (50-100 remedies) covering the most common remedies for acute conditions so you have what you need when you need it.
- Join an online homeopathy support group where parents and practitioners help one another find remedies and continue to learn and grow.

- Find a homeopath to work with, preferably one specializing in children and open to your active involvement in the process. NCH and NASH are two homeopathic organizations offering directories of practitioners, and you can find more referrals at my website, www.intuitivehomeopathy.com.

Homeopathy can be overwhelming. There is so much information to explore! To ease this complexity, let your heart-led intuition help you to see the big picture by asking, "Is this remedy going to bring healing, and if so, in what potency?" Or, "What is the most important remedy to start with?" Opening your heart to love and compassion and using this field of awareness to intuit remedies will make your journey much smoother. Just close your eyes, feel love in your heart, connect to the soul of the child, and let the child be your teacher. When a child progresses, parents may realize that their own issues and blocks in life start to dissolve. This is because we ARE our children. Healing children means healing ourselves, our parents, our grandparents, and beyond that, the whole human collective.

Acknowledgements

This book exists because of the hundreds of mothers whose "heart-broken-open" compassion led us down the path of learning together. It was birthed from their interest in learning and a desire to combine their preexisting skill sets as intuitive healers with the breadth of knowledge available in the world of homeopathy. In 2014, a group of twenty moms whose children recovered using intuitive homeopathy asked me to teach them more in-depth classes on homeopathy, and for this purpose I compiled a simple photocopied handbook of charts titled *The Book of Life*. In reality it was an extension of Rajan Sankaran's well known collection of homeopathy charts, *Sankaran's Schema,* with my own additions gleaned from my clinical practice detailing how these remedies applied to special-needs children. The charts in *The Book of Life* were used successfully by my students and clients in helping them prescribe for their own families, and many of my students went on to practice homeopathy themselves and continued to utilize this handbook.

I began teaching another two-year homeopathy course in early 2019 and one of my students, Bridget Biscotti Bradley, who happened to be a book author and editor, insisted my handbook of charts be expanded into a published book and made available to parents outside of my practice and classes. Thank you, Bridget for the ease and grace you brought to the creation of this project. Thank you also to Susan Budge, who offered to help us edit it, and to André and Kate Swartley, who offered to publish it. I also deeply appreciate the time of my colleagues Ryan Robbins, ND; Julie Mann, CFHom; Jane Rees; Colleen Hill; Sarah Valentini, BHSc; and Kim Elia, who reviewed the manuscript.

I have so much gratitude for my community of mothers, healers, and homeopaths who have explored with me what is possible through intuitive homeopathy, including Laura Aranjani; Jeanne Bain; Flavia Bazzon; Wendy Beers; Heather Mulligan Begley; Judith Bianco; Christie Biesold; Pamela Brown; Aimee Burns; Virginie Claire; Gretchen Colon; Helen Koronides Conroy; Lori Congdon; Colleen Cox; Janice Doyle; Tami Duncan; Jo-Ann Eccher; Jessica Sauls Eliason; Lisa Fox; Jessica Galligani; Stacy Grant; Katrina Horn; Barbara Howe; Sasha Hughes; Katrina Iiams-Hauser, ND; Jadranka Ivanovic; Anaheed Jackson, ND; Amy Johnson-Kidd; Crystal Johnston; Zoe Jones; Abbe Lange; Jeni Leonard; Pamela H. Lialias; Erika von Loewe; Kristin Maloney, ND; B. G. Mancini; Nathalie Laforest Mathers; Ashlee Maroney; Mallory McClelland; Sonya McLeod, DCH; Melinda McCauley; Brooke McReynolds; Angelique Mercier; Samanta Batra Mehta; Jaimee Miller; Beth Monterosso; Stephanie Newton; Jill Oja; Kerry Persad; Natalie Peterson; Katie Pizer; Jessie D Ray; Sue Rigg; Anne-Marie Rizzuto; Heather Patricia Stafford; Susan Sanders; Jennifer Salcido, ND; Sandra Seaman; Michelle Voss Stephens; Heather Stewart; Kate Branam Swartley; Kimberly Swabsin; Erin Tullius; Silke Weiss; and Stephanie Whitzell.

Thank you to my beloved husband Ryan for your never-ending support, and my daughter Eva for your joy and beauty. Thank you to my homeopathy teachers and mentors: Julie Mann, CFHom; Nancy Mercer, ND; Paul Herscu, ND; Amy Rothenberg, ND; Pierre Fontaine, RsHom; Jan Scholten; and Dr. Rajan Sankaran.

Appendix

 Sources for Additional Information
on Homeopathy and Intuition

Basic Home Guides

Desktop Companion to Physical Pathology by Roger Morrison
Everybody's Guide to Homeopathic Medicines by Stephen Cummings and
Dana Ullman
Homeopathic Self Care: The Quick and Easy Guide for the Whole Family by
Robert Ullman and Judyth Reichenberg-Ullman
Homeopathy for Pregnancy, Birth and Your Baby's First Year by Miranda
Castro

Philosophy

A Guide to the Methodologies of Homeopathy by Ian Watson
Impossible Cure by Amy Lanksy
Method by Alastair Grey
The Organon of the Medical Art by Samuel Hahnemann
The Science of Homeopathy by George Vithoulkas

Materia Medica

Clinical Observations of Children's Remedies by Farokh Master
Concordant Materia Medica by Frans Vermeulen
Desktop Guide to Keynotes and Confirmatory Symptoms by Roger Morrison
Homeopathic Psychology by Phillip Bailey

Homeopathy and the Elements by Jan Sholten
Julian's Materia Medica of Nosodes with Repertory by O.A. Julian
Lectures on Homeopathic Materia Medica by James Tyler Kent
Monera by Frans Vermeulen
Nature's Materia Medica by Robin Murphy
Portraits of Homeopathic Medicines Vol 1, 2, 3 by Catherine Coulter
Prisma by Frans Vermeulen
The Homeopathic Treatment of Children by Paul Herscu
The Matridonal Remedies by Melissa Assilem
The Periodic Table in Homeopathy by Ulrich Welte
The Soul of Remedies by Rajan Sankaran
Fighting Fire with Fire by Ton Jansen
Sankaran's Schema by Rajan Sankaran
The Complete Practitioner's Manual of Homeoprophylaxis by Isaac Golden
The Thesis of Immunization Impossible by Torako Yui

Intuition

A Course in Miracles by Foundation for Inner Peace
Charts for Homeopathy—A Book of Muscle Testing and Dowsing Charts by Willow Thomson (sold on ETSY)
Creative Visualization by Shakti Gawain
Innerwise The Complete Healing System by Uwe Albrecht
Intuition on Demand: A step-by-step guide to powerful intuition you can trust by Lisa K
The Emotion Code by Bradley Nelson

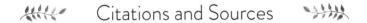 Citations and Sources

Chapter 2: The History and Practice of Homeopathy

1. Ullman, Dana. *Discovering Homeopathy: Medicine for the 21st Century,* North Atlantic Books. https://homeopathic.com/a-condensed-history-of-homeopathy/
2. Winston, Julian. "Treatment of Epidemics with Homeopathy - A History." https://www.homeopathycenter.org/treatment-epidemics-homeopathy-history
3. Winston, Julian. Influenza-1918: Homeopathy to the Rescue. *The New England Journal of Homeopathy.* Spring/Summer 1998, Vol.7 No.1

4. Ullman, Dana. *Discovering Homeopathy: Medicine for the 21st Century*, North Atlantic Books. https://homeopathic.com/a-condensed-history-of-homeopathy/

5. Homeopathy Research Institute. "Homeopathy use around the world." https://www.hri-research.org/resources/essentialevidence/use-of-homeopathy-across-the-world/

6. "What is the HPUS?" The Homœopathic Pharmacopœia of the United States. http://www.hpus.com/what-is-the-hpus.php

7. Speight, Phyllis. *A Study Course in Homeopathy.* CW Daniels UK; 2nd Edition (January 1, 1996). Page 145

8. The rigid application of Hering's law has been put to question by Dr. Andre Saine in his article, "Hering's Law: Law, Rule or Dogma?" https://www.homeopathy.ca/articles_det12.shtml

9. http://www.impossiblecure.com/referrals.php

10. Gray, Alastair. *Method.* B Jain Archibel. 2011. Page 249

11. Smits, Tinus. "CEASE Therapy". http://www.cease-therapy.com

12. www.homeopathy.com/college-sequential-therapy

13. "Free and Healthy Children." freeandhealthychildren.com

14. Journal of International Medical Research, 2017 Vol 45(2) 407-408. https://journals.sagepub.com/doi/pdf/10.1177/0300060517693423

Chapter 3: Miasms

1. Morrell, P. *Journal of Medical Ethics: Medical Humanities 2003*; 29:22-32.

2. https://mh.bmj.com/content/medhum/29/1/22.full.pd

3. https://hpathy.com/organon-philosophy/summary-sankarans-miasms/

4. Sankaran, Rajan. *Sankaran's Schema.* Homeopathic Medical Publishers, 2006.

5. https://www.cdc.gov/tb/statistics/reports/2017/default.htm

6. Morrell, "P. Hahnemann's Miasm Theory and Miasm Remedies"

7. http://www.homeoint.org/morrell/articles/pm_miasm.htm

Chapter 4: Animal Remedies

1. Lee, Alicia. *Homeopathic Mind Maps – Remedies of the Class Aves – Birds.* Narayana Verlag. Vol 4. 2013.

2. LeRoux, Patricia. *Butterflies. An innovative guide to the use of butterfly remedies in homeopathy.* Narayana Publishers. 2009.

3. Master, Farokh. *Clinical Observations of Children's Remedies.* Lutra

Services BV. 2006.

4. Murphy, Robin. *Nature's Materia Medica: 1,400 Homeopathic and Herbal Remedies.* Lotus Health Institute, 2006.

5. Sankaran, Rajan. *Sankaran's Schema.* Homoeopathic Medical Publishers, 2006.

6. Shore, Jonathan, et al. *Birds: Homeopathic Remedies from the Avian Realm.* Homeopathy West, 2004.

Chapter 5: Plant Remedies

1. Daisy family Scholten Quote: Scholten, Jan. *Wonderful Plants.* Narayana Publishers, 2014. Page 751.

2. Heather family Scholten Quote: Scholten, Jan. *Wonderful Plants.* Narayana Publishers, 2014. Page 583.

3. Lily family quote: Scholten, Jan. *Wonderful Plants.* Narayana Publishers, 2014. Page 193.

4. Magnolia family quote: Scholten, Jan. *Wonderful Plants.* Narayana Publishers, 2014. Page 96.

5. Nightshade family section, refer to: Herscu, Paul. *Stramonium.* New England School of Homeopathy Press. 1996.

6. Orchid family section: Klein, Lou. *Orchids in Homeopathy.* Naryana Publishing. 2014. Pages 65-72.

Other reference material for this chapter includes:

• Morrison, Roger. *Desktop Guide to Keynotes and Confirmatory Symptoms.* Hahnemann Clinic Publishing. 1993.

• Murphy, Robin. *Nature's Materia Medica: 1,400 Homeopathic and Herbal Remedies.* Lotus Health Institute, 2006.

• Sankaran, Rajan. *Sankaran's Schema.* Homoeopathic Medical Publishers, 2006.

• Sankaran, Rajan. *An Insight Into Plants Volumes 1-3.* Homoeopathic Medical Publishers; 2007.

• Vermeulen, Frans, and Linda Johnston. *Plants: Homeopathic and Medicinal Uses from a Botanical Family Perspective.* Saltire Books, 2011.

• Vermeulen, Frans. *Concordant Materia Medica.* Emryss Publishers. 1994.

• Vermeulen, Frans. *Fungi: Kingdom Fungi.* Emryss Publishers, 2007.

Chapter 6: Mineral Remedies

1. http://www.interhomeopathy.org/the-elements-of-life-carbon-series

Other reference material for this chapter includes:

- Herscu, Paul. *The Homeopathic Treatment of Children*. North Atlantic Books, 1991.
- Le Roux, Patricia. *Metals in Homeopathy*. Core essences and Paediatric cases for all the elements of Iron, Silver and Gold series. Naryana Publishers. 2009.
- Master, Farokh. *Clinical Observations of Children's Remedies*. Lutra Services BV. 2006
- Morrison, Roger, and Julie Bernard. *Carbon: Organic and Hydrocarbon Remedies in Homeopathy*. Hahnemann Clinic Pub., 2006.
- Scholten, Jan. *Homoeopathy and Minerals*. Stichting Alonnissos, 1999.
- Scholten, Jan. *The Lanthanides: Rare Earth Remedies for Our Time*. Narayana Publishers, 2012.
- Tumminello, Peter. *Twelve Jewels*, Southwood Press, Australia, 2005.
- Welte, Ulrich. *The Periodic Table in Homeopathy, The Silver Series*. Narayana Publishers. 2010.

Chapter 7: Nosodes

1. https://www.webmd.com/a-to-z-guides/bacterial-and-viral-infections
2. https://www.mayoclinic.org/diseases-conditions/c-difficile/symptoms-causes/syc-20351691
3. Winston J., *The Faces of Homeopathy*. Tawa, New Zealand: Great Auk Publishing 1991:236-238
4. *British Homoeopathic Journal*, volume XXVII, no 6
5. https://www.mdedge.com/dermatology/article/178644/pediatrics/hand-foot-and-mouth-disease-caused-coxsackievirus-a6-rise
6. Vermeulen, Frans. Wheeler and Kenyon. *Monera: Kingdom Bacteria & Viruses*. Emryss, 2005. Ref Works.
7. Vermeulen, Frans, Wheeler and Kenyon. *Monera: Kingdom Bacteria & Viruses*. Emryss, 2005. Ref Works.
8. https://blog.seattlepi.com/naturalnotes/2009/04/30/a-good-homeopathy-resource-on-flu/
9. Zimmer, Carl. *Parasite Rex: Inside the Bizarre World of Nature's Most Dangerous Creatures*. Atria Books 2000. Page 16.
10. Golden, Isaac PhD, Bracho, Gustavo, "A Reevaluation of

the Effectiveness of Homoeoprophylaxis Against Leptospirosis in Cuba in 2007 and 2008," March 11, 2014. https://doi.org/10.1177/2156587214525402

11. Riefer, Marco. *Exploited, Defenseless, Sucked Dry. Spectrum of Homeopathy*. No 3, 2015. ISSN 1869-3091. Page 20.

Other reference material for this chapter includes:

• Alex, Peter. *The Homeopathic Treatment of Lyme Disease.* Homeopathy West. 2005.
• Riefer, Marco. "Exploited, Defenseless, Sucked Dry, Parasitic aspects in the lives of patients suffering from borreliosis." *Spectrum of Homeopathy*. No 3. 2015, page 20.

Chapter 8: Sarcodes

1. Johnson, Geoff. "Sensational Sarcodes." www.interhomeopathy.org/sensational-sarcodes
2. Colin Griffith. *New Materia Medica: Key Remedies for the Future of Homoeopathy*. Duncan Baird Publishers. 2012. Location 9101 of 9980.
3. Assilem, Melissa. *Matridonal Remedies of the Humanum Family: Gifts of the Mother*. Idolatry, Inc., 2009. Page 5.
4. Smits, Tinus. "Lac Maternum" www.tinussmits.com/3871/lac-maternum.aspx

Chapter 9: Tautopathy

1. Vithoulkas, George. *Science of Homeopathy*. Grove Press. 1980, page 111.
2. https://www.focusforhealth.org/chronic-illnesses-and-the-state-of-our-childrens-health/
3. Murphy, Robin. *Nature's Materia Medica: 1,400 Homeopathic and Herbal Remedies*. Lotus Health Institute, 2006. Ref Works.
4. Ibid. Ref Works.
5. Griffith, Colin (2011-10-27). *New Materia Medica Volume II: Further Key Remedies for the Future of Homoeopathy: 2* (Location 4664-4666). Duncan Baird Publishers.

Index

A

Abandonment, 93, 106, 107, 175
Abies nigra, 180, 375
Abrotanum, 85, 153, 388
Absinthium, 287, 381
Abuse. *See also* sexual abuse
  bird remedies, 114–115
  Folliculinum, 316
  generational impact, 68
  insect remedies, 108
  mammal remedies, 89, 92, 94
  mollusc remedies, 122
Acer saccharum, 162–163
Acetaminophen clear, 336
Acetylcholine, 317
Acid remedies, 192, 289
Aconite, 39, 61, 90
  acute rage and panic, 349
  birth trauma, children with, 388
  head trauma, children with, 388
  highly anxious children, 350
  Lyme pain, 291
  for parents, 393
  qualities, 141
  remedies compared to, 117, 176
  symptoms, 141
Acorus calamus, 188
Actea spicata, 291
Actinide. *See* Uranium/Actinide
  series

Acute miasm, 69, 348–350
Acute rage and panic, children with,
    348–350
  characteristics, 348–349
  diseases, 348–349
  medications, 349
  remedies, 349–350
  symptoms, 348
Adamas (diamond), 196, 361
ADHD, 96, 99, 177, 262, 295, 385
Adrenal gland, 309, 317, 318
Adrenalinum (Epinephrine), 172,
    317, 349, 385
Aethusa, 375, 391
Agaricus muscarius (Mushroom),
    75, 158, 270, 368, 381
Age regression, 249
Aggravations, 54, 55, 57, 62–63,
    331
Aggression symptoms, 173, 256,
    281
AIDS, 263, 268–269, 271
Alcoholism, 82, 134, 158, 183, 196
Alcoholus, 196
Alex, Peter, 290–291
Allergies. *See also* environmental
    symptoms; food allergies
  Agaricus, 75
  Apis, 44, 62, 75, 106
  Blatta, 75
  enuresis, 38

C

D

M

T